Current Developments in Hematology

Current Developments in Hematology

Edited by **Martha Roper**

hayle
medical

New York

Published by Hayle Medical,
30 West, 37th Street, Suite 612,
New York, NY 10018, USA
www.haylemedical.com

Current Developments in Hematology
Edited by Martha Roper

International Standard Book Number: 978-1-63241-389-5 (Hardback)

Printed in the United States of America.

Contents

Preface

Every book is a source of knowledge and this one is no exception. The idea that led to the conceptualization of this book was the fact that the world is advancing rapidly; which makes it crucial to document the progress in every field. I am aware that a lot of data is already available, yet, there is a lot more to learn. Hence, I accepted the responsibility of editing this book and contributing my knowledge to the community.

Hematology is the study of blood, its production and the diseases related to it. There are different kinds of conditions and issues related to blood such as myeloma, hemophilia, anemia, bleeding disorders and problems related with blood cancer. The scope of hematology ranges from blood, red blood cells, white blood cells, platelets, reticuloendothelial system, lymphatic system, blood transfusion, hematosis to globulins. The aim of this book is to present researches that have transformed this discipline and aided its advancement. Different approaches, techniques and advanced studies in this field have been included in this text. For all readers who are interested in hematology, the case studies included in this book will serve as an excellent guide to develop a comprehensive understanding.

While editing this book, I had multiple visions for it. Then I finally narrowed down to make every chapter a sole standing text explaining a particular topic, so that they can be used independently. However, the umbrella subject sinews them into a common theme. This makes the book a unique platform of knowledge.

I would like to give the major credit of this book to the experts from every corner of the world, who took the time to share their expertise with us. Also, I owe the completion of this book to the never-ending support of my family, who supported me throughout the project.

Editor

AML with Additional Cytogenetic Abnormalities to t(8: 21) has Poorer Survival than that with Isolated t(8;21): A Retrospective Multicenter Cohort Study

Nahla Ahmad Bahgat Abdulateef[1,2*], Manar Mohammad Ismail[2,3],
Soha Aly Elmorsy[4,5], Aziza F. ALswayyed[6], Essam Hamed Abdou[2,9]
and Omima Elemam[7,8]

[1]Laboratory and Blood Bank Department, King Abdullah Medical City, Makkah, Kingdom of Saudi Arabia.
[2]Clinical Pathology Department, National Cancer Institute, Cairo University, Cairo, Egypt.
[3]Laboratory Medicine Department, Faculty of Applied Medical Science, Um Al-Qura University, Makkah, Kingdom of Saudi Arabia.
[4]Pharmacology Department, Faculty of Medicine Cairo University, Egypt.
[5]Research Center, KAMC, Makkah, Kingdom of Saudi Arabia.
[6]Laboratory and Blood Bank ,KFMC, Riyadh, Kingdom of Saudi Arabia,
[7]Oncology Center, KAMC, Makkah, Kingdom of Saudi Arabia.
[8]Medical Oncology, Oncology Center, Mansoura University, Mansoura, Egypt.
[9]Clinical pathology Consultant, SGH, KSA, Jeddah, Kingdom of Saudi Arabia.

Authors' contributions

This work was carried out in collaboration between all authors. Author NABA performed lab analysis at KAMC, designed the study, wrote the protocol, managed the literature searches and wrote the manuscript. Author MMI designed the study, wrote the protocol, and wrote the manuscript. Author SAE performed the statistical analysis and revised the manuscript. Author AFA performed lab analysis at KFMC. Author EHA collected patient data and perform lab analysis at NCI. Author OE collected clinical data and revised the manuscript. All authors read and approved the final manuscript.

<u>Editor(s):</u>
(1) Tadeusz Robak, Medical University of Lodz, Copernicus Memorial Hospital, Poland.
<u>Reviewers:</u>
(1) Anonymous, Taiwan.
(2) Anonymous, India.

Corresponding author: E-mail: BahjatAbdullateef.N@kamc.med.sa, bahgatnahla@yahoo.com

ABSTRACT

Aim of the Study: To investigate the poor prognostic factors incriminated in AML with t (8; 21), particularly additional cytogenetic findings, clinicopathological presentation and their impact on survival rate in Egyptian and Saudi patients.

Study Design: Patients were collected from three centers: 9 cases from King Abdullah Medical City in Makah, between 2010 and 2013, 16 from King Fahad Medical City in Riyadh, Saudi Arabia between 2007 and 2013 and 16 patients from National Cancer Institute, Cairo University, Egypt 2010 and 2013.

Methodology: We studied 41 cases with t (8; 21). Immunophenotyping was performed using BD-FACS System. Conventional karyotypic analysis was done using standard culturing and banding techniques. Clinicopathological and cytogenetic data were correlated with disease outcome.

Results: There was no statistically significant difference between Egyptian and Saudi patients concerning the hematological parameters or immunophenotype markers expression, Thirty four (82.9%) out of 41 patients achieved complete remission. The follow up period for the whole group ranged from 2.1 to 170.3 weeks. The median survival was 146 weeks. The overall survival rate was 80% at one year and 70% at two years. Regarding the cytogenetic profile 33/41(80.5%) had isolated t(8;21) and 8 patients (19.5%) had a chromosomal aberration in addition to t(8;21); the commonest of which was + 8 that was found in 5 patients. The median overall survival of those 8 patients was 28.4 compared to 146.7 weeks in cases with isolated t (8; 21) p=0.002. Also, they had a lower one year overall survival rate (44%) than those with isolated t (8; 21) (86%) and their two years overall survival was zero.

Conclusion: AML associated with additional cytogenetic abnormalities to t (8;21) has poorer survival than that with isolated t(8;21). Trisomy 8 is mostly incriminated for this being the most commonly encountered in this study.

Keywords: AML; cytogenetic; t (8; 21); FLT3; survival.

1. INTRODUCTION

Acute myeloid leukemia (AML) with t (8; 21) (q22; q22) is usually associated with a good response to chemotherapy and a high complete remission rate with long term disease free survival [1]. Translocation (8; 21) abnormality is found in approximately 5-10% of all AML cases and 10 - 22% of AML cases with maturation corresponding to the previous FAB class M2 [2,3].

Translocation 8; 21 with breaks at 8q22 and 21q22.3 was first reported by Dr Janet Rowley in 1973 during the analysis of a leukemia patient sample, and today it offers a unique example of how a cytogenetic abnormality is used to define a distinct subgroup of patients [4]. The translocation fuses the AML1 gene (also called RUNX1) on chromosome 21 which encodes the alpha subunit of core-binding factor (CBF) that is essential for normal hematopoiesis with the ETO gene (also referred to as the RUNX1T1 or MTG8 gene) on chromosome 8, producing a novel chimeric gene, AML1–ETO which disrupts the CBF transcription complex and initiates the first step of leukemogenesis [5]. The AML1–ETO fusion protein is a multifunctional cellular protein

that affects cell differentiation, proliferation, apoptosis and self-renewal. Evidences suggest that additional cytogenetic aberrations may act synergistically with AML–ETO in leukemogenesis [6].

The t (8; 21) abnormality is often detected together with additional cytogenetic or molecular genetic abnormalities. These abnormalities are often numerical, but other translocations or deletions can also be detected. The most common chromosomal abnormalities are loss of sex chromosome, del (9q), trisomy 8 and complex abnormalities while molecular abnormalities include c-KIT mutations and FLT3-ITD [7,8].

AML with t (8; 21)(q22;q22) is considered to have a favorable prognosis, however some patients rapidly giving in to the disease within a few months of diagnosis despite chemotherapy [9,10]. In patients with poor outcome, several adverse prognostic indicators have been suggested as possible explanations. Among these are additional cytogenetic aberrations, leukocytosis, CD56 expression and extramedullary manifestations. In the medical literature some suggested indicators, most notably CD56 [11] and extramedullary involvement [12] were identified in relatively small studies. Identification of other indicators was based on groups of patients treated with different protocols [13,14] or groups of patients that included some secondary leukemia cases [15] rendering the conclusions liable to confounding.

1.1 Aim of the Study

To investigate the poor prognostic factors incriminated in AML with t (8; 21), particularly additional cytogenetic findings, CD56 expression and the overall clinicopathological presentation and their impact on survival rate in Egyptian and Saudi patients.

2. METHODS

2.1 Patient Selection

We searched the files of all newly diagnosed AML cases and selected only the cases that carried t (8; 21) (q22; q22) either as the sole cytogentic abnormality or combined with other abnormalities. All patients who had secondary leukemia or diagnosed as relapsed cases when first seen in these centers were excluded.

All the patients received induction protocol 3+7 that consisted of Idarubicin 12 mg/m^2 IV bolus daily or daunorubicin 60 mg/m^2 IV from day 1 to day 3. Cytarabine 100 mg/m^2/d continuous IV infusion from day 1 to day 7. Bone marrow aspiration and biopsy were done on day 14 where treatment is proceeded accordingly: In case of aplasia or severe hypoplasia (BM blasts <5%); await recovery, and in case of significant residual blasts (cellularity > 15%) a salvage Protocol will be used, and if significant cytoreduction (cellularity < 15%) with low % residual blasts, Re-induction with 3 & 7 protocol. All patients who achieved complete remission received HiDAC (High dose Ara-C) protocol as a part of their post-remission consolidation for 3-4 cycles [16,17].

Diagnosis was based on WHO criteria in addition to FAB classification. All cases had representative bone marrow aspiration together with trephine core biopsy specimens for evaluation, EDTA peripheral blood or bone marrow aspirate specimens for flow cytometry analysis of surface and cytoplasmic markers, and heparinised sample for cytogenetic study.

2.2 Immunophenotyping (IPT)

It was performed using BD- FACS-Canto II System or FACS Caliber cytometer (BD- Bio Science) and reagent system (BD- FACS Setup) as previously described [18]. A panel of monoclonal antibodies was performed, including the myeloid markers (MPO, CD13, CD33, CD14, CD 15 & CD 64) in addition to CD3, CD7, CD10, CD19, CD20, CD34 and CD117, as well as HLA-DR and TdT (terminal deoxynucleotidyl tansferase). CD56 was also performed in a subset of cases. Cell populations were designated as positive for a particular surface antigen if expressed in ≥ 20% of blasts events (stained beyond an appropriate isotype cutoff) and for intracellular antigen ≥ 10% [18].

2.3 Cytogentic Analysis

Conventional karyotypic analysis was performed on metaphase cells using standard culturing and G -banding techniques (Fig. 1), results were reported in accordance to the International System for Human Cytogenetics Nomenclature [19].

2.4 Statistical Analysis

Data were analyzed using SPSS statistical package version 21.0. Numerical data were expressed as mean ± SD or as the median, minimum and maximum according to the distribution of the values. Qualitative data were expressed as frequency and percentage. For comparisons between Egyptian and Saudi patients and between isolated t(8;21) and t(8;21) with other genetic aberrations, the Chi square test was used to compare categorical variables and the independent "t" test or the Mann Whitney test was used to compare numeric variables according to the type of data distribution.

Overall survival (OS) was measured from the date of diagnosis until death from any cause with observations being censored at the date of last contact for patients last known to be alive. The OS and impact of additional cytogenetic aberrations on survival were analyzed using the Kaplan–Meier method. A multivariate Cox proportional hazard model was used to analyze the impact of clinicopathological variables e.g. (age, gender, leukocyte count as well as CD19 or CD56 expression) on survival. For all comparisons, a two-sided alpha value was set at 0.05. Significance tests and confidence intervals were not adjusted for multiple testing due to the exploratory nature of the study.

3. RESULTS

We had 41 cases fulfilling the previous criteria in the three centers: 9 cases from King Abdullah Medical City (KAMC) in Makah, diagnosed between 2010 and 2013, 16 patients from King Fahad Medical City (KFMC) in Riyadh, Saudi Arabia diagnosed between 2007 and 2013 and 16 patients from National Cancer Institute (NCI), Cairo University, Egypt seen 2010 and 2013. Data from Saudi Arabian patients were combined together, the patients being from the same genetic and ethnic background.

Clinicopathological data of the studied patients is shown in (Table 1). Egyptian patients had significantly higher incidence of hepatomegaly, splenomegaly, fatigue and pallor (P value = .009, .001, .05 and .05 respectively) while the Saudi patients had higher incidence of bleeding tendency (P =.006). Otherwise there were no significant differences between the two groups regarding the hematological parameters or marker expression by IPT.

Regarding the genetic profile, it was noted that all of the Egyptian patients had isolated t (8; 21) whereas 32% of Saudi patients had an additional genetic abnormality with their t (8; 21). None of the studied cases showed Internal Tandam Duplication (ITD) of FLT3 gene and the gene was in the wild type in all cases; Egyptians and Saudis. Thirty four out of 41(82.9%) patients achieved complete remission.

Secondly, the whole studied group were divided into two subgroups according to cytogenetic aberration for analysis of prognosis , group 1: isolated t(8;21); 33 cases (80.5%) and group 2: t(8;21) plus other cytogenetic aberrations; 8 cases (19.5%), these accompanying cytogenetic abnormalities were in the form of trisomy 8 in 5 cases, trisomy 7 in one case, trisomy 8 and other abnormalities in 2 cases [XX, t(8;21) ,+8,-5,-7, t(10;11)] and [XX t(8;21),+8,5q-,+19,+22] (Table 2). It is worthy to mention that there is a statistically significant higher achievement of complete remission and longer overall survival in group1 than group 2, P = 0.002. Otherwise there

was no difference between the two groups regarding symptoms at clinical presentation, hematological findings or immunophenotyping markers.

Table 1. Clinicopathological features of the whole studied patients

Variable	Egyptian N=16	Saudi N=25	P-value
Age(mean ± SD)	22.6±18.3	27.8±14.6	0.32
Age category [no (%)]			
15 years or less	6(37.5%)	2(8.0%)	0.02
15 years more	10(62.5)	23(92.0%)	
Gender [no (%)]			
Male	9(56.2%)	10(40.0%)	0.29
Female	7(43.8%)	15(60.0%)	
*Clinical presentation [no (%)]			
Hepatomegaly	9(56.2%)	3(15%)*	0.009
Splenomegaly	10(62.5%)	2(10%)*	0.001
Fever	12(75%)	10(50%)*	0.126
Fatigue	16(100%)	7(77.8%)*	0.05
Bleeding	2(12.5%)	7(63.6%) *	0.006
Pallor	16(100%)	7(77.8%)*	0.05
Hematological variables (mean ±SD)			
Total Leukocyte Count	14.6±9.8	26.6±29.9	0.08
Hb	8.1±1.2	8.1±2.2	0.91
Platelets	46.7±36.	38.7±32.4	0.47
Bone marrow blasts	59.5±24.9	66.1±24.9	0.42
FAB subtype [no (%)]			
M1	1(6.3%)	2(8.0%)	
M2	15(93.7%)	21(84.0%)	0.22
M4	-	2(8.0%)	
Cellularity [no (%)]			
Normocellular	0%	1(4.0%)	
Hypocellular	0%	2(8.0%)	0.32
Hypercellular	16(100%)	22(88.0%)	
*Selected Immunophenotyping markers [no (%)]			
MPO	16(100%)	25(100%)	0.39
CD13	16(100%)	18(72%)	0.04
CD33	16(100%)	21 (84%)	0.13
CD34	14(87.5%)	20(83.3%)*	0.63
CD117	11(78.6%)*	22(95.6%)*	0.27
CD7	0(0%)	2(8%)	0.37
CD19	4(25%)	10(43.5%)*	0.23
Cytogenetics			
T(8;21)	16(100%)	17(68%)	0.012
T(8;21)with other cytogenetic aberrations	0	8(32%)	
Complete remission	15/34(44%)	19/34(56%)	0.77

* Denominators used to calculate these percentages represent the numbers of cases with available data.
N.B.: p values refer to comparisons between Egyptian and Saudi patients

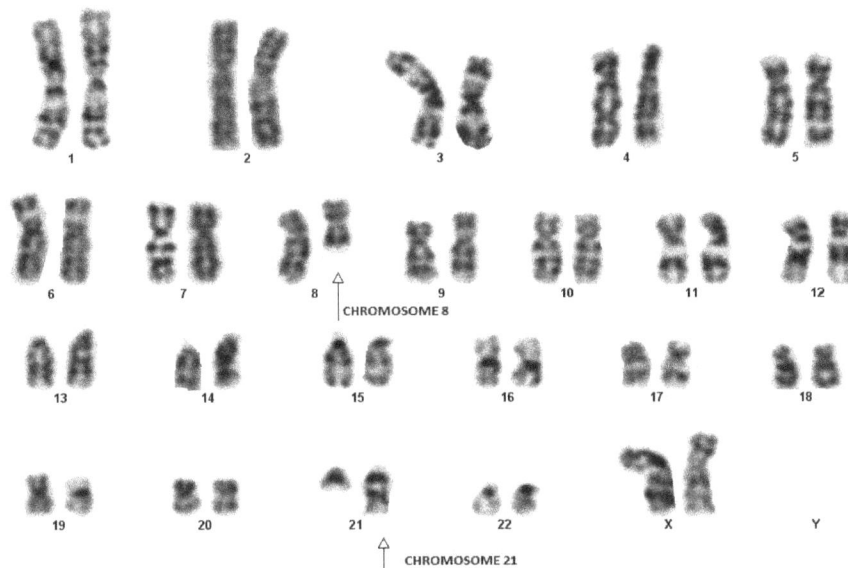

Fig. 1. Conventional karyotypic analysis performed on metaphase cells using standard culturing and banding techniques showing chromosome 8; 21 translocation

3.1 CD19 and CD56 Expression

CD19 was expressed in 14/41 (34.1%), with M2 FAB subtype.

Because this study is a retrospective study, CD56 was not available for most Egyptian patients as it was not part of the routine protocol for the time frame of collected data. Regarding the Saudi cases CD56 was expressed in 14/25(56%) with FAB subtype M2. Co expression of both CD19 and CD56 was noticed in 8 cases; 6 patients were M2 with isolated t (8; 21), while the other two patients had additional trisomy 8. Neither the expression of CD19 nor CD56 predicted the OS based on Cox Regression ($P=0.5$ and 0.4 respectively).

3.2 Survival Analysis

The follow up period for the whole group ranged from 2.14 to 170.3 weeks, with a median of 27.7 weeks. The median overall survival (OS) was 146 weeks. The one year overall survival rate was 80% with 95% confidence interval (95% CI) of 64.3-95.7%. The two years overall survival rate was 70% (95% CI: 52.4-87.6%) (Fig. 2).

Survival analysis stratified by the type of cytogenetic abnormality shows that the median OS was 146.7 and 28.4 for the group with isolated t (8; 21) (Group 1) and that with t (8; 21)

plus other cytogenetic aberrations (Group 2) respectively with P=0.002. The one year OS rate was 94 % (95% CI: 82.8-105.2%) for group 1 and 44% (95%CI: 7.0-80.8%) for group 2. The two years OS rate was 86% (95% CI: 68.0-104.0%) for group 1 and zero for group 2 (Fig. 3).

Neither age nor gender predicted OS, nor did the blast % ($P=.57$, $.48$, and $.45$ respectively). Neither leucocytosis nor the expression of CD19 or that of CD56 correlated with the survival outcome ($P=.16$, $.51$ and $.43$ respectively).

4. DISCUSSION

AML with t (8; 21) (q22;q22) is recognized as a distinct type of AML in the WHO classification [20]. Several adverse prognostic factors reported in AML with t (8:21) include leukocytosis, secondary cytogenetic aberrations, extramedullary manifestation and CD19 and CD56 expression. Many earlier studies were limited by small sample size or heterogeneous patient composition rendering it difficult to draw conclusions, especially regarding the role of secondary cytogenetic aberrations [21].

This study included 41 patients from three centers in Saudi Arabia and Egypt that were comparable to each other regarding hematological data, bone marrow (BM) cellularity, FAB subtypes, immunophenotyping marker expression and FLT3. All the cases were newly diagnosed de novo AML cases and received the same treatment. Considering also the ethnic Arab background we could consider them as a homogenous group.

In the current work 36/41 (87.8%) cases were AML-M2 subtype, which is in accordance with the proportions reported in several other studies [20,21]. In this study, blasts were expressing CD19 in 14/41(34.1%) of cases in addition to the expression of myeloid markers. Aberrant expression of CD19 in AML with t (8;21) has been reported by several authors with different frequencies; the high rates were 54% and 66% [21,22] while lower rates were detected by others (20.9% and 14%) [23,24].

Table 2. comparison between cases with isolated t (8; 21) and cases with t(8;21) plus other cytogenetic aberrations in relation to the clinicopathological parameters

Variable	Isolated t (8;21) No (%) =33(80.5%)	t (8;21) with other cytogenetic aberrations No (%) = 8(19.5%)	P-value
Age category			
15 years or less	8	0	0.12
15 years more	25	8	
Gender			
Male	16	3	0.57
Female	17	5	
***Clinical presentation**			
Hepatomegaly	11(37.9%)	1(14.3%)	0.23
Splenomegaly	10(34.5)	2(28.6%)	0.76
Fever	19(65.5%)	3(42.9%)	0.27
Fatigue	18(94.7%)	5(83.3%)	0.36
Bleeding	6(28.6%)	3(50%)	0.32
Pallor	18(94.7%)	5(83.3%)	0.36
Hematological variables (mean ±SD)			
Total Leukocyte Count	22.1±24.7	17.4±21.2	0.62
Hb	8.3±1.8	7.9±2.2	0.61
Platelets	42.7±35.7	49.2±37.8	0.64
Bone marrow blasts	64.4±25.4	55.7±22.7	0.38
FAB subtype			
M1	2	1	
M2	31	5	0.05
M4	0	2	
BM Cellularity			
Normocellular	0	1(12.5%)	
Hypocellular	0	2(25%)	0.001
Hypercellular	33(100%)	5(62.5)	
***Immunophenotyping (selected markers)**			
MPO	33(100%)	8(100%)	0.47
CD13	29(87.9)	5(71.4)	0.26
CD33	31(93.9%)	6(75.0%)	0.10
CD34	28(87.5%)	6(75.0%)	0.37
CD117	25(80.6%)	8(100%)	0.17
CD7	1(3.1%)	1(14.3%)	0.22
CD19	11(33.3%)	3(37.5%)	0.82
CD56[a]	10(55.6%)	4(50%)	0.79
Complete remission	30	4	0.002
Overall survival (weeks)	146.7±46	28.4±1.6	0.002

* Denominators used to calculate these percentages represent the numbers of cases with available data.
[a] CD56 was done in 25 Saudi cases

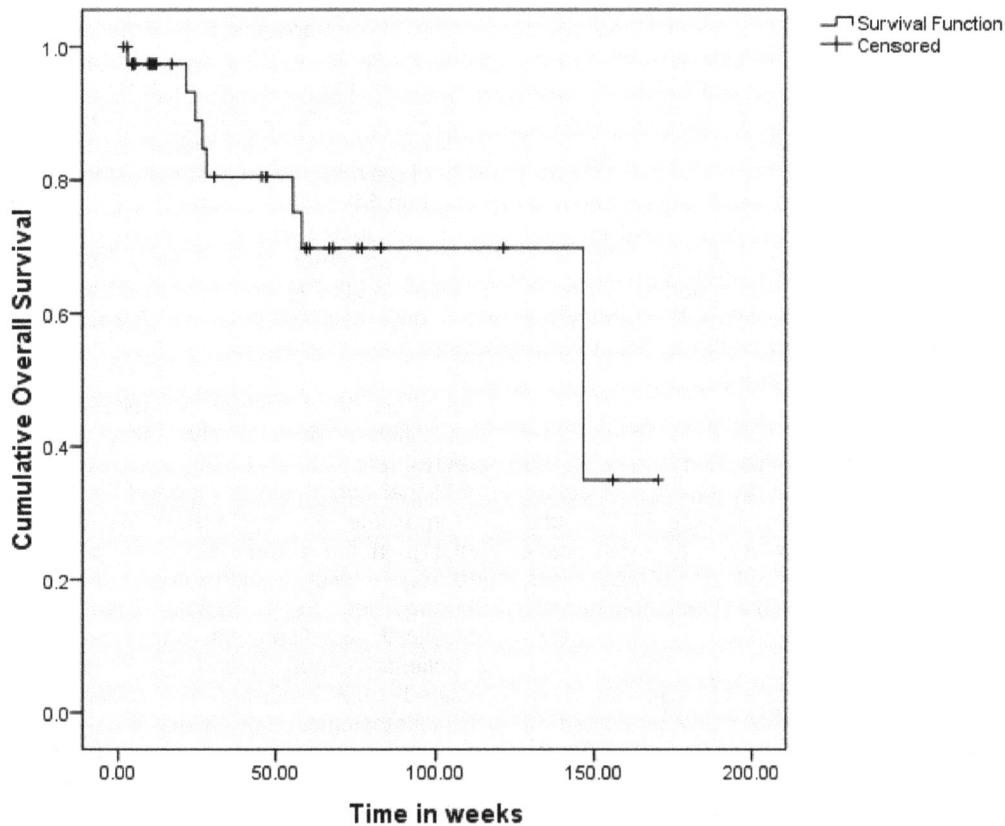

Fig. 2. Overall survival of studied patients N=41, the median survival was 146 weeks; the two years overall survival was 70%

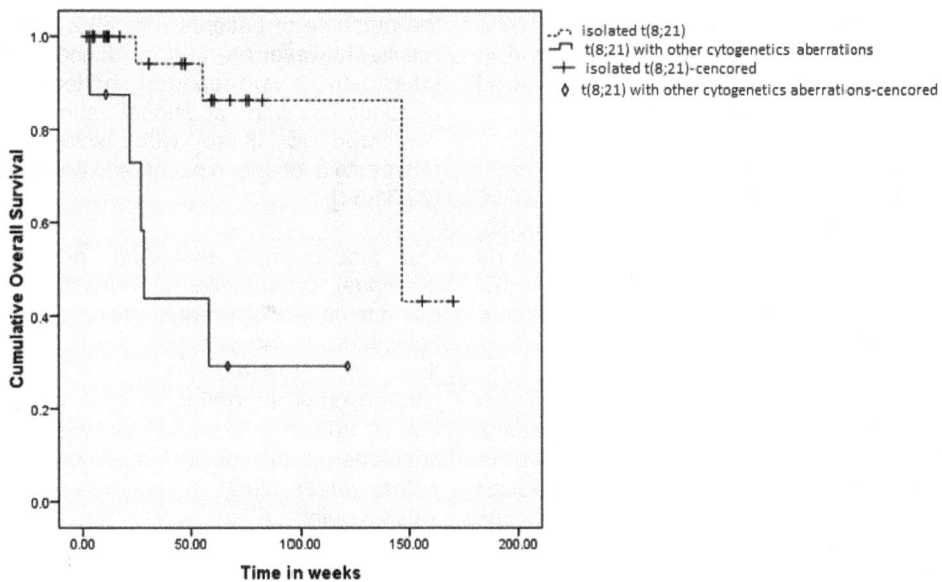

Fig. 3. Impact of cytogenetic aberrations on survival in AML studied cases

Regarding the Saudi patients in this study, CD56 was expressed in 14/25(56%) with FAB subtypes M2. This is in line with the findings of Fan et al. [22] and Chen Sw et al. [24] that showed CD56 expression in 66.7% and 58% of their t (8:21) - AML patients respectively.

In the current study the positive rate of stem cell markers of CD34, CD117, and HLA-DR were 85%, 84.6%, and 95% respectively. This also was comparable to what was reported by Fan et al. [22] who found the positive rate of the same stem cell markers respectively in 87.2%, 97.9%, and 95.7% of his studied cases.

The complete remission (CR) rate achieved by the patients included in this study was 82.9% which was comparable to the findings of earlier studies that reported rates of 96%, 82.7% and 95% [21,23,25]. However, a statistically significant higher achievement of CR was detected in patients with t(8;21) as a solo genetic abnormalities.

In this study we did not detect FLT3 (ITD); these results are in keeping with a study conducted on 20 patients with complex variants of t (8;21) by Xia [26]. A lower percentage of FLT3 detection (3.4%) was found by Kuchenbauer [27]. However several other studies showed higher percentages of 7.5%, 11%, and 10% [21,25,28].

The two years overall survival rate was 70% in our cases which was in accordance with the findings of Parihar et al. and Wu J et al., who reported 69% and 72% two years survival in their work [21,29]. A lower survival rate (56%) however, was reported by Pei Lin [28].

Further analysis could not confirm that age, leukocytosis, or expression of CD19 or CD56 was associated with poor survival in our patients, although this was suggested by other reports [23,29]. This could be due to the regular consolidation chemotherapy applied to our studied patients after CR.

We report here 8 cases with t(8:21) who had also been found to have additional chromosomal aberrations (19.5% of our cohort), with +8 as the most common additional aberration being found in 5 cases, trisomy 7 in one patient, and complex abnormality in the last two. In the literature, additional chromosomal aberrations are reported in different frequencies. In a study by Schoch et al. [30] it was found that (41/51) (80%) of their studied AML patients with t(8;21) had additional chromosomal abnormalities. They had detected a gain of chromosome 8 in 3 patients (6%) in addition to loss of a sex chromosome and deletion of the long arm of chromosome 9. In another more recent study by Parihar et al. [21] additional chromosomal aberrations were seen in 88% of patients with, trisomy of chromosome 8 in less than 5% of the total patients. In yet another study conducted by Pei Lin et al., most patients (60%) had other chromosomal aberrations in addition to t(8; 21), with trisomy 8 being detected in 4 patients (7%) and with 7 patients having complex karyotypes [28].

The effect of secondary cytogenetic aberration has different aspects and influences on the survival rate [30]. The main associated recurrent additional abnormalities reported are loss of sex chromosome, del (9q), trisomy 4 and trisomy 8 [28,31]. In the current work, we had 8 cases (19.5%) with additional chromosomal abnormalities to t (8;21). There were no statistically significant differences between those 8 patients (Group 2) and the 33 patients with isolated t(8;21) (Group 1) regarding their clinicopathological   features   (including hematological   and   immunophenotyping parameters), while there was a statistically significant higher achievement of complete remission in group1 than group 2, P = 0.002. The two years OS rate for Group 1 was 86% while none of the patients in Group 2 survived for two years. Some series demonstrate no deleterious effect of additional chromosomal aberrations on the outcome of patients with t(8:21) [32,33]. Our results, however are in accordance with those of other authors who reported shorter survival time of patients with additional abnormalities as compared to those with isolated t (8:21) irrespective of the type of additional aberration [23,31,34].

Our results show that AML associated with additional cytogenetic abnormalities to t(8;21) has a relatively lower rates of complete remission achievement and poorer survival outcome than that with isolated t(8;21). The additional chromosomal aberration mostly incriminated for this is trisomy 8 being the most commonly encountered in our group of patients and a further larger study is recommended to prove these results.

CONSENT

Not applicable.

ETHICAL APPROVAL

All authors hereby declare that all experiments have been examined and approved by the appropriate ethics committee.

The study was approved by KAMC IRB registered at National Biomedical Ethics committee, King abdulaziz city Science and Technology on 14-07-1433 (registration No.H-02-K-001) with IRB number 12-027.

COMPETING INTERESTS

Authors have declared that no competing interests exist.

REFERENCES

1. Arber DA, Vardiman JW, Brunning RD, Porwit A, Le Beau MM, Thiele J, et al. World Health Organization Classification of Tumors of Haematopoietic and Bloomfield CD. Acute myeloid leukemia with recurrent genetic abnormalities, In: Swerdlow SH, Campo E, Harris NL, Jaffe ES, Pileri SA, Stein H, Thiele J, Vardiman JW (eds). WHO Classification of Tumours of Hematopoietic and Lymphoid Tissue. International Agency for Research on Cancer (IARC), Lyon, France, 4th edition. 2008;111.

2. Arber DA, Stein AS, Carter NH, Ikle D, Forman SJ, Slovak ML. Prognostic impact of acute myeloid leukemia classification: Importance of detection of recurring cytogenetic abnormalities and multilineage dysplasia on survival. American Journal of Clinical Pathology. 2003;119(5):672–80.

3. Klaus M, Haferlach T, Schnittger S, Kern W, Hiddemann W, Schoch C. Cytogenetic profile in de novo acute myeloid leukemia with FAB subtypes M0, M1 and M2: A study based on 652 cases analyzed with morphology, cytogenetics and fluorescence in situ hybridization. Cancer Genetics and Cytogenetics. 2004; 155(1):47–56.

4. Rowley JD. Identification of a translocation with quinacrine fluorescence in a patient with acute leukemia. Annales de Genetique. 1973;16(2):109–112.

5. Peterson LF, Zhang DE. The 8;21 translocation in leukemogenesis. Oncogene. 2004;23(24):4255–62.

6. Peterson LF, Boyapati A, Ahn EY, Biggs JR, Okumura AJ, Lo MC, et al. Acute myeloid leukemia with the 8q22; 21q 22 translocation: Second- ary mutational events and alternative t(8;21) tran- scripts. Blood. 2007;1(110):799–805.

7. Liu XP, Xue YP, Liu SH, Mi YC, Han MZ, Xiao ZJ, et al. An analysis of cytogenetic characteristics and prognosis of 189 t(8;21) acute myeloid leukemia patients. Zhonghua Nei Ke Za Zhi. 2006;45(110;918-21 (abstract).

8. Reikvam H, Hatfield KJ, Kittang AO, Hovland R, Bruserud Ø. Acute Myeloid Leukemia with the t(8;21) Translocation: Clinical Consequences and Biological Implications. Journal of Biomedicine and Biotechnology. 2011;104631. DOI: 10.1155/2011/104631.

9. O'Brien S, Kantarjian HM, Keating M, Gagnon G, Cork A, Trujillo J, et al. Association of granulocytosis with poor prognosis in patients with acute myelogenous leukemia and translocation of chromosomes 8 and 21. J Clin Oncol. 1989;7(8):1081–86.

10. Lee KW, Choi IS, Roh EY, Kim DY, Yun T, Lee DS, et al. Adult patients with t(8;21) acute myeloid leukemia had no superior treatment outcome to those without t(8;21): a single institution's experience. Ann Hematol. 2004;83(4):218–24.

11. Baer MR, Stewart CC, Lawrence D, Arthur DC, Byrd JC, Davey FR, et al. Expression of the neural cell adhesion molecule CD56 is associated with short remission duration and survival in acute myeloid leukemia with t(8;21)(q22;q22). Blood. 1997; 90(4):1643–48.

12. Byrd JC, Weiss RB, Arthur DC, Lawrence D, Baer MR, Davey F, et al. Extramedullary leukemia adversely affects hematologic complete re- mission rate and overall survival in patients with t(8;21)(q22;q22): Results from Cancer and Leukemia Group B 8461. J Clin Oncol. 1997;15(2):466–75.

13. Byrd JC, Mrozek K, Dodge RK, Carroll AJ, Edwards CG, Arthur DC, et al. Pretreatment cytogenetic abnormalities are predictive of induction success, cumulative incidence of relapse, and overall survival in adult patients with de novo acute myeloid leukemia: Results from Cancer and Leukemia Group B (CALGB 8461). Blood. 2002;100(13):4325–36.

14. Schlenk RF, Benner A, Krauter J, Büchner T, Sauerland C, et al. Individual patient data-based meta-analysis of patients aged 16 to 60 years with core binding factor acute myeloid leukemia: A survey of the German Acute Myeloid Leukemia Intergroup. J Clin Oncol. 2004; 22(18):3741–50.

15. Appelbaum FR, Kopecky KJ, Tallman MS, Slovak ML, Gundacker HM, Kim HT, et al. The clinical spectrum of adult acute myeloid leukaemia associated with core binding factor translocations. Br J Haematol. 2006;135(2):165–73.

16. Wiernik PH, Banks PL, Case DC Jr, Arlin ZA, Periman PO, Todd MB, et al. Cytarabine plus idarubicin or daunorubicin as induction and consolidation therapy for previously untreated adult patients with acute myeloid leukemia. Blood. 1992;79(2):313-9.

17. Preisler H, Davis RB, Kirshner J, Dupre E, Richards F3rd, Hoagland HC, et al. Comparison of three remission induction regimens and two postinduction strategies for the treatment of acute nonlymphocytic leukemia: A Cancer and Leukemia Group B study. Blood. 1987;69(5):1441-9.

18. Ludwig WD, Rieder H, Bartram CR, Heinze B, Schwartz S, Gassmann W, et al. Immunophenotypic and genotypic features, clinical characteristics and treatment outcome of adult pro-B acute lymphoblastic leukemia: Results of the German multicenter trials GMALL 03/87 and 04/89. Blood. 1998;92(6):1898-909.

19. ISCN. An international system of human cytogenetic nomenclature. Report of the Standing Committee on Human Cytogenetic Nomenclature. Birth Defects Origi Artic Ser. 1985;21:1-117.

20. Huang L, Abruzzo LV, Valbuena JR, Medeiros LJ, Lin P. Acute myeloid leukemia associated with variant t(8;21) detected by conventional cytogenetic and molecular studies. Am J Clin Pathol. 2006;125(2):267-72.

21. Parihar M, Kumar JA, Sitaram U, Balasubramanian P, Abraham A, Viswabandya A, et al. Cytogenetic analysis of acute myeloid leukemia with t(8;21) from a tertiary care center in India with correlation between clinicopathological characteristics and molecular analysis leuk lymphoma. 2012;53(1):103-9.

22. Fan L, Wu YJ, Zhang JF, Qiu HR, Qiao C, Wang R, et al. Immunophenotypic analysis of acute myeloid leukemia with t(8;21). Zhongguo Shi Yan Xue Ye Xue Za Zhi. 2010;18(6):1410-3.

23. Lai YY, Qiu JY ,Jiang B, Lu XJ, Huang XJ, Zhang Y, et al. Characteristics and prognostic factors of acute myeloid leukemia with t (8;21) (q22;q22). Zhongguo Shi Yan Xue Ye Xue Za Zhi. 2005;13(5):733-40.

24. Chen Sw, Li CF, Chuang SS, Tzeng CC, Hsieh YC, Lee PS, et al. Aberrant co-expression of CD19 and CD56 as surrogate markers of acute myeloid leukemia with t (8;21) in Taiwan. Int J Lab Hematol. 2008;30(2):133-8.

25. Gustafson SA, Lin P, Chen SS, Chen L, Abruzzo LV, Luthra R, et al. Therapy – related acute myeloid leukemia with t(8:21) (q22:q22) shares many features with De Novo Acute Myeloid leukemia with t(8:21) (q22:q22) but Does Not have a favorable outcome. American J Clin Pathol. 2009;131(5):647-655.

26. Xia J, Chen SN, Pan JL, Wang QR, Wu YF, Wang Y, et al. Clinical and experimental characteristics of 20 patients with acute myeloid leukemia with complex variant of t(8;21). Z hongguo Shi Yan Xue Ye Xue Za Zhi. 2013;21(4):815-20.

27. Kuchenbauer F, Schnittger S, look T, Gilliland G, Tenen D, Haferlach T, etal.Identification of additional cytogenetic and molecular genetic abnormalities in acute myeloid leukemia with t(8;21) / AML1-ETO. Br J Haematol. 2006; 134 (6):616-19.

28. Lin P, Chen L, Luthra R, Konoplev SN, Wang X , Medeiros LJ. Acute myeloid leukemia harboring t(8;21)(q22:q22): A heterogeneous disease with poor outcome in a subset of patients unrelated to secondary cytogenetic aberrations. Modern pathology. 2008;21(8):1029-36.

29. Wu J , Zhang LP, Lu AD, Wang B, Cheng YF, Liu GL. Clinical features and prognosis of t(8;21)/AML1-ETO- positive childhood acute myeloid leukemia. Zhongguo Dang Dai Er Ke Za Zhi. 2011;13(12):931-5.

30. Schoch C, Haase D, Haferlach T, Gudat H ,Buchner T, Freund M, et al. Fifty –one patients with acute myeloid leukemia and translocation t(8;21) (q22;q22): An additional deletion in 9q is an adverse prognostic factor. Leukemia. 1996; 10(8):1288-95.

31. Lai YY, Qiu JY, Jiang B, Lu XJ, Huang XJ, Liu YR, et al. Analysis of characteristics of

72 cases of t (8; 21) acute myeloid leukemia. Beijing Da Xue Xue Bao. 2005;37(3):245-8.

32 Appelbaum FR, Kopecky KJ, Tallman MS, Slovak ML, Gundacker HM, Kim HT, et al. The clinical spectrum of adult acute myeloid leukaemia associated with core binding factor translocations. Br J Haematol. 2006;135(2):165–73.

33 Marcucci G, Mrózek K, Ruppert AS, Maharry K, Kolitz JE, Moore JO, et al. Prognostic factors and outcome of core binding factor acute myeloid leukemia

patients with t(8;21) differ from those of patients with inv(16): A Cancer and Leukemia Group B study. J Clin Oncol. 2005;23(24):5705–17.

34 Rege K, Swansbury GJ, Atra AA, Horton C, Min T, Dainton MG, et al. Disease features in acute myeloid leukemia with t(8:21) (q22:q22). Influence of age, secondary karyotype abnormalities, CD19 status and extramedullary leukemia on survival. Leuk lymphoma. 2000;40(1-2):67-77.

Palliative Radiotherapy for Spinal Extramedullary Hematopoiesis in Thalassemia Major

Feryal Karaca[1], Cigdem Usul Afsar[2*], Fatma Sert[3], Sebnem Izmir Guner[4],
Vehbi Ercolak[5], Erkut Erkurt[6] and Candas Tunali[6]

[1]*Department of Radiation Oncology, Van Regional Training and Research Hospital, Van, Turkey.*
[2]*Department of Medical Oncology, Tekirdag Corlu State Hospital, Tekirdag, Turkey.*
[3]*Department of Radiation Oncology, Faculty of Medical, Ege University, Izmir, Turkey.*
[4]*Department of Hematology, Bahcelievler Medical Park Hospital, Istanbul, Turkey.*
[5]*Department of Medical Oncology, Faculty of Medical, Harran University, Sanlıurfa, Turkey.*
[6]*Department of Radiation Oncology, Faculty of Medicine, Cukurova University, Adana, Turkey.*

Authors' contributions

This work was carried out in collaboration between all authors. Author FK designed the study and wrote the protocol. Author CUA wrote the first draft of the manuscript and managed the literature search. All authors read and approved the final manuscript.

Editor(s):
(1) Dharmesh Chandra Sharma, Blood Component and Aphaeresis Unit, G. R. Medical College, Gwalior, India.
Reviewers:
(1) Celso Eduardo Olivier, Department of Allergy and Immunology, Instituto Alergoimuno de Americana, Brazil.
(2) Golam Hafiz, Department of Pediatric Hematology and Oncology, Bangabandhu Sheikh Mujib Medical University, Bangladesh.
(3) Luiz Arthur Calheiros Leite, Biophisic Departament, Federal University of Pernambuco, Brazil.
(4) Anonymous, Romania.

ABSTRACT

Introduction: Non-hepatosplenic Extramedullary Hematopoiesis (NHEMH) is seen as a compensation mechanism in the patients with hematologic dysfunction. Thalassemia is an autosomal recessive hematologic disorder. The tissue involvement is seen very rarely in thalasemia major.

Case: A 45-years old patient diagnosed with thalassemia major was presented in this case report. The patient had splenectomy after 12 years from diagnosis and he was followed with continuous blood transfusions. Due to the newly emerged chest pain and dyspnea, he was evaluated with computed tomography. The operation was done for paraspinal masses caused by NHEMH. But

---

*Corresponding author: E-mail: cigdemusul@yahoo.com

same complaints were seen after 5 years from the operation. Paraspinal and sacral recurrences were detected in screening examinations. External palliative radiotherapy (ERT) was given to the patient with 3000 cGy total doses. Both clinical and radiological response was obtained with ERT. **Conclusion:** Radiotherapy might be considered as an efficient palliative treatment option for the thalassemia major patients with NHEMH masses recurring after operation.

Keywords: Thalassemia; extramedullary hematopoiesis; radiotherapy.

1. INTRODUCTION

Thalassemia is an autosomal recessive hematologic disease and its characteristic finding is a genetic defect in globin chain of hemoglobin. It is commonly seen in Southern Iran society. The most common manifestation of the disease is anemia. It is divided into two subgroups according to the location of deficient chain as α-thalassemia and β-thalassemia. Only one allele mutation in β globin chain is called β-thalassemia minor and two allele mutations in the same chain is called β-thalassemia major. Additionally, thalassemia intermedia cover the groups which are located between above mentioned groups [1].

Non-Hepatosplenic Extramedullary Hematopoiesis (NHEMH) is commonly seen in patients with thalassemia major, thalassemia intermedia and sickle cell anemia as a result of hematologic dysfunction [1]. The patients with thalassemia intermedia include heterogeneous groups in terms of clinic and genetic features [1]. High hemoglobin levels in some patients are due to extensive NHEMH [2]. Heterotrophic bone marrow can commonly occur due to the erythropoietic stress. The development and growth of unexpected masses outside of bone marrow is called NHEMH tissue (NHEMHT). EMH appears as a compensation mechanism to hematologic dysfunction in thalassemia major, thalassemia intermedia and sickle cell anemia [3]. EMH is commonly seen in liver, spleen and lymph nodes which are providing hematopoiesis in the embryologic period. EMH occurring outside of hematopoietic system is associated with myelofibrosis caused by myeloid metaplasia [4]. Intra-thoracic NHEMH is rare and usually has an asymptomatic course. Intra-thoracic NHEMH does not need treatment except the symptoms such as massive hemothorax, symptomatic pleural effusion and spinal cord compression [5]. Fine needle biopsy and radionuclide screening are appropriate for the diagnosis of NHEMH. Computed Tomography (CT) and/or Magnetic Resonance Imaging (MRI) are required for the patients with NHEMH symptoms [6,7].

Spinal NHEMH tissue is seen rarely and the hypothesis for spinal NHEMHT occurrence is spreading with trabecular bone of vertebral corpus or proximal costa. Hematopoietic tissue caused by anemia obtains extra branches including intercostal veins [6]. In early evaluation, immature erythroid and myeloid cells in dilated sinusoids are seen which are located in paraspinal NHEMHT. Also, iron depots are found in adipose tissue and in massive fibrotic tissue. These small intraspinal NHEMHT causes cord compressions.

While NHEMHT is seen in 20% of thalassemia intermedia, the rate of NHEMHT is <1% for the patients with thalassemia major requiring frequent blood transfusion. Paraspinal hematopoiesis has 11-15 % incidence rate between all NHEMH cases [6]. Paraspinal masses have usually asymptomatic clinic progress. The major symptom is spinal compression which can be shown in CT easily. Neurologic symptoms appear in 3rd-4th decade of disease due to the chronic progress of the pathogenesis [8-10]. Very few cases are diagnosed in early age. It is five times more frequent in males than females [11,12]. Our presented case is important in terms of being thalassemia major and obtaining great benefit from irradiation.

2. CASE

A 45-years-old male patient was diagnosed with thalassemia major due to his physical examination and hemoglobin electrophoresis in 1983. His laboratory findings were as WBC: 11.800/mm3 Hemoglobin: 9,6 mg/dL HCT: 29.2% HbA1: 0%, HbA2: 2.4%, HbF: 97.6%. The patient had blood transfusion during 12 years for 2-3 times in a week. In 1995, splenectomy operation was done for painful splenomegaly. In 2008, he had operation from paravertebral NHEMHT. Because of his high iron status, he was followed with folic acid and deferasirox treatment till 2011. His serologic markers for hepatitis and HIV (human immuno-deficiency virus) were negative. Whole body tomography screening was done in 2011 because of ongoing complaints of chest pain and dyspnea. Multifocal soft tissue lesions located in paravertebral area were detected in the CT and lesions were compatible with NHEMH focuses starting from upper level of mediastinum and continuing in pelvic and the presacral area. Bilateral paravertebral nodules were more marked on the left than the right side. The maximum size of them was 3x2 cm. Pelvic masses were bigger than the paravertebral ones and their maximum size was 6x4.7 cm. Masses located in posterior mediastinum and the presacral area, which were defined as NHEMHT, were shown in Figs. 1-3. His laboratory findings for homovanillic acid and vanilmandelic acid were negative. The patient was evaluated and external palliative radiotherapy (RT) was planned to be given to those postoperative recurrent masses for obtaining symptomatic improvement. Palliative RT, consisting of 18 MV photons, was given with 15 fractions, 2 Gy daily doses and totally 30 Gy. Paravertebral field was planned bilaterally on the other hand; box field was accepted suitable for pelvic irradiation field. Complete clinical response was obtained after palliative RT and partial radiological response was seen in control CT after 18-months follow-up period (Figs. 4 and 5).

NHEMHTs, which are located in the paraspinal area, can trigger neurologic complications as a result of spinal cord compression. Target hemoglobin level is usually >10 g/dl in thalassemia major treatment. Significant difference at hemoglobin levels draws attention after the operation of NHEMHTs. Additionally, oxygenation of the postoperative tissues differentiates and this is useful for the improvement of neurological symptoms caused from paraspinal masses [14,15].

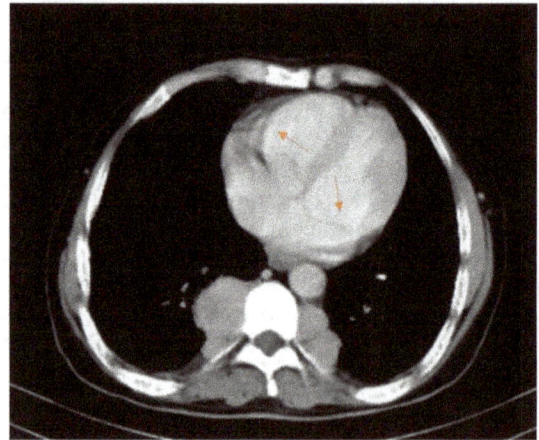

Fig. 2. Soft tissue lesions located at the paravertebral area in computed tomography

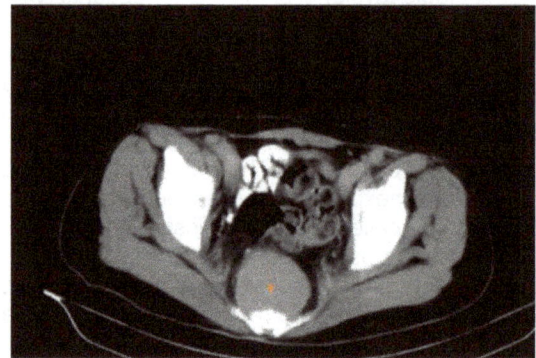

Fig. 3. Soft tissue lesion located at the sacral area in computed tomography

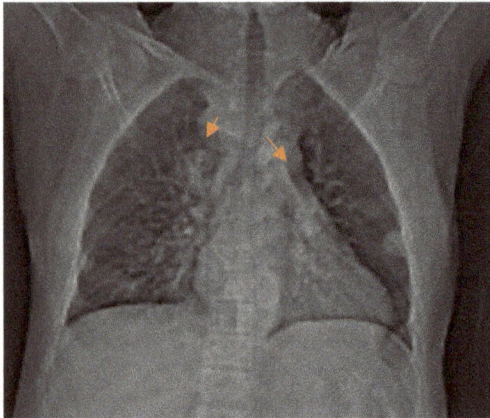

Fig. 1. Bilaterally located paravertebral masses in the chest radiograph of the patient

3. DISCUSSION

NHEMH is very rarely seen in thalassemia major. The main treatment of thalassemia major is blood transfusion. Surgery and RT options are suggested for NHEMHT treatment. Clinically symptomatic masses require treatment immediately. Chronic anemia and continuous blood transfusions can cause and facilitate the occurrence of NHEMHT [13].

Surgery is the main treatment for symptomatic NHEMHTs. It is stated that obtaining normal hemoglobin level in case of progressive clinical status is contingent with clinic decompression. Nevertheless, the risk of recurrence is high for diffuse mature masses. Briefly, it is cited that surgery provides improvement for the patient with acute, progressive disease and with symptomatic neurologic deficits [16]. The treatment results of blood transfusion and RT combination is promising.

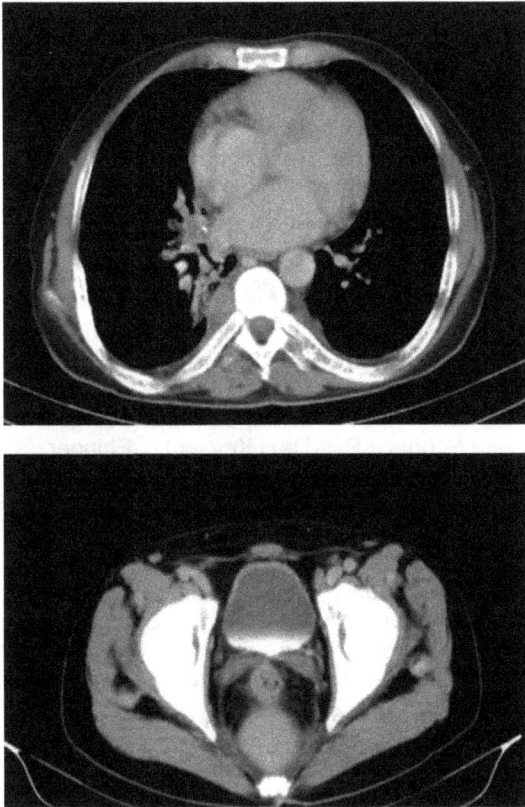

Fig. 4-5. Partial regression of the masses were seen in thoracic and pelvic computed tomography screening

It was shown that neurologic deficits could recover with low dose RT in approximately 50 % of patients after 3-7 months from therapy. Hematopoietic tissues are quite sensitive to RT. Hematopoietic tissue volume is reduced by 16.4 % after RT. The doses between 900 and 3500 cGy were seen effective [17]. On the other hand, there is a high (19-37 %) recurrence risk after RT. It is suggested that RT and operation should be considered to use concomitantly. It was seen that the recurrence risk with RT applied after laminectomy was lower than the RT alone option [18-21]. Therefore, immediate palliative RT should be preferred for the patient with neurologic symptoms which have favorable response to RT. Furthermore, it is reported that combined treatment of low dose RT with blood transfusion and hydroxyurea represents excellent results [22,23]. There is a review for complete recovery from paraparesis by emergency RT in literature [24].

Neurologic symptoms may get worse at the beginning of RT as a result of tissue edema. Additionally, it should be kept on mind that RT is a common factor for occurring pancytopenia due to its immunosuppressive effect. Blood count should be followed continuously during RT [19].

Another treatment option is the drug called hydroxyurea. Hydroxyurea is a kind of ribonucleotide enzyme inhibitor which is used to treat the patients with paraspinal NHEMHTs [25,26].

4. CONCLUSION

Management of the patients with NHEMH changes from patient to patient. The treatment algorithms will be maturated with the help of understanding the molecular, clinical and pathologic characteristics of thalassemia major. Single or combined treatment modalities are experienced for the patient with NHEMHT located in the paraspinal and pelvic area. Our case is important in terms of presenting a good radiological and clinical response with the use of RT.

CONSENT

It is not applicable.

ETHICS STATEMENT

The patient's informed consent was taken for publication.

COMPETING INTERESTS

Authors have declared that no competing interests exist.

REFERENCES

1.   Bayat N, Farashi S, Hafezi-Nejad N, Faramarzi N, Ashki M, Vakili S, et al. Novel mutations responsible for α-thalassemia in Iranian families. Hemoglobin. 2013;37(2): 148-159.

2.   Haidar R, Mhaidli H, Taher AT. Paraspinal extramedullary hematopoiesis in patients with thalassemia intermedia. Eur Spine J. 2010;19(6):871-8.

3.   Alam R, Padmanabhan K, Rao H. Paravertebral mass in a patient with thalassemia intermedia. Chest. 1997;112 (1):265-267.

4. Hijikata Y, Ando T, Inagaki T, Watanabe H, Ito M, Sobue G. Spinal cord compression due to extramedullary hematopoiesis in a patient with myelofibrosis. Rinsho Shinkeigaku. 2014;54(1):27-31.

5. Xiros N, Economopoulos T, Papageorgiou E, Mantzios G, Raptis S. Massive hemothorax due to intrathoracic extramedullary hematopoiesis in a patient with hereditary spherocytosis. Ann Hematol. 2001;80(1):38-40.

6. Alorainy IA, Al-Asmi AR, delCarpio R. MRI features of epidural extramedullary hematopoiesis. Eur J Radiol. 2000;35(1):8-11.

7. Zhu G, Wu X, Zhang X, Wu M, Zeng Q, Li X. Clinical and imaging findings in thalassemia patients with extramedullary hematopoiesis. Clinical Imaging. 2012;36 (5):475-482.

8. Zafeiriou DI, Economou M, Athanasiou-Metaxa M. Neurological complications in β-thalassemia. Brain and Development. 2006;28(8): 477-481.

9. Alam MR, Habib MS, Dhakal GP, Khan MR, Rahim MA, Chowdhury AJ, et al. Extramedullary hematopoiesis and paraplegia in a patient with hemoglobin e-Beta thalassemia. Mymensingh Med J. 2010;19(3): 452-457.

10. Haidar R, Mhaidli H, Musallam KM, Taher AT. The spine in β-thalassemia syndromes. Spine (Phila Pa 1976). 2012;37(4): 334-339.

11. Shin KH, Sharma S, Gregoritch SJ, Lifeso RM, Bettigole R, et al. Combined radiotherapeutic and surgical management of a spinal cord compression by extramedullary hematopoiesis in a patient with hemoglobin E beta thalassemia. Acta Haematol. 1994;91(3):154-157.

12. Ileri T, Azik F, Ertem M, Uysal Z, Gozdasoglu S. Extramedullary hematopoiesis with spinal cord compression in a child with thalassemia intermedia. J Pediatr Hematol Oncol. 2009; 31(9):681-683.

13. Munn RK, Kramer CA, Arnold SM. Spinal cord compression due to extramedullary hematopoiesis in beta-thalassemia intermedia. Int J Radiat Oncol Biol Phys. 1998;42(3):607-609.

14. Salehi SA, Koski T, Ondra SL. Spinal cord compression in beta thalassemia: case report and review of the literature. Spinal Cord. 2004;42(2):117-123.

15. Atmaca HU, Akbas F, Karagoz Y, Sametoglu F. Spinal cord compression due to Extramedullary Hematopoiesis (EMH) in a subject with beta thalassemia. Eur J Int Med. 2013;24(1):168-169.

16. PistevouGompaki K, Skaragas G, Papaskevopoulos P, Kotsa K, Repanta E. Extramedullary haematopoiesis in thalassemia: results of radiotherapy: a report of three patients. Clin Oncol (R Coll Radiol). 1996;8(2):120-122.

17. Jackson DV Jr, Randall ME, Richards F 2nd. Spinal cord compression due to extramedullary hematopoiesis in thalassemia: long-term follow-up after radiotherapy. Surg Neurol. 1988;29(5):389-392.

18. De Klippel N, Dehou MF, Bourgain C, Schots R, De KeyserJ, Ebinger G. Progressive paraparesis due to thoracic extramedullary hematopoiesis in myelofibrosis. Case report. J Neurosurg. 1993;79(1):125-127.

19. Phupong V, Uerpairojkij B, Limpongsanurak S. Spinal cord compression: a rareness in pregnant thalassemic woman. J Obstet Gynaecol Res. 2000;26(2):117-120.

20. Mattei TA, Higgins M, Joseph F, Mendel E. Ectopic extramedullary hematopoiesis: evaluation and treatment of a rare and benign paraspinal/epidural tumor. J Neurosurg Spine. 2013;18(3):236-242.

21. Papavasiliou C. Clinical expressions of the expansion of the bone marrow in the chronic anemias: The role of radiotherapy. Int J Radiat Oncol Biol Physics. 1994;28 (3):605-612.

22. Hassoun H, Lawn-Tsao L, Langevin ER, Lathi ES, Palek J. Spinal cord compression secondary to extramedullary hematopoiesis: a non-invasive management based on MRI. Am J Hematol. 1991;37(3):201-203.

23. Karimi M, Cohan N, Pishdad P. Hydroxyurea as a first-line treatment of extramedullary hematopoiesis in patients with beta thalassemia: Four case reports. Hematology. 2015;20(1): 53-57.

24. RuoRedda MG, Allis S, Reali A, Bartoncini S, Roggero S, Anglesio SM, et al. Complete recovery from paraparesis in spinal cord compression due to extramedullary haemopoiesis in beta-thalassemia by emergency radiation therapy. Intern Med J. 2014;44(4):409-412.

25. Cario H, Wegener M, Debatin KM, Kohne E. Treatment with hydroxyurea in thalassemia intermedia with paravertebral pseudotumors of extramedullary hematopoiesis. Ann Hematol. 2002;81(8): 478-482.

26. Cianciulli P, Sorrentino F, Morino L, Massa A, Sergiacomi GL, Donato V, et al. Radiotherapy combined with erythropoietin for the treatment of extramedullary hematopoiesis in an alloimmunized patient with thalassemia intermedia. Ann Hematol. 1996;72(6):379-381.

Blood Donors Status of HIV, HBV and HCV in Central Blood Bank in Tripoli, Libya

**Basma Doro[1*], Wajdi M. Zawia[2], Walid M. Ramadan Husien[3],
Nagi Meftah Gerbil Abdalla[2], Adam M. Rifai[2], Enase Dourou[4], Fatma J. Amar[2]
and Abdulwahab N. Aboughress[2]**

[1]Department of Microbiology and Immunology, Faculty of Pharmacy, University of Tripoli,
Tripoli, Libya.
[2]Central Blood Bank, Tripoli, Libya.
[3]Department of Microbiology and Immunology, Medical Faculty, University of Tripoli,
Central Blood Bank, Tripoli, Libya.
[4]Department of Community Medicine, Medical Faculty, University of Tripoli, Libya.

Authors' contributions

This work was carried out in collaboration between all authors. Authors BD and WMZ designed the study, wrote the protocol, and wrote the first draft of the manuscript. Authors NMGA and WMRH managed the literature searches; analyses of the study performed the spectroscopy analysis. Authors ED and BD done the analyses of the study with help of statisticians. Authors AMR, ANA and FJA done and supervised the laboratory work. All authors read and approved the final manuscript.

<u>Editor(s):</u>
(1) Anamika Dhyani, Laboratory of Biochemistry & Molecular and Cellular Biology Hemocentro-UNICAMP, Brazil.
(2) Armel Hervé Nwabo Kamdje, University of Ngaoundere, Cameroon, Ngaoundere, Cameroon.
<u>Reviewers:</u>
(1) Prabhuswami Hiremath, Krishna Institute of Medical Sciences University, India.
(2) Mathew Folaranmi Olaniyan, Achievers University, Owo, Nigeria.
(3) Paul C. Inyang-Etoh, University of Calabar, Nigeria.

ABSTRACT

Background: Post transfusion infections such as hepatitis and human immunodeficiency virus infection continues to be an important public health concern with regard to blood transfusion in Libya and in Africa. This concern is related to the screening test.
Objectives: The main aim of this study to investigate the blood donors samples for HIV, HBV and HCV infections in Tripoli-Libya, North Africa during the first five months of 2015.
Methods: The total of 686 blood samples obtained from healthy blood donors who attended

Corresponding author: E-mail: basmadoro@yahoo.co.uk

Tripoli's central blood bank, were tested for HBsAg, HCV and HIV using the VITROS® 3600 Immunodiagnostic System.

Results: From the 686 samples examined, the frequency of HBsAg positive cases was 0.8%, the number of anti-HBc positive samples was found to be particularly high in the age group 29 and 36 years ($p = 0.0001$). The number of anti-HBc positive samples was found to be particularly high in the age group 30-39 years ($p=0.01$). Most occupation that had positivity with anti-HBc and HBV-DNA were free workers and was less in students. Most positive cases were from east of Tripoli the capital (Tagora, Soq-Aljomaha).

Conclusion: The frequency of HBsAg positive blood donors and anti-HBc among this sample was 0.8% and 0.7% respectively, which is low compared with the international findings. The current study estimated the expected exclusion rate of anti-HBc and HBsAg positive donated blood, as this would be an important factor to consider before donation.

Keywords: Hepatitis B virus; blood donors; HBsAg; anti-HBc; HIV; Libya.

ABBREVIATIONS

HBsAg: Hepatitis B Surface Antigen; HIV: Human Immunodeficiency Virus; HBV: Hepatitis B Virus; HCV: Hepatitis C Virus.

1. INTRODUCTION

Transfusion of blood and blood product is a life saving measurement and benefits numerous patients worldwide. At the same time blood transfusion is an important mode of transmission of infection to the recipients. Blood donation is a process involving the collection, testing, preparing, and storing of blood and blood components. Transfusion plays an important role in the supportive care of medical and surgical patients. Transfusion-transmitted infectious diseases remain a major topic of interest for those involved in blood safety [1].

Blood-borne infections have been recognized as an occupational hazard for nearly 50 years. However, it is only in the last 20 years that there has been a widespread recognition of the specific risk posed to health care workers by blood-borne viruses such as hepatitis B virus, hepatitis C virus and human immunodeficiency virus [2]. To avoid infection by blood transfusion, safety is very important. Blood transfusion is an integral part of medical and surgical therapy. Blood transfusion can cause infection of HIV, Hepatitis, Syphilis, malaria and other viral infections. To avoid this, the tests for HIV, HBV, HCV Syphilis and Malaria are mandatory in the blood bank [3].

The risk of transmitting hepatitis through transfusions of blood and blood products has been known since 1950. In 1965, Blumberg reported on the discovery of the hepatitis B surface antigen (HBsAg) [4]. Hepattis B virus (HBV) is the most common cause of serious liver infection in the world and is said to have infected more than two billion people [5]. The World Health Organization (WHO) reports that approximately 350 million people are chronically infected with the hepatitis B virus and 170 million people carry the hepatitis C virus worldwide[6]. The hepatitis C virus was discovered in 1989 as the major causative agent of non A and non B hepatitis. The hepatitis C virus is transmitted via blood and blood products, both parenterally and through sexual contact [7].

A national serological survey for HBV and HCV infections among the general population was performed in Libya during 2003 and revealed prevalences of 2.2% and 1.2% for HBV and HCV, respectively [8]. Other local surveys reported that the rate of HBsAg positivity among blood donors ranged from 1.3% to 4.6% [9], while the rate of HCV antibodies was 1.2% [10]. The present study has been conducted to screen the HIV, HBV and HCV in blood donors in western Libya (Tripoli area), as well as to estimate the correlation risk factors in blood donor samples. This would be an important factor for the health authorities to consider in blood donor bank.

2. MATERIALS AND METHODS

2.1 Study Design

The study was a Cross sectional study.

2.2 Study Area

North West of Libya, Tripoli the capital. Blood donors were from different regions of the Tripoli metropolitan area like Tagora, Soq Aljomaha in the east, Alfernag, Almadina Alrithia in the center and Alsrage, Hayalandlas in the west.

2.3 Period of Study

The samples were collected in 2015 form January to May.

2.4 Ethical Consideration

The study protocol was reviewed and approved by the Ethical Committees of National Authority for Scientific Research (NASR) of Libya. All participants endorsed a written informed consent form.

2.5 Study Population, Design and Sample Size

The total of 686 blood samples were obtained from healthy blood donors who attended Tripoli's central blood bank during the period from the first of January to end of May of 2015. This blood bank serves neighboring cities as well as Tripoli. All the donors were interviewed and medically examined by consultant before donation; as per the blood bank's standard operating protocol; any donors who were anemic, or who had low body weight or low blood pressure at the time of donation, were excluded. All the donors were counseled and informed about the study, and consent was obtained from each donor to collect an Anonymous questionnaires were completed by each donor, which included personal and demographic data.

2.6 Serological Analysis

All mandatory screening tests for blood transmitted infections, such as HBsAg, anti-HCV and anti-HIV (anti-HIV-1 and -2), were performed in the central blood bank using the VITROS® 3600 Immunodiagnostic System (France) which is fully automated serologic analyzer.

2.7 Data Statistical Analysis

Data was analysed using Statistical Package for Social Science (SPSS) computer software (Version 19, SPSS Inc. USA). The contributing blood donors were divided into age groups. Data

were presented and described by using mean, mode, standard deviation, cross tabulations and graphical presentations. A chi-square test was performed to examine and compare the seroprevalence of anti-HBV, HCV between age groups and blood group.

3. RESULTS

The total of 686 donors blood samples form January to May in Tripoli blood bank were screened for HIV, HBV and HCV, their age were ranged from 16 to 93 years old (mean age 33.5±8.5) (Fig. 1). The majority of the donors were males (683, or 99.6%) and only 3 donors (0.4%) were females (Table 1). Donors occupations were concentrated mainly in free workers and less in students (Fig. 2). The donors were from different regions of the Tripoli metropolitan area like Tagora, Soq Aljomaha in the east, Alfernag, Almadina Alrithia in the center and Alsrage, Hayalandlas in the west (Fig. 3). The total 344 (50.1%) were donors who had non-tested before and have very high risk to transfer hepatitis to others, if not diagnosed during the window gap, and 342 (49.9%) were tested before, who are less dangers because they are repeaters of blood donation (Table 2).

Table 1. Distribution of blood donors according to sex

Gender	Frequency	Percent
Male	683	99.6
Female	3	0.4
Total	686	100

Table 2. The screening of denoting before

Tested before	Frequency	Percentage
Yes	342	49.9%
No	344	50.1%
Total	686	100%

The majority of donors had Rh+ve 82.6% (Table 3). Furthermore, the percentages of blood group O positive were highest (40%) followed by A positive (25.4 %). Whereas, the donors with blood group AB negative was the least (1.3%) (Fig. 4). Additionally, the blood pressure for most of donors was normal to high blood pressure, whilst the percentage of the hypotensive donor was 13.5% (Fig. 5).

The age groups and infections were statistically associated with each other. All 6 HBsAg positive blood donors were in age between 29 and 36 (p=0.0001). All of seropositive donors were found to negative HIV as result of our donation clinic investigation.

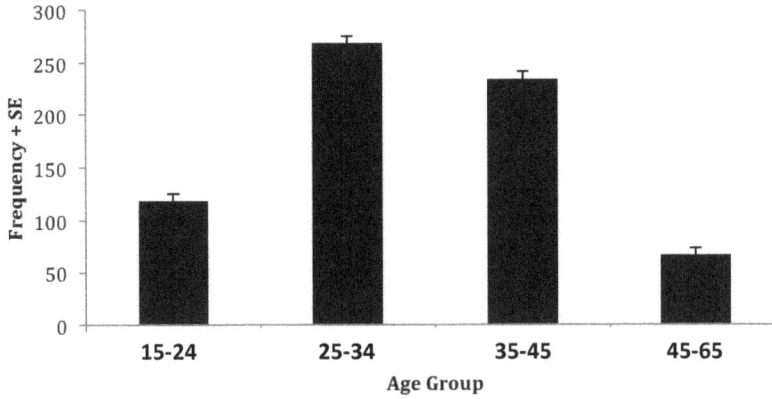

Fig. 1. The age group distribution of blood donor from the total of 686 samples form January to May in Tripoli blood bank

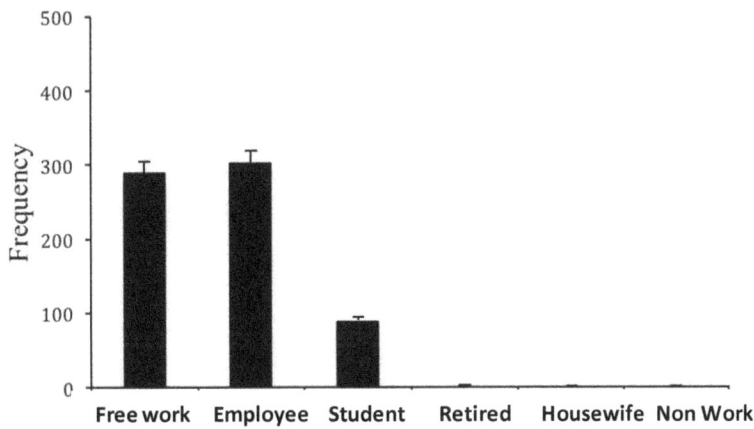

Fig. 2. The frequency of donor occupation that donor blood in Tripoli bank center from of blood donor from January to May

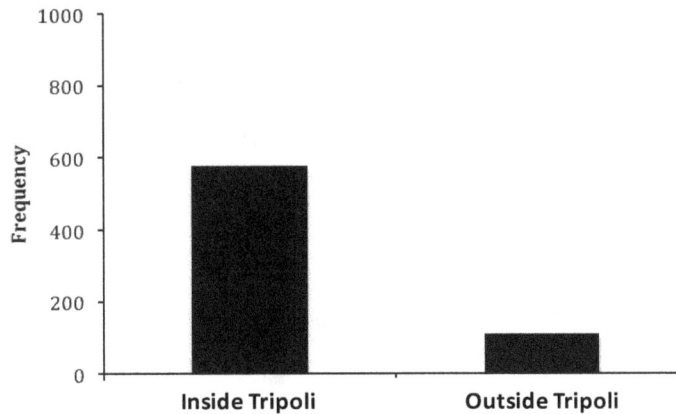

Fig. 3. The address of the donor of blood donor in Tripoli blood bank form January to May 2015

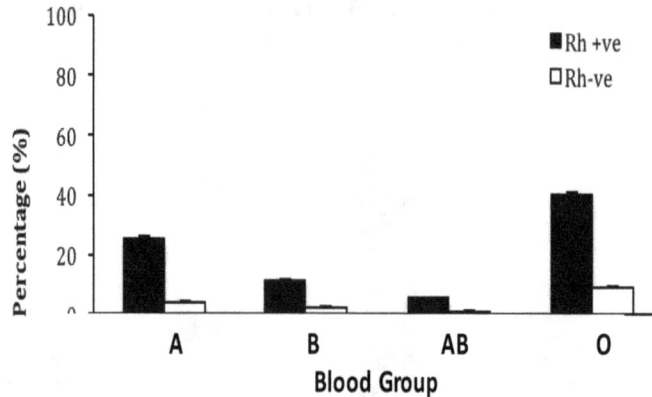

Fig. 4. Frequency of the blood group of blood donor from the total of 686 samples form January to May 2015 in Tripoli blood bank

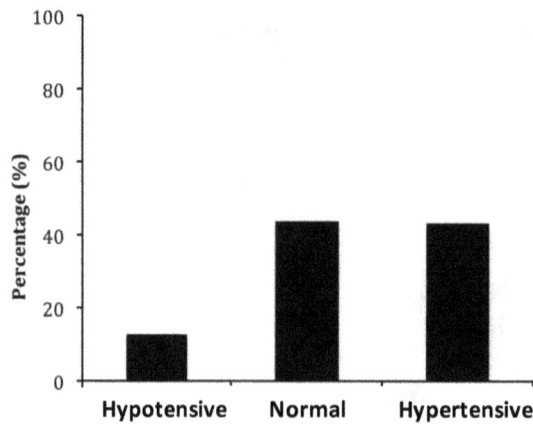

Fig. 5. The blood pressure distribution about donor in Tripoli blood bank center

Table 3. Distribution Rh positive/Rh negative among blood donor

Blood group	Blood donor
Rh positive	82.6%
Rh negative	17.4 %

Anti-HBc screening was performed simultaneously with the other mandatory screening tests for blood-transmitted infections; 5 samples gave positive results for anti-HBc, giving an overall prevalence 0.7%. The frequency of anti-HBc positive cases among the donors was 5 persons (Table 4). In contrast to HBsAg-positive blood donors, the number of anti-HBc positive samples was found to be particularly high in the older age group 30-39 years (44.7%) (p=0.002). Most occupations had positivity with anti-HBc and HBV-DNA were free workers but less in students. Most positive cases were from east of Tripoli the capital (Tagora, Soq Aljomaha).

4. DISCUSSION

HIV, HBV and HCV infections occurrence among blood donors in a rural setting was determined by serological methods and the results were compared to assess the trends in five consecutive months in 2014.

Table 4. Percentage of anti-HBsAg among different age groups

Test	HBsAg		HCV		HIV	
	Frequency	Percentage	Frequency	Percentage	Frequency	Percentage
Positive	6	0.8%	5	0.7%	0	0%
Negative	680	99.2%	681	99.3%	686	100%

The prevalence of viral carrier rates in the blood donors appears in the data with a decrease in HBV and HCV and no HIV. Total 686 donors were screened in five months in 2015 in our blood bank of Tripoli for HIV, HBV and HCV. In current study group the blood donors were majorly belong to 24-45 years and majority of them were Rh-positive males. In present study there are no seroprevalence of HIV. In current study, none of the donors had a confirmed positive result for HIV infections.

Importantly, this present study showed a low frequency of HBV and HCV. This could be explained by the fact that families of blood receipts search for "physically healthy" blood donors. The frequency of anti-HBc among this sample was 5 (0.7%). This percentage was low in comparison with the findings of a previous pilot study (15.6%) that was conducted in the same region, though this difference may be due to the difference in study size [11]. However, the percentage was similar to the results of a preliminary study (9.8%) conducted by the authors in the same place earlier in 2014 [12].

In general, the prevalence rates of hepatitis B and C were lower among young donors than older donors. This confirms the results reported earlier by other investigators [13]. In contrast, most of the blood donors in this study are young men (25-34 years of age). It is recognized that this age group is generally involved in misusing of drug, insecure sex, and other misbehavior habits for the transmission of the virus. Furthermore, The comparisons of the prevalence of transfusion viruses among different sex blood donors may not be applicable because of high proportion of male donors; this is due to low hemoglobulin in females and the fact that Libyan women are less willing to donate blood as the most of the donors (99.3%) were male, which is in consistency with preceding studies [14,15].

In the present study, the prevalence of HBsAg and anti-HCV antibodies was 0.8% and 0.7% respectively. These prevalence rates can be compared with other provincial studies from Central Tripoli Hospital and from Libyan National Center for Infectious diseases were 2.2%, 1.2% [16] and others studies 22.7% was reported with HCV infection through blood transfusion [17]. Moreover, the prevalence of HBV and HCV between blood donors was lower than it is in other countries, for example, the prevalence of hepatitis B among blood donors was 3.8% in Syria [17,18], 9.8% in Yemen [19], 2.1% in Egypt

[20], more than 5.0% in Sudan [21]. Similarly, the prevalence of HCV was 2% in Yemen[19], and high in Egypt 13.6% [20]. The other infectious agent of blood transfusion is HIV causes major health problem in sub Saharan Africa where the prevalence of HIV among blood donors ranges between 2-20% in Kenya [22] and 5.9% in Ethiopia [23]. However, our results showed no confirmed HIV in the analyzed blood donors.

The decreasing trend of HBV and HCV could be due to the fact that screening of blood donors for HBsAg and anti-HCV does not totally eliminate the risk of HBV and HCV infection through blood transfusion since donors with occult HBV and HCV infection that lacked detectable levels of HBsAg and anti-HCV [24] were screened as negative.

It is generally accepted that the diagnosis of infection by HBV is based on the presence of the HBsAg in the bloodstream [25]. However, screening of blood bank donors for HBsAg does not totally eliminate the risk of HBV infection through blood transfusion [26,27], since the absence of this marker in the serum does not exclude the presence of HBV DNA [28]. It is possible that, donors with occult HBV infection, who lacked detectable HBsAg but whose exposure to HBV infection was indicated by a positive anti-HBc and HBV DNA, are a potential source of HBV infection [29]. This emphasizes the need for a more sensitive and stringent screening algorithm of blood donations to improve blood safety. Finally, a national study, including a statistically significant number of blood donors from different blood donation centers across the Libya, should determine whether screening for anti-HBc in addition to HBsAg detection and introduction of PCR based screenings like NAT should also be considered for the libyan blood donors. In the meantime, blood transfusion should only be given when the benefit clearly outweighs the risk.

5. CONCLUSION

Among blood donors that were screened for seroprevalence, only few blood donors were found to be positive for HBV and HCV, there was no HIV cases. A donor requires an effective donor education and high quality selection programme especially during big blood donation camps. Adding of testing for HIV antigen will also reduce risk of HIV infection on a large scale. Even though there is low prevalence of infectious diseases like HBV and HCV in local area, continuous surveillance through strict selection of blood donors and comprehensive screening of donor's blood using standard methods are highly recommended to ensure the safety of blood for recipients in future. Health education and motivation of females is also needed in this area in order to ensure adequate availability of donated blood in cases of emergency. Lastly, strategies should be put in place to take care of infected blood donors.

6. STRENGTHS AND LIMITATIONS OF THE STUDY

It is the first Libyan laboratory based study that used anti-HBc and HBsAg to detect the positivity of hepatitis B disease among blood donors in Libya. Moreover, it uses enough sample size, thus, the result produced from this study reflect the real situation in the Libyan populations living in the capital Tripoli but cannot be generalized among the whole general blood donors of Libya.

7. RECOMMENDATION

To do other studies to measure HIV, anti-HBc and HBsAg in other parts of Libya specially the South. As there is a high level of immigration status in that area.

COMPETING INTERESTS

Authors have declared that no competing interests exist.

REFERENCES

1.   Marcucci C, Madjdpour C, Spahn DR. Allogeneic blood transfusions: Benefit, risks and clinical indications in countries with a low or high human development index. Br Med Bull. 2004;70:15-28.
2.   Alqahtani JM, Abu-Eshy SA, Mahfouz AA, El-Mekki AA, Asaad AM. Seroprevalence of hepatitis B and C virus infections among health students and health care workers in the Najran region, southwestern Saudi Arabia: The need for national guidelines for health students. BMC Public Health. 2014; 14:577.
3.   Anuradha M, Rh E. Seroprevalence of transfusion-transmissible infections HIV, HBV and HCV among Blood Donors in Perambalur, Tamilnadu. IJHSR. 2014;4(5): 76-81.
4.   Manesis EK, Papatheodoridis GV, Tiniakos DG, Hadziyannis ES, Agelopoulou OP, Syminelaki T, Papaioannou C, Nastos T, Karayiannis P. Hepatitis B surface antigen: relation to hepatitis B replication parameters in HBeAg-negative chronic hepatitis B. J Hepatol. 2011;55(1): 61-8.
5.   Lavanchy D. Hepatitis B virus epidemiology, disease burden, treatment, and current and emerging prevention and control measures. J Viral Hepat. 2004; 11(2): 97-107.
6.   Parry J. At last a global response to viral hepatitis. Bull World Health Organ. 2010; 88(11): 801-2.
7.   Alberti A, et al. The interaction between hepatitis B virus and hepatitis C virus in acute and chronic liver disease. J Hepatol. 1995;22(1):38-41.
8.   Elzouki A, E.M, Samod M, Abonaja A, Alagi B, Daw M. Prevalence of hepatitis B, C and HIV infection in Libya: A population-based nationwide seropepidemiological study. Liver Int. 2006;26-20.
9.   An E. Hepatitis B infection in Libya: The magnitude of the problem. The Libyan Journal of Infectious Diseases. 2008;2(1): 20-25.
10.   Daw MA, E.M., Drah AM, Werfalli MM, Mihat AA, Siala IM. Prevalence of hepatitis C virus antibodies among different populations of relative and attributable risk. Saudi Med J. 2002;23(11):1356–1360.
11.   Ismail F, S.M., Aboutwerat A, Elbackush M. Serological and molecular characterization of total hepatitis B core antibodies in blood donors in Tripoli, Libya. The Libyan Journal of Infectious Diseases. 2010;4: 24-30.
12.   Mohamed Kaled A. Shambesh EAF, Faisal Fathalla Ismail, K.A.A.a.F.A. Nagi Meftah Gebril, Anti-HBc and HBV-DNA among Blood Donors inNorth Africa; Western Libya. International Blood Research & Reviews. 2015;3(4):152-159.
13.   Rao P, A.K. HIV status of blood donors and patients admitted in KEM Hospital Pune. Indian J Hemat Blood Transf. 1994; 12:174-176.
14.   Saeed AA, F.D., Al-Admawi AM, Bacchus R, Osoba A, Al-Rasheed A, et al. Hepatitis C virus in Saudi Arabia - a preliminary survey. Saudi Med J. 1990;11:331-332.
15.   Arora D, A.B., Khetarpal A. Seroprevalence of HIV, HBV, HCV and Syphilis in blood donors in Southern

Haryana. Indian J Pathol Microbial. 2010; 53(2):308-309.

16. Nilima Sawke, Chawala SG. Seroprevalence of common transfusion-Transmitted infections among blood donors. People's. Journal of Scientific Research. 2013;1:5-7.

17. Abudher A, E.M., Sammud M, Elzouki A, Tashani O, El-Gadi S. Prevalence of hepatitis B, C and HIV infections in Libya how big are the problem. In XVII International AIDS Conference. Mexico City; 2008.

18. Sarkodie F, A.M., Adu-Sarkodie Y, Candotti D, Acheampong JW, Allain JP. Screening for viral markers in volunteer and replacement blood donors in West Africa. Vox Sang. 2001;80:142-147.

19. NA H. Prevalence of hepatitis B and hepatitis C in blood donors and high riskgroups in Hajjah, Yemen Republic 2. Saudi Med. J. 2002;23:1090-94.

20. Darwish MA, R.T., Rushdy P, Constantine NT, Rao MR, Edelman R. Risk factors associated with a high seroprevalence of hepatitis C virus infection in Egyptian blood donors. Am J Trop Med Hyg. 1993;49: 440-447.

21. Mahgoub, Hepatitis B virus infection and recombination between HBV Genotypes Dand in Asymptomatic Blood Donors from khartoum, Sudan. JCl in Microbiol. 2011; 49(1):298-309.

22. Moore A, H.G., Nyamongo J, Lackritz E, Granade T, Nahlen B, Oloo A, Opondo G., Estimated risk of HIV transmission by blood transfusion in Kenya. Lancet. 2001; 358: 657-60.

23. Sentjens R, S.Y., Vrielink H, Kebede D, Ader HJ, Leckie G, Prevalence of and risk factors for HIV infection in blood donors and various population subgroups in Ethiopia. Epidemiol Infect. 2002;128: 221-228.

24. Allain JP. Occult hepatitis B virus infection: implications in transfusion. Vox Sang. 2004;86(2):83-91.

25. Badur S, A.A. Diagnosis of hepatitis B infections and monitoring of treatment. J Clin Virol. 2001;21:229-237.

26. Conjeevaram HS, L.A. Occult hepatitis B virus infection: A hidden menace. Hepatology. 2001;34:204-206.

27. JP A. Occult hepatitis B virus infection Transfus Clin Biol. 2004;11:18-25.

28. Wang JT, L.C., Chen PJ, Wang TH, Chen DS. Transfusion-transmitted HBV infection in an endemic area: The necessity of more sensitive screening for HBV carriers. Transfusion. 2002;42:1592-1597.

29. Dreier J, K.M., Diekmann J, Götting C, Kleesiek K. Low-level viraemia of hepatitis B virus in an anti-HBc- and anti-HBs-positive blood donor. Transfus Med. 2004; 14:97-103.

4

Complications of Allogeneic Blood Transfusion: Current Approach to Diagnosis and Management

Ademola S. Adewoyin[1*] and Olayinka A. Oyewale[2]

[1]Department of Haematology and Blood Transfusion, University of Benin Teaching Hospital, P.M.B.1111, Benin City, Edo State, Nigeria.
[2]Department of Anaesthesiology, University of Benin Teaching Hospital, P.M.B.1111, Benin City, Edo State, Nigeria.

Authors' contributions

This work was carried out in collaboration between both authors. Author ASA conceived the study and wrote the first draft of the manuscript. Author OAO participated in literature search and performed critical appraisal of the content. Both authors read and approved the final manuscript.

Editor(s):
(1) Dharmesh Chandra Sharma, Incharge Blood Component & Aphaeresis Unit, G. R. Medical College, Gwalior, India.
Reviewers:
(1) Celso Eduardo Olivier, Department of Allergy and Immunology, Instituto Alergoimuno de Americana, Brazil.
(2) Anonymous, Medical University, Poland.
(3) Mario Bernardo-Filho, Universidade do Estado do Rio de Janeiro, Brazil.
(4) Yakubu abdulrahaman, Haematology Department, Usmanu Danfodiyo University, Sokoto, Nigeria.

ABSTRACT

Introduction: Blood transfusion remains a vital component of modern medicine, as yet artificial blood or blood substitute is still widely promising. In well-organized health care systems, with standard transfusion services/facilities and safe practices, the risk associated with infusion of allogeneic blood components is minimal or negligible. However, in most developing nations, significant morbidity is still associated with allogeneic blood transfusion.
Objective: This article is a review on diagnosis of transfusion reactions and modalities for treatment, aimed at promoting interest and awareness as well as, providing current knowledge regarding blood transfusion complications among clinical staff involved in transfusion care.
Methodology: Relevant literatures were searched using search engines such as PubMed and Google Scholar, as well as standard textbooks in transfusion medicine. Results were summarized in appropriate sections.
Results: There are several complications associated with allogeneic blood transfusion. Many of

Corresponding author: E-mail: drademola@yahoo.com

these complications can be prevented and controlled through effective donor and recipient haemovigilance, as well as training and re-training of both clinical and blood bank staff.

Conclusion: Improved knowledge regarding these complications, as well as current treatment guidelines is a crucial strategy to their prevention and control in developing nations. This will invariably increase the capacity and ability of the attending clinical staff (physicians/nurses) to correctly identify, manage and report these adverse transfusion reactions.

Keywords: Blood transfusion; transfusion reactions; complications; allogeneic blood; developing countries; diagnosis and management; prevention of transfusion reactions.

1. INTRODUCTION

Blood transfusion refers to therapeutic infusion of blood, blood components and blood products into an individual in order to meet a specific physiologic need. As yet, laboratory synthesis or culture of blood components is still neither practically possible nor commercially available, safe transfer of blood from the donor to the recipient must be ensured [1–3]. While researches are directed at commercial production of artificial blood, current practices must aim at zero tolerance for blood transfusion reactions [1-3]. There is therefore a need for effective haemovigilance system particularly in developing nations.

There are several notable complications of allogeneic blood transfusion. Since the inception of transfusion practices, transfusion safety has been a major concern and challenge. Earliest attempts at blood transfusion were fraught with life-threatening complications such as acute haemolytic transfusion reactions [4,5]. However, the discovery of ABO blood group system by Karl Landsteiner in 1901 provided the much needed clinical insights into the immunologic basis of transfusion reactions [6,7]. This paved the way for today's routine immune pre-compatibility testing of blood units. However, transfusion reactions were not limited to immunologic causes alone. In the 1970s prior to routine viral screening of blood components and prior to discovery of HIV in 1983, a significant proportion of haemophiliacs and other patients regularly transfused with blood components developed acquired immunodeficiency syndrome (AIDS) [8-10]. These observations propelled the quest for invention of reliable methods of detecting and curbing transfusion transmissible infections (TTIs) [11]. Up until this moment, myriad of complications have been reported and described in association with blood transfusion. Incidence of many of these complications has been controlled to the barest minimum in most developed nations [12-15]. Conversely,

haemovigilance systems in developing African/Asian nations including Nigeria are poor or even non-existent [16]. On a global scale, the incidence of transfusion reactions range from less than 1% in US to as high as 8.7% in developing countries [17-19].

In view of the burden and potential hazards associated with blood transfusion especially in developing nations, it is pertinent to review the current definitions and differential diagnosis of blood transfusion-related complications, their treatment and prevention. Improved knowledge among hospital clinical staff (transfusionist) will foster better awareness and improved transfusion care, especially in developing nations. As well, it provides a practical framework for developing local/institutional protocols that are geared towards implementing a more effective haemovigilance system.

Relevant local and foreign literatures on epidemiology, diagnosis and management of transfusion reactions were sought, collated and summarized in appropriate sections of this manuscript. Searches were performed using search engines such as google scholar, PubMed, as well as standard textbooks in transfusion medicine. Search words such as complications, allogeneic blood, transfusion medicine and epidemiology were used.

2. CURRENT TRENDS IN TRANSFUSION MEDICINE

The current scope of transfusion medicine goes beyond the traditional infusion of blood to include infusions of peripheral stem cells, recombinant coagulation proteins and use of haemopoiesis stimulating drugs such as erythropoietin and aphaeresis technology [20,21]. In today's practice, infusion of whole blood is hardly indicated except cases of significant acute blood loss, autologous blood transfusions, as well as neonatal/intrauterine transfusions. Blood components are therapeutic components of blood intended for transfusion. Blood product refers to therapeutic products, derived from blood or plasma, produced through a manufacturing process [21].

In today's transfusion practice, whole blood therapy is hardly utilized. However, this may not be the case in most developing nations, including Nigeria. Ideally, specialist blood components such as red cell concentrates, platelets, fresh frozen plasma (FFP) and cryoprecipitate are administered to individual patients as indicated. Even where multiple transfusion needs are present as in a patient with symptomatic severe pancytopenia, each specific component is administered. The practice of blood component therapy (BCT) is associated with improved utility of blood (a single whole blood unit may be separated into three different components for possible use by three different patients) [22]. Further to this, BCT reduce unnecessary patient exposure to non-therapeutic fractions of the whole blood being transfused, resulting in fewer complications. In the long run, BCT if well practiced reduces blood supply needs and the overall cost of transfusion practice [23].

Blood components are prepared through centrifugation technique or aphaeresis [24]. Aphaeresis refers to extraction of specific cells from a blood donor using a programmed machine. Aphaeresis components are more effective and preferable to red cells/platelets prepared by cold centrifugation. The major therapeutic benefits of aphaeresis include automation, reduced recipient exposure to multiple donors, thus reducing the risk of immunologic transfusion reactions and TTIs [24,25].

3. COMPLICATIONS OF BLOOD TRANSFUSION

These are undesirable and unintended response or effects during or after administration of blood, blood components or blood products, that can be associated with a said product. Simply put, they are adverse transfusion reactions or hazards of blood transfusion [20]. Transfusion reactions are categorized based on the timing of onset or its underlying pathophysiologic mechanisms, as shown in Table 1. A transfusion reaction is said to be acute if it occurs during or within 24 hours of transfusion or delayed if it occurs beyond 24 hours up to 4 weeks after transfusion. Acute transfusion reactions (ATR) occur at a rate of 0.5–3% [26]. Long-term complications such as iron overload, TTIs occurs and persists for months or years after transfusion episodes. Transfusion reactions may also be immune mediated or non-immunologic [20].

Table 1. Complications of blood transfusion

ACUTE COMPLICATIONS	DELAYED/LONG-TERM COMPLICATIONS
IMMUNOLOGIC • Allergic reactions • Febrile non-haemolytic transfusion reactions • Anaphylactic reaction • Transfusion related acute lung injury • Acute haemolytic transfusion reaction	**IMMUNOLOGIC** • Delayed haemolytic transfusion reaction • Delayed serologic transfusion reaction • Allo-immunization • Transfusion associated Graft Versus Host Disease • Post transfusion purpura
NON-IMMUNOLOGIC • Bacterial contamination/sepsis • Transfusion associated circulatory overload • Clotting abnormalities • Metabolic complications: citrate toxicity, hyperkalaemia, hypocalcaemia, hypothermia, etc Others: Air embolism	**NON IMMUNOLOGIC** • Transfusion transmissible infections • Thrombophlebitis • Iron overload

4. ACUTE COMPLICATIONS AND TREATMENT GUIDELINES

4.1 Febrile Non-haemolytic Transfusion Reactions

Febrile non-haemolytic transfusion reaction (FNHTR) is the commonest immediate complication of blood transfusion [19,20,27,28]. It is almost always associated with infusion of cellular components and rarely plasma components. Its incidence is higher with transfusion of whole blood derived platelet concentrates (4.6%) compared to red cell transfusions (0.33%) [29]. FNHTR is more frequent in multi-transfused persons as well as multi-parous women. Immune and non-immune mechanisms are implicated in its aetiology. FNHTR is considered a form of systemic inflammatory response syndrome (SIRS) which results from exposure to antigenic stimuli in the donor blood. In most settings, the recipient has been sensitized to the implicating antigen usually HLA antigens on leucocytes or less frequently human platelet antigens and neutrophil specific antigens, that are lacking in the recipient [20]. The resultant antigen-antibody interaction triggers systemic inflammation with release of pyrogenic cytokines such as interleukin-1 (IL-1) and tumor necrosis factor (TNF). With increasing length of storage, the levels of cytokines in stored components also increase, explaining why FNHTR is more frequent in stored blood components [29]. Clinically, patients with FNHTR develop fever (at least 38°C) or at least 1°C rise above baseline, within 30 to 90 minutes of commencement of transfusion. Fever may be associated with chills, rigors and headaches [20]. Diagnosis of FNHTR requires exclusion of other causes of fever including pre-transfusion morbidities, life threatening transfusion reactions such as septic transfusion reactions, transfusion related acute lung injury (TRALI) and acute haemolytic transfusion reaction (AHTR). Often times, FNHTR are more troublesome than dangerous especially in situations mediated by very potent lymphocytotoxic HLA antibodies. Treatment guidelines for FNHTR are suggested in Table 2 below [29-31].

Although, there are strong arguments for and against universal leucoreduction of blood products [35], the potential benefits in support of universal leucodepletion as practiced in some nations is related to preventing transmission of prions and cytomegalovirus, prevention of transfusion related immune-modulation (TRIM), asides reducing the incidence of FNHTR. However, cost-benefit analysis suggests that leucodepletion does not have a favorable cost effectiveness ratio in relation to the incidence of FNHTR [36].

Table 2. Treatment of febrile non-haemolytic transfusion reactions

1.	The goal of treatment is to relieve symptoms and prevent recurrences.
2.	Patients with prior history of FNHTR should be pre-medicated with antipyretics before onset of transfusions
3.	At the outset of FNHTR, blood transfusion should be temporarily discontinued until life threatening differentials of transfusion pyrexia such as AHTR is excluded.
4.	Intravenous access should be maintained with isotonic saline.
5.	Antipyretics should be administered immediately in order to relieve the fever. Oral acetaminophen should be given at a dose of 500–1000mg in adults or 10–15 mg/kg in children. NSAIDS should be avoided.
6.	If rigor is persistent, it may be controlled with morphine 2–4 mg intravenously (IV) stat. Meperidine (pethidine) 25–50 mg IV should be avoided due to its potentials for neurotoxicity.
7.	If there is inter-current allergies/urticaria, antihistamines such as diphenhydramine, chlorpheniramine or promethazine should be administered.
8.	In patients that are refractory to the above regimen, gluco-corticoids are indicated. Hydrocortisone IV should be administered at a dose of 100 mg stat (adults) or 1–2 mg/kg in children.
9.	If symptoms are controlled within 30 minutes to an hour, transfusion should be resumed at a slower rate.
10.	In patients with prior history of FNHTR, pre-medication with hydrocortisone 100 mg IV 4–6 hours before commencement of transfusion and or other antipyretics prevents FNHTR.
11.	Transfusion should be administered at a slow rate after symptoms abate.
12.	Pre-storage leucodepletion of blood component reduces the risk of FNHTR [32-34].

Due to its lack of cost-effectiveness, universal leuco-depletion of blood components may not be practical in most developing nations. However, leucodepletion should be favourably considered in selected cases including neonatal transfusions, history of prior FNHTR and haemopoietic stem cell transplant (HSCT) recipients.

4.2 Acute Haemolytic Transfusion Reaction

Acute haemolytic transfusion reaction (AHTR) is the most dangerous early complication of blood transfusion. It is frequently associated with human errors such as mislabeling of samples, patient misidentification, erroneous interpretation of tests, misrecording/transcription errors and other clerical issues. Incidence is about 1 per 600,000 red cell transfusions, with mortality rate of about 5 to 10%. Overall, the incidence of haemolytic transfusion reaction is in the range of 1 per 10000 to 50000 blood components transfused [37–39]. Often times, AHTR is associated with ABO antigens and majority of AHTR are caused by mismatch blood transfusions [12]. Non-ABO antigens such as Rh and Kell antigens are also implicated, especially in the extravascular forms. AHTR may be intravascular or extravascular. Typically, haemolysis occurs within 24 hours of blood transfusion. Intravascular haemolysis mediated by ABO antibodies is the most dramatic and is potentially life-threatening if prompt treatment is not instituted. In ABO mismatch transfusion reactions, interaction of naturally occurring anti-A and anti-B with corresponding antigens in the recipient circulation provokes full complement activation. Membrane attack complexes (C5b-C9) are deposited on the red cell membranes, causing intravascular haemolysis. The degree of haemolysis depends on the site of haemolysis, class or subclass of the implicating antibody, volume of blood unit transfused and patient's clinical state [20]. It is most severe in the setting of an O recipient with high titre of anti–A and anti–B receiving A, B or AB blood unit. It is less severe when A red cells is given to B recipient or vice versa or where O plasma is infused into A, B, or AB recipient. The host inflammatory response to the foreign antigen and the massive haemolysis underlies the symtomatology of AHTR. Affected patients may complain of pain/heat at the infusion site/cannulated vein, feeling of impending doom, chest tightness, loin pain or nausea [20]. The patient develops fever, associated with chills, rigors, tachycardia or hypotension which may progress to shock. Massive intravascular haemolysis may precipitate a pre-renal acute kidney injury (AKI). Release of pro-coagulant substances from red cell stroma may trigger activation of systemic intravascular coagulation, culminating in disseminated intravascular coagulopathy (DIC). Diagnosis of AHTR in an unconscious patient requires a high index of suspicion; the only pointers may be hypotension, haemoglobinuria or oozing from the infusion site. AHTR may mimic hyper-haemolytic crisis in sickle cell disease.

Treatment of AHTR is presented in Table 3 below [30,31,39,40].

4.3 Allergic Reactions

Allergic transfusion reactions are also common. It occurs in about 1–3% of all transfusions and is more frequent in atopic individuals [41]. It is a type 1 hypersensitivity reactions mediated by IgE bound basophils and mast cells in previously sensitized blood recipients. When re-exposed to implicating allergens (most often plasma proteins) in the donor blood, antigen-antibody interaction causes cross-linking of bound-immunoglobulins on mast cells, hence degranulation. Preformed vaso-active amines (principally histamine and serotonin) in mast cells and basophils are released [20,42]. As a late response, leukotrienes, slow release substances of anaphylaxis are also released. Typically, patient develops a localized or systemic urticarial rash with erythema and pruritus [29]. In severe allergies or anaphylactic reactions, other organs systems such as the chest, cardiovascular and gastro-intestinal are involved. Generally, allergies are more troublesome than dangerous. Allergies do not always recur in subsequent transfusions and is not associated with fever. Treatment modalities include temporary cessation of blood transfusion, relief of allergy and completion of transfusion after symptoms abate. For control of symptoms, H-1 blocking antihistamines such as diphenhydramine 25–50 mg IV or oral should be administered. Newer antihistamines such as cetirizine and loratidine are less sedating. H2 blocking antihistamines may speed up resolution of symptoms. Transfusion should be resumed after 30 minutes if symptoms abate. In severe allergies or refractory cases, transfusion of the index blood unit should be stopped completely. In patients with laryngeal/facial oedema or even hypotension, adrenaline (subcutaneous) at 0.2–0.5 ml (1:1000 dilution 0.2–0.5 mg) should be administered [29]. For subsequent transfusions, pre-medications with anti-histamines are recommended. Saline washed red cells is indicated in subsequent transfusion of patients with two or more serious allergic reactions that were unresponsive to HI and H2 blockers. Incidence of allergic reactions is not reduced by leucocyte reduction [43].

4.4 Anaphylactic/Anaphylactoid Reactions

Anaphylactic reaction is a severe of allergy mediated by Ig E antibodies which induce cross linking of basophils and mast cells on re-exposure to the allergens in the donor blood unit. Asides preformed mediators including serotonin and histamine, newly synthesized chemical mediators such as platelet activating factors (PAF), prostaglandins and leukotrienes are also released. PAF is believed to play a major/central role in anaphylaxis. PAF induces up-regulation of nitric oxide production, leading to widespread vessel dilatation and shock [29].

Anaphylactoid reactions are not mediated by Ig E antibodies. The classic anaphylactoid transfusion reaction occurs in the setting of an Ig A deficient blood recipient transfused with Ig A containing blood component.

Table 3. Treatment of acute haemolytic transfusion reaction

1.	AHTR is suspected in a patient with transfusion-related fever which may be associated with loin pains/tachycardia/hypotension, drop in haemoglobin level within 24 hours of transfusion and evidence of haemolysis (elevated serum bilirubin, LDH and low haptoglobin levels).
2.	AHTR is a haematologic emergency and should be treated as such.
3.	Blood transfusion must be stopped immediately, while intravenous access is maintained with isotonic saline using a new infusion giving set. The patient's identity, blood bag label and compatibility form must be re-checked for any form of mismatch or clerical errors.
4.	The discontinued blood unit, along with its tubing and the patient's post-transfusion blood sample should be sent to the blood bank. Repeat grouping with cross-matching must be performed on patient's pre- and post-transfusion samples. A direct anti-globulin test is usually positive.
5.	Urine should be examined for haemoglobinuria. Blood chemistries including renal function test (serum electrolytes, urea and creatinine), markers of haemolysis such as serum bilirubin levels, LDH and haptoglobin levels, should be performed.
6.	Patient's blood sample and the blood in the bag should be sent for microbiologic culture.
7.	In suspected DIC cases, it is necessary to do coagulation studies including prothrombin time, activated partial thromboplastin time, thrombin time and plasma fibrinogen levels, D-dimers or FDPs. A full blood count may reveal neutrophilia, thrombocytopenia (in consumptive coagulopathy) and anaemia.
8.	Patients with organ system damages such shock, renal shut-down should be co-managed with appropriate specialist teams in the intensive care units (ICU) or high dependency units.
9.	Other supportive cares include adequate hydration to maintain normal blood pressure and good urinary output (at least 1 ml/kg/hr or 100 ml/hour).
10.	If patient is oliguric, renal challenge with furosemide 40–80 mg IV stat (1–2 mg/kg in children) is given, with later doses adjusted to maintain adequate urine output. Dialysis is necessary if oliguria persists after 2 to 3 hours of renal challenge, further fluid and furosemide therapy may be contra-indicated.
11.	Oxygen therapy should be administered if indicated. Antipyretics are given to control the fever.
12.	Hypotension should be controlled with dopamine infusion 2–5 ug/kg/min. Other pressor drugs such as adrenaline, nor-adrenaline and high dose dopamine should be avoided since they reduce renal perfusion.
13.	For an established DIC, replacement therapy should be offered. Fresh frozen plasma (FFP) at a dose of 10–15 ml/kg should be infused if PT or APTT ratio exceeds 1.5. Similarly, 1.5 Unit per 10 kg of cryoprecipitate is given if plasma fibrinogen level is less than 1 g/l. An adult therapeutic dose of platelet concentrate is given if counts drop below 50,000/ul.
14.	Close monitoring of the patient's coagulation profile is necessary until the disease wanes.
15.	Patient's haemoglobin level should be optimized with group identical blood units.

It is a rare entity. Ig A deficiency occurs with a frequency of about 1 per 700 persons [44]. However, most affected persons do not develop anti-Ig A. For individuals who develop anti-Ig A antibodies, upon transfusion of an Ig A containing blood component, Ig A anti-Ig A complexes are formed which trigger classical complement pathways, inducing massive release of anaphylatoxins, C3a, C4a and C5a. There is massive dilatation of peripheral vessels, increased vascular permeability and pooling of blood in the peripheral, culminating in shock (cardiovascular collapse) [20,29,42]. Typically, the onset of symptoms occurs rapidly within seconds and minutes of transfusion and multiple systems are involved including cutaneous, respiratory, cardio-vascular and gastro-intestinal manifestations [29,42]. The patient develops rapid onset of laryngeal oedema and bronchospasm with stridor, wheezing, coughing and respiratory distress. Other symptoms include generalized urticarial, erythema, tachycardia, hypotension, nausea, vomiting, diarrhoea, cramping abdominal or pelvic pain [42,45]. Severe reactions lead to shock, syncope, respiratory failure and death. Anaphylaxis is an emergency and should be managed by experienced staff in an ICU setting. Subcutaneous dose of 0.2–0.5 ml of 1:1000 epinephrine solutions (1 mg/ml) should be administered in adults (0.01 ml/kg body weight in children). This may be repeated every 15–30 minutes as needed. Further infusion may be titrated based on Blood Pressure. If isystolic blood pressure drops below 60mmhg, IV epinephrine is given at a dose of 1–5 ml of a 1:10000 solution (0.1 mg/ml) in adults and 0.1 ml/kg IV push in children, over 2–5 minutes. A central venous pressure (CVP) line may be used to monitor the effectiveness of fluid replacement and pressor infusion. For respiratory distress, supplemental oxygen at 4 Litres/min is given in adults [29]. Endotracheal intubation is given in laryngeal oedema with obstruction (stridor is a sign of larygngeal oedema). Endotracheal intubation with mechanical ventilation is instituted if PaCO2>65 mmHg. If intubation is difficult or impossible, cricothyrotomy or tracheostomy is indicated. Wheezing is controlled with nebulized albuterol and IV aminophylline [29,42]. Urticaria/angioedema/GI distress is managed with antihistamine, diphenhydramine 50 mg IV (in children 1–2 mg/kg IV). Intravenous hydrocortisone 200 mg 6 hourly is given to control late inflammatory responses. For subsequent transfusions, washed red cells are given. If plasma transfusions are needed, Ig A deficient plasma must be administered [29,42].

4.5 Transfusion Related Acute Lung Injury (TRALI)

TRALI is defined as a new acute lung injury that develops with a clear temporal relationship to transfusion in patients without alternate risk factors for acute lung injury [46]. TRALI is non-cardiogenic, rare and is associated with infusion of plasma containing blood components. Transfusion related acute lung injury (TRALI) is a rare complication of blood transfusion. Its incidence is about 1 in 5,000–10,000 transfusions. It is a leading cause of transfusion related fatality [47]. It occurs more frequently in the setting of blood donations from multiparous women. Its aetiology is attended by the presence of leucoagglutinins in donor blood, causing agglutination of leucocytes (often times, that of the recipients, less frequently donor leucocytes or both) in the recipient pulmonary microcirculation. The resultant endothelial and epithelial injury, alveolar damage and inflammatory changes cause adult respiratory distress (ARD) like symptoms [48]. Most cases are mild-moderate and may be missed. Typically, the patients develops respiratory distress, associated with fever, chills, cough, usually within two hours of transfusion, but sometimes up to 6 hours. Chest radiography shows new bilateral pulmonary infiltrates. There may be associated hypotension. Treatment essentially is supportive and patients may require high dependency unit (HDU) care [48]. Supportive therapy includes antipyretics and oxygen support [48]. Mortality rate is about 5 to 10% and most cases resolve within 72 to 96 hours [49]. TRALI is not improved by diuretic therapy. Transfusion of blood units from male donors reduces the risk.

4.6 Septic Transfusion Reaction

Septic transfusion reaction (STR) is a potentially life-threatening complication that results from bacterial contamination of a blood unit. Bacterial contamination may be due to asymptomatic bacteraemia in the donor or contamination by skin commensals during the blood collection process [50]. STR is commoner with platelet transfusion than red cell transfusions due to room temperature storage of platelets [41]. Psychrophilic organisms such as *Yersinia enterolitica*, is associated with red cell contamination. Commonly implicated organisms in platelet transfusions include *Staphyoloccus aureus*, coagulase negative *staphylococci*, diphtheroids and other skin commensals [50,51]. Depending on specie and load of the implicating bacteria in the blood component, the patient develops fever (usually above 39°C) with chills and rigors, tachycardia, hypotension, dyspnoea, gastro-intestinal tract disturbances and may progress to DIC. Symptoms usually evolve during the transfusion process, usually within the first 15 minutes.

In cases of suspected acute transfusion reaction due to bacterial contamination, the blood unit should be stopped immediately. The blood bank should be notified immediately so that other components from same donor can be traced and withdraw before use. Microbiologic testing should be commenced immediately. Samples for blood culture should be taken from the blood unit and the patient and sent for appropriate testings [52]. Treatment involves commencement of broad spectrum antibiotics before culture results are made available. Patient should be monitored closely with aggressive supportive care for fever, shock and DIC as indicated [45].

STR can be prevented by applying measures that reduce or eliminate bacterial contamination of blood components. Proper donor arm cleansing and diversion of the first 20–30 mls of blood reduces the risk of bacterial contamination by up to 77% [53–55]. Donated units should intermittently be checked and cultured for bacterial contamination. Visual checks of every blood unit should be performed before transfusion [52]. Visible growth in the bag, flocculation and discoloration are signs of bacterial contamination. Storage of platelet units should not exceed 5 days except in settings where bacterial detection systems are available and monitoring/bacterial culture is performed between days 2 and 3 [52,56].

4.7 Transfusion Associated Circulatory Overload

Transfusion associated circulatory overload (TACO) is a potentially fatal complication, with incidence of about 0.1 to 1% of all transfusions. Neonates, elderly patients, patients with cardiac or renal disease are at particular risk. TACO is caused by pulmonary oedema induced by volume overload during large volume transfusions or infusion of blood products with high osmotic load. Clinical features of TACO include cough, dyspnoea, raised jugular venous

pressure (JVP), bibasal crepitations, tachycardia, hypertension and widened pulse pressure [41]. Elevated Brain Natiuretic peptide, BNP, a peptide secreted from the ventricules in response to increased filling pressures, may assist in diagnosis [57]. In patients with TACO, transfusion should be discontinued immediately and treatment for heart failure commenced. Typically, furosemide 20 –40 mg IV is given and patient is nursed with cardiac position. Oxygen therapy may also be required.

In at risk patients, transfusion should be administered at a slower pace at longer intervals except in emergencies. Premedication with a diuretic, furosemide 20–40 mg IV stat should be given. For patient requiring immediate reversal of warfarin overdose, prothrombin complex concentrate (PCC) is preferred to infusion of large volumes of FFP. Packed red cells or red cell concentrate is the appropriate component.

4.8 Complications of Massive Blood Transfusion

Massive blood transfusion is said to occur when a blood recipient has received at least one blood volume within a 24 hours period. This is often associated with conditions of acute blood loss following trauma or obstetric complications. With replacement of one blood volume, dilutional coagulopathy sets. With replacement of 1.5 times blood volume, dilutional thrombocytopenia set in. Complications of massive blood transfusion are related to biochemical and metabolic changes that accompany blood storage, as well as dilutional effects of large volume transfusion. They include metabolic and coagulopathic complications. Metabolic complications include citrate toxicity with resultant hypocalcaemia, hyperkalaemia and hypothermia [40]. Symptomatic hypocalcaemia manifests as peri-oral tingling, facial numbness, muscle twitching and cardiac arrhythmias in extreme cases. With prolonged storage of red cells, intracellular potassium leaks out of the cells into the suspending plasma, hence hyperkalaemia. This particularly significant in neonates receiving EBT with stored blood or patients with renal disease. Most anticoagulants in routine use are citrate based and they act by chelating calcium ions. Infusion of large volumes of citrated plasma induces hypocalcaemia. Blood is stored at 2–6°C. Transfusion of several cold units of blood induces hypothermia and increases risk for cardiac arrest and DIC. Massive transfusion is associated with clotting abnormalities from dilutional effects, attended by hypothermia. In current practice, an expectant approach often denoted as massive transfusion protocol is usually engaged in massive transfusion [14,58]. Treatment guideline depicted in Table 4 below is recommended in patients enduring massive blood transfusion.

5. DELAYED/LONG-TERM COMPLICATIONS AND TREATMENT GUIDELINES

5.1 Delayed Haemolytic Transfusion Reactions

Delayed haemolytic transfusion reactions (DHTR) may be secondary or primary. Secondary forms occur in individuals that have been previously sensitized during prior transfusion or pregnancies but have low (undetectable) antibody titre which was missed during routine compatibility testings. However, upon re-exposure to the antigens during transfusion, there is a brisk anamnestic response with production of high titre Ig G allo-antibodies. Delayed haemolysis ensues and may occur up to 1 to 2 weeks post transfusion. Primary forms occur without prior antigenic sensitization and occurs up to 28 days. DHTRs are mediated by Ig G antibodies. Rh, Kell and Kidd antibodies are frequently implicated. DHTRs are often missed since most patients are often asymtoptomatic or may develop slight fever. In the absence of clinical evidence and only serologic confirmation, the term Delayed serologic transfusion reaction (DSTR) is used. As such, the actual incidence may be difficult to estimate. Some authors put its incidence at about 1 in 1500 transfusions [60,61]. The clinical suspicion of DHTR may be raised by a triad of fever, hyperbilirubinaemia (jaundice) and drop in post-transfusion haemoglobin levels. Diagnosis is confirmed by a positive post-transfusion DAT. Significant DHTRs are treated in a similar form to AHTRs. DHTR is not totally preventable or predictable. However, it is recommended that fresh serum samples should be used for pre-compatibility testing if last transfusion occurred more than 72 hours [20].

5.2 Red Cell Allo-immunisation

Allo-immunization is a potentially fatal immunologic disease characterized by development of allo-antibodies against non-self antigens following exposure through transfusion, pregnancy, deliberate injection of immunogenic materials or transplant [62]. Clinical sequelae of red cell allo-immunisation may include delayed haemolytic transfusion reaction, acute haemolytic transfusion reaction and haemolytic disease of the fetus and newborn [63,64].

Table 4. Massive transfusion protocol (MTP)

1. There must be a clear trigger for activation of an MTP. This presupposes that every transfusion service/unit should develop appropriate guidelines and protocols.
2. There should be a single person/co-ordinator saddled with the responsibility of establishing continuous communication and collaboration between the blood bank, clinical unit and other requisite services.
3. A porter/runner should be designated for prompt transfer of blood components and samples when necessary.
4. Targets include an haemoglobin level of 10 g/dl, prothromin time ratio/APTT ratio of at most 1.5, platelet count in excess of 50,000/ul (100,000/ul in polytrauma/ CNS trauma) and, plasma fibrinogen level greater than 1g/L. pH>7.2, base excess<6, lactate<4 mmol/l, ionized calcium>1.1 mmol/l should be maintained.
5. Monitoring of patient's full blood count and coagulation studies should be repeated every 3 to 6 hours and at every instance after infusion of plasma components.
6. Fresh frozen plasma should be given at 10–15 ml/kg if PT/APTT Ratio is greater than 1.5, or 1 blood volume (~10 units) has been replaced.
7. Cryoprecipitate is given at a dose of 1.5 unit/10kg if fibrinogen is less than 1 g/l.
8. Platelet concentrate is administered if counts are less than targets or after 1.5 times blood volume (~12 units) has been replaced.
9. Hypothermia (core temperature <35ºC) must be counteracted. Blood and resuscitation fluids should be pre-warmed using temperature controlled blood warmers or warm air blankets. Warming blood to 33–35ºC, not only prevents hypothermia, but also improve blood flow up to 50% by reducing viscosity [59].

Red cell allo-immunisation also accounts for difficulties in selecting appropriate antigen negative units for transfusion especially in the setting of multiple allo-antibodies. However, allo-immunisation rate is higher in patients with history of multiple transfusions or patients on chronic blood transfusion therapy such as thalassemia major and sickle cell disease [65–67]. In most developed centres worldwide (UK and US), routine allo-antibody screening of blood recipients and donated blood units or donors is carried out. This allows detection of atypical antibodies in potential blood recipients. Allo-antibody screening if positive must be followed by antibody identification. When the specificity of the implicating antibody is known, the transfusion laboratory must ensure the selection and provision of antigen-negative blood units (or the least incompatible) for all future transfusions [20].

Incidence of erythrocyte allo-immunisation among at-risk patients may be reduced or prevented by a closer donor–recipient matching, especially in settings of multiple or chronic blood transfusions. Antenatal and postnatal Anti-D prophylaxis should be offered to Rh D negative mother carrying Rh D positive babies.

5.3 Platelet Allo-immunisation

Repeated transfusion places the recipients at risk of allo-antibody formation. Platelet allo-immunisation is most frequently associated with HLA antigens. Occasionally, platelet specific antibodies are implicated. The clinical sequela of platelet allo-immunisation is refractoriness to platelet transfusions. It is noteworthy that platelet refractoriness may also be due to non-immune causes such as fever, splenomegaly, sepsis, occult or obvious bleeding, DIC or ITP or certain drugs [25,68].

Platelet refractoriness is assessed with the corrected count increment (CCI). Non immune causes of platelet refractoriness are commonest and should be excluded in suspected cases. CCI is estimated using 15 minutes to 1 hour post-transfusion platelet count, patient's body surface area and the platelet yield. CCI less than 7.5 at 1 hour or less than 4.5 at 24 hours on at least two occasions is in keeping with platelet refractoriness [68–70]. In refractory patients suspected to be due to platelet allo-immunisation, platelet cross match is needed to identify and provide compatible units. In the alternative, HLA matched platelet units should be

transfused [25,68,69]. Such patients should be regularly monitored with CCI [68–70].

5.4 Post-transfusion Purpura

Post transfusion purpura (PTP) is a rare immunologic complication. It is thought to arise as a result of recipient allo-antibodies against platelet antigens, most commonly human platelet antigen (HPA) 1a and HPA 5b [71]. PTP is more common in multi-parous women due to sensitization from previous pregnancies. PTP occurs about 5 to 10 days after transfusion of red cells, platelets or plasma. Immunologic destruction of transfused platelets results in severe thrombocytopenia, manifesting as purpura. PTP should be suspected in patient presenting with purpura up to 12 days after transfusion. Diagnosis is confirmed by the presence of platelet allo-antibodies (usually anti-HPA 1a), detection of its antithetical antigen in the donor or by a positive platelet cross-match. In severe symptomatic cases, treatment requires intravenous immunoglobulins or plasmapheresis as second option [41,72].

For subsequent transfusions, HPA-1a negative red cell or platelet component is preferable. If not available, a leucodepleted component should be given [20,41].

5.5 Transfusion Associated Graft vs Host Disease

Transfusion associated Graft vs Host disease (TA-GvHD) occurs up to about 1 to 6 weeks following blood transfusion. Its pathophysiology is consequent upon immune attack of host tissues (predominantly the liver, the skin, the gastro-intestinal tract) by immune-competent donor T lymphocytes [73]. Engraftment and proliferation of the foreign clone of T lymphocytes occur in the setting of an immune-compromised recipient or directed donation from a close relative with homozygous expression of HLA antigens for which the recipient is heterozygous. Other risk factors for TA-GvHD include bone marrow transplantation, intrauterine transfusion, congenital immunodeficiency states and HLA matched platelet transfusions [73–75].

Ta-GvHD should be suspected in a patient presenting with fever, rash, diarrhoea, liver dysfunction, cytopenia, within 1 to 6 weeks of blood transfusion, for which no other apparent cause has been found. Diagnosis is confirmed by tissue biopsy of affected organs (Skin biopsy, liver biopsy or bone marrow aspiration) and genetic studies to show chimerism of both donor and recipient lymphocytes [74]. Though rare, Ta-GVHD is a dreaded complication, with very high mortality of over 90%, especially when diagnosis is delayed [74–76]. Treatment is largely supportive. TA-GvHD is unresponsive to immunosuppressive therapy. Leucodepletion does not eliminate the risk of TA-GVHD. Prevention of TA-GVHD rests on irradiation of all cellular products at a minimum recommended dose of 25Gy for all high risk patients [73,77,78].

5.6 Transfusion Siderosis

One unit of red cell transfusion contains about 200 to 250 mg of elemental iron. There is no exact physiologic mechanism for excretion of excess iron from the body. Plasma iron levels and storage iron is regulated by hepcidin regulated release of enterocytes and iron laden macrophages. Daily body iron requirement vary by age, sex and other related conditions such as pregnancy. In an average adult, about 1–3 mg of iron is required daily [79]. Iron losses occur through sloughing off of skin and other epithelial surfaces and menstruation in females. As such, patients receiving multiple transfusions or chronic transfusions are at particular risk of iron overload [80]. Patients with conditions associated with some form of transfusion dependence such as myelodysplastic syndrome, aplastic anaemia, refractory anaemia, myelofibrosis are at particular risk of transfusional iron overload. Such patients should be closely monitored. Serum ferritin level gives a reflection of iron stores. However, serum ferritin level is falsely elevated in chronic inflammatory states such as infections and cancers, pregnancy and surgery and should be interpreted cautiously. Normal serum ferritin levels is about 15–300 ug/l. most authorities recommend commencement of iron chelation therapy when ferritin level is in excess of 1000 ng/ml. a patient that has received about 20 to 30 units of red cells (equivalent to about 4 – 6 gm of iron) is likely to be iron overloaded. Definitive diagnosis is liver biopsy. Liver iron in excess of 7 mg/g in adults and 4 mg/g in children is confirmatory [80,81]. Non-invasive evaluation using sequential quantum interference device (SQUID) is also reliable but relatively unavailable [82–84].

Iron overload induces tissue damage in major organs such as the liver, heart and endocrine glands. Such patients may present with liver cirrhosis with risk of transformation to hepatocellular carcinoma, cardiomyopathy, skin hyperpigmentation (bronze diabetis), diabetis mellitus, hypothyroidism, hypogonadism and other endocrine dysfunctions. Therapy requires iron chelation. Traditionally, intravenous desferrioxamine is used; however newer oral agents such as deferasirox (exjade, asunra) are currently available [85].

5.7 Transfusion Transmissible Infections

In developed areas of the world (UK and US), the risk of TTIs is very low or perhaps negligible due to development of sophisticated testings for infectious pathogens (such as Nucleic Acid Testing, NAT), strict adherence to donor selection criteria and pathogen inactivation techniques [86–89]. In Nigeria and other sub-Saharan African countries, significant infectious risk is still associated with blood transfusion [90–94].

TTIs may be bacterial, viral or parasitic. Bacterial contamination of blood components has been discussed earlier. Known transfusion transmissible viral infections include Hepatitis viruses, HIV, HTLV-1 and HTLV-2 [13]. Parasitic infections such as *Plasmodium* spp, *Babesia* spp, *Leishmania* spp, *Trypanosoma* spp, *Toxoplasma* spp, and microfilaria are also transmissible through blood transfusions. Emerging pathogens, particularly viruses such as SEN V virus, Hepatitis G virus, West Nile Virus, human Herpes Virus – 8 (HHV-8) have also been described [95]. There is also a risk for transmission of prion diseases through blood transfusion [96,97]. However, for economic reasons, all known viral, bacterial or parasitic agents are not routinely tested in blood donors, particularly in developing countries. However, most countries have minimum standard (mandatory screening) measures which often depend on the regional burden/prevalence of these infectious agents (epidemiological patterns), availability of requisite technology and cost of blood supply. As a counter measure (for prion diseases), all fractionated pooled plasma products used in the UK are sourced outside UK (from the US) since 1999 [20].

5.8 Mistransfusions/Overtransfusion/ Under-transfusion

The term, 'mistransfusion' implies transfusion of a unit of blood to the wrong recipient and is often due to mis-identification errors. In the SHOT haemovigilance system, the category termed, 'incorrect blood component transfused' compasses both cases of mistransfusions and inappropriate blood use [12].

Over-transfusion refers to a practice where blood components are transfused in excess of patients estimated transfusion needs [98]. Whereas, under-transfusion is when blood in transfused in a volume less than required to meet to physiologic needs. Under-transfusion may be associated with some benefits including lower risk of TTI, reduced incidence of acute transfusion reactions and less cost to the patient [98].

6. RECOMMENDATIONS

Strategies to improve blood transfusion safety as recommended by WHO include a well organised blood transfusion services, prioritization of blood donation from VNRBDs, screening of donated blood for at least the four major TTIs with quality assured system, rational use of blood and implementation of effective quality control systems [99].

Authors recommend that hospital transfusion committees should design and implement well designed protocols for management of transfusion reactions. These protocols should be distributed to all transfusion units in the hospital and should be updated regularly. As well, medical and nurse practitioners as well as blood bank staff should undergo regular training and retraining of diagnosis and treatment of complications of blood transfusion.

Autotransfusion as well as other alternatives to allogeneic transfusion should be explored where necessary. It is recommended that hospital blood banks should have a system for reporting suspected transfusion reactions. This should be carried out in consonance with the regional and national haemo-vigilance system to ensure adequate co-ordination.

7. CONCLUSION

The complications of blood transfusion are myriad. Good clinical practice is found on morally right and sound ethical principles of autonomy, beneficence, non-maleficence and justice [100]. Therefore, ensuring safe blood transfusions in healthcare systems remains an onus, not an option. Safety of blood transfusions in every transfusion service must be pursued and ensured by relevant stakeholders particularly those in developing nations. Blood systems in developing nations such as Nigeria should be upgraded to meet international standards.

Furthermore, there is need for development of local /institutional protocols and guidelines for management of complications of blood transfusion in Nigeria, especially protocols for investigation and management of acute transfusion reactions. Such protocols should reflect best current practices, should be clear and readily accessible. All clinical staff involved in patient care should undergo training and retraining in relevant clinical areas of transfusion medicine. Improved awareness and knowledge regarding transfusion reactions is a critical step and leverage for successful implementation of institutional, regional and national haemovigilance systems.

CONSENT

It is not applicable.

ETHICAL APPROVAL

It is not applicable.

COMPETING INTERESTS

Authors have declared that no competing interests exist.

REFERENCES

1. Parvajani P, Patel K, Sindhi K, Patel D, Jain H, Pradhan P. Artificial blood: The blood surrogate. Novus International Journal of Pharmaceutical Technology. 2012;1(3):1–9.

2. Shalini S. A review on artificial blood. International Journal of Pharmacy Practice and Drug Research. 2012;2(1):8–16.

3. Habler O, Pape A. Alternatives to allogeneic blood transfusions. Best Practice & Research Clinical Anaesthesiology. 2007;(21)2:221–239. DOI: 10.1016/j.bpa.2007.02.004.

4. Blundell J. Experiments on the transfusion of blood by the syringe. Med Chir Trans. 1818;9:56.

5. Ottenberg R, Kaliski DJ. Accidents in transfusion. Their prevention by preliminary blood examination: Based on

experience of one hundred and twenty-eight transfusions. JAMA. 1913;61:2138.

6. Landsteiner K, Levine P. A new agglutinable factor differentiating individual human bloods. Proc. Soc. Exp. Biol. 1927; 24:600–2.

7. Landsteiner K. On agglutination of normal human blood. Transfusion. 1961;1:5-8.

8. Kleinman SH, Niland JC, Azen SP, et al. And the Transfusion Safety Study Group. Prevalence of antibodies to human immunodeficiency virus type 1 among blood donors prior to screening: The Transfusion Safety Study/NHLBI donor repository. Transfusion. 1989;29:572–580.

9. Donegan E, Stuart M, Niland JC, et al. And the Transfusion Safety Study Group. Infection with human immunodeficiency virus type 1 (HIV–1) among recipients of antibody-positive blood donations. Ann Intern Med. 1990;113:733–1739.

10. Gjerset GF, Clements MJ, Counts RB, et al. Treatment type and amount influenced human immunodeficiency virus seroprevalence of patients with congenital bleeding disorders. Blood. 1991;78:1623.

11. Pankaj Abrol, Harbans Lal. Transfusion transmitted bacterial, viral and protozoal infections. In: Kochhar P (ed). Blood transfusion in clinical practice. InTech Publisher, Rijeka Croatia; 2012. Available:http://www.intechopen.com/books/blood-transfusion-in-clinical-practice/transfusion-transmitted-bacterial-viral-and-protozoal-infections

12. The serious hazards of transfusion steering group. SHOT annual report 2012. manchester, UK: SHOT office; 2012. Available:www.shotuk.org/wp-content/uploads/.../SHOT-Annual-Report-2012.pdf. (Accessed on 09 – 03 – 2014).

13. Fida AH, Mohsin S. Blood transfusion complications and their Prevention. Haematology. Updates. 2011;95–107.

14. Maxwell MJ, Wilson MJA. Complications of blood transfusion. Continuing Education in Anaesthesia, Critical Care & Pain. 2006; 6(6):225–229. DOI: 10.1093/bjaceaccp/mkl053.

15. Australian Haemovigilance report. National Blood Authority Haemovigilance Advisory Committee; 2013.

16. World Health Organisation. Report on global consultation on Haemovigilance. WHO; 2013.

17. The national blood collection and utilization survey report. Report of the U.S. Department of Health and Human Services; 2011. Available:http://www.hhs.gov/ash/bloodsafety/2011-nbcus.pdf (Accessed October 15, 2014).

18. Arewa PO, Akinola NO, Salawu L. Blood transfusion reactions; evaluation of 462 transfusions at a tertiary hospital in Nigeria. African Journal of Medicine and Medical Sciences. 2009;38(2):143–148.

19. Gwaram BA, Borodo MM, Dutse AI, Kuliya-Gwarzo A. Pattern of acute blood transfusion reactions in Kano, North-Western Nigeria. Niger J. Basic Clin Sci. 2012;9:27–32.

20. Contreras M, Taylor Clare PF, Barbara JA. Clinical blood transfusion. In: Hoffbrand AV, Catovsky D, et al. (eds.). Postgraduate haematology, 6 ed. west sussex. Wiley-Blackwell. 2011;16:268–299.

21. U.K. Blood Services. McCelland DBL, (ed). Handbook of transfusion medicine 4ed, TSO, London; 2007.

22. World Health Organisation. The clinical Use of Blood. WHO Blood Transfusion Safety Geneva; 2001.

23. Gurevitz SA. Update and utilization of component therapy in blood transfusions. Labmedicine. 2011;42(4):235–240.

24. Devine DV, Serrano K. Preparation of blood products for transfusion: Is there a best method? Biologicals. 2012;40:187–190.

25. Stroncek DF, Rebulla P. Platelet transfusions. Lancet. 2007;370:427–438.

26. Fry JL, Arnold D, Clase C, Crowther M, Holbrook, Traore A, et al. Transfusion premedication to prevent acute transfusion reactions: A retrospective observational study to assess current practices. Transfusion. 2010;50:1722–1730.

27. Ibrahim UN, Garba N, Tilde IM. Acute blood transfusion reactions in pregnancy, an observational study from North Eastern Nigeria. J. Blood Disorders Transf. 2013; 4:145. DOI:10.4172/2155-9864.1000145.

28. Bhattacharya P, Marwaha N, Dhawan HK, Roy P, Sharma RR. Transfusion-related adverse events at the tertiary care center in North India: An institutional hemovigilance effort. Asian Journal of Transfusion Science. 2011;5(2):1641-1670.

29. Pomper GJ. Febrile, allergic and nonimmune transfusion reactions. In: Simon TL, et al. (eds.). Rossi's principles of Transfusion Medicine. West Sussex. Wiley-Blackwell. 2009;53:826–846.

30. Arewa OP. Evaluation of transfusion pyrexia: A review of differential diagnosis and management. ISRN Hematology; 2012.
DOI: 10.5402/2012/524040.

31. Tinegate H, Birchall J, Gray A, Haggas R, Massey E, Norfolk D, et al. Guideline on the investigation of acute transfusion reactions prepared by the british committee for standards in haematology blood transfusion task force. British Journal of Haematology. 2012;152:35–51.

32. King KEE, Shirey RS, Thoman SK, Bensen-Kennedy D, Tanz WS, Ness PM. Universal leukodepletion decreases the incidence of febrile nonhaemolytic transfusion reactiosn to RBCs. Transfusion. 2004;44:25–29.

33. Yazer MH, Podlosky L, Clarke G, Nahirmak SM. The effect of pre-storage WBC reduction on the rates of febrile nonhaemolytic transfusion reactions to platelet concentrates and RBC. Transfusion. 2004;44:10–15.

34. Kumar H, Gupta PK, Mishra DK, Sarkar RS, Jaiprakash BM. Leucodepletion and Blood Products. MJAFI. 2006;62:174-177.

35. Eleftherios C. Vamvakas. The abandoned controversy surrounding universal white blood cell reduction. Blood Transfus. 2014;12:143-5.
DOI:10.2450/2014.0009-14.

36. Tsantes AE, Kyriakou E, Nikolopoulos GK, Stylos D, Sidhom M, Bonovas S, et al. Cost-effectiveness of leucoreduction for prevention of febrile non-haemolytic transfusion reactions. Blood Transfus. 2014;12:232-7.
DOI:10.2450/2014.0263-13.

37. Lichtiger B, Perry-Thomton E. Hemolytic transfusion reactions in oncology patients; experience in a large cancer center. J. Clinl Oncol. 1984;2:438–442.

38. Pineda AA, Brzica SM. Jr, Taswell HF. Haemolytic transfusion reaction. Recent experience in a large blood bank. Mayo Clin Proc. 1978;53:378–390.

39. Linden JV, Wagner K, Voytovich AE, Sheehan J. Transfusion errors in New York State: An analysis of 10 years' experience. Transfusion. 2000;40:1207–1213.

40. Ogedegbe HO. A Review of non-immune mediated transfusion reactions. Laboratory Medicine. 2002;33(5):380–385.

41. Hendrickson JE, Hillyer CD. Non-infectious serious hazards of transfusion. Anesthesia and Analgesia. 2009;108(3):759–69.

42. Mertes PM, Bazin A, Alla F, Bienvenu J, Caldani C, Lamy B, Laroche D, et al. Hypersensitivity reactions to blood components: Document Issued by the allergy committee of the french medicines and healthcare products regulatory agency. J. Investig Allergol Clin Immunol. 2011;21(3):171–178.

43. Paglino J, Pomper G, Fisch G, Champion M, Snyder E. Reduction of febrile but not allergic reactions to RBCs and platelets after conversion to universal prestorage leukoreduction. Transfusion. 2004;44:16–24.

44. Latiff A, Kerr M. The clinical significance of IgA deficiency, Ann Clin Biochem. 2007;44:131–139.

45. Torres R, Kenney B, Tormey CA. Diagnosis, Treatment and reporting of adverse effects of transfusion. Lab Medicine. 2012;43(5):217–231.

46. Toy P, Popovsky MA, Abraham E, Ambruso DR, Holness LG, Kopko PM, McFarland JG, Nathens AB, Silliman CC, Stroncek D. National Heart lung, blood institute working group on TRALI. Transfusion related acute lung injury: Definition and review. Crit Care Med. 2005;33:721–726.

47. Williams A. Transfusion related acute lung injury: Issue summary for blood products advisory committee.
Available:http://www.fda.gov/ohrms/dockets/AC/07/briefing/2007-4300B2-01.htm (Gaithersburg, MD).

48. Triulzi DJ. Transfusion-Related acute lung injury: Current concepts for the clinician. Anesth Analg. 2009;108:770–776.

49. Webert KE, Blajchman MA. Transfusion-related acute lung injury. Curr Opin Hematol. 2005;12:480–487.

50. Korsak J. Transfusion-associated Bacterial Sepsis. In: Fernandez R, (ed.). Severe Sepsis and septic shock-understanding a serious killer. InTech Publishers, Rijeka Croatia. 2012;3:47–68.

Available:http://www.intechopen.com/books/severe-sepsis-and-septic-shock-understanding-a-serious-killer/transfusion-associated-sepsis

51. Brecher ME, Hay SN. Bacterial contamination of blood components. Clin Microbiol Rev. 2005;18:193–204.

52. Eder AF, Goldman M. How do I investigate septic transfusion reactions and blood donors with culture-positive platelet donations? Transfusion. 2011;51:1662–1668. DOI:10.1111/j.1537-2995.2011.03083.x.

53. Wagner SJ, Robinette D, Friedman LI, Miripol J. Diversion of initial blood flow to prevent whole-blood contamination by skin surface bacteria: An *in vitro* model. Transfusion. 2000;40(3):335–338.

54. deKorte D, Marcelis JH, Verhoeven AJ, Soeterboek AM. Diversion of first blood volume results in a reduction of bacterial contamination for whole-blood collections. Vox Sang. 2002;83(1):13–16.

55. Chassaigne M, Vassort-Bruneau C, Allouch P, Audurier A, Boulard G, Grosdhomme F, Noel L, Gulian C, Janus G, Perez P. Reduction of bacterial load by predonation sampling. Transfus Apher Sci. 2001;24(3):253.

56. Brecher ME, Means N, Jere CS, et al. Evaluation of an automated culture system for detecting bacterial contamination of platelets: An analysis with 15 contaminating organisms. Transfusion. 2001;41:477–482.

57. Zhou L, Giacherio D, Cooling L, Davenport RD. Use of B-natriuretic peptide as a diagnostic marker in the differential diagnosis of transfusion-associated circulatory overload. Transfusion. 2005; 45:1056–1063.

58. Donaldson MDJ, Seaman MJ, Park GR. Massive blood transfusion. Br J. Anaesth. 1992;69:621–630.

59. Iserson KV, Huestis DW. Blood warming: Current applications and techniques. Transfusion. 1991;31(6):558–571.

60. Ness PM, Shirey RS, Thoman SK, Buck SA. The differentiation of delayed serologic and delayed haemolytic transfusion reactions: Incidence, long-term serologic findings and clinical significance. Transfusion. 1999;30:688–693.

61. Pineda AA, Vamvakas EC, Gorden LD, Winters JL, Moore SB. Trends in the incidence of delayed haemolytic and delayed serologic transfusion reactions. [Erratum Appears in Transfusion. 2000;40:891]. Transfusion. 1999;39:1097–1103.

62. Contreras M, Daniels G. Red cell immunohaematology: An introduction. In: Hoffbrand AV, Catovsky D, et al. (eds.). Postgraduate haematology, 6 ed. west sussex. Wiley-Blackwell. 2011;14:226–243.

63. Ramasethu J, Luban NLC. Allo-immune Haemolytic disease of newborn. In: Lichtman MA, Kipps TJ, et al. (eds.). William's haematology 8 ed. New York, McGraw Hill. 2010;54:985–1005.

64. Hauck-Dlimi B, Achenbach S, Strobel J, Eckstein R, Zimmermann R. Prevention and management of transfusion-induced alloimmunization: Current perspectives. International Journal of Clinical Transfusion Medicine. 2014;2:59–63.

65. Dhawan HK, Kumawat V, Marwaha N, Sharma RR, Sachdev S, Bansal D, Marwaha RK, Arora S. Alloimmunization and autoimmunization in transfusion dependent thalassemia major patients: Study on 319 patients. Asian J. Transfus Sci. 2014;8:84–88.

66. Vinchinsky EP, Earles A, Johnson RA, Hoag MS, Williams A, Lubin B. Alloimmunisation in sickle cell anaemia and transfusion of racially unmatched blood. New England Journal of Medicine. 1990;322(23):1617–1621.

67. Chou ST, Jackson T, Vege S, Smith-Whitley K, Friedman DF, Westhoff CM. High prevalence of red blood cell allo-immunisation in sickle cell disease despite transfusion from Rh matched minority donors. Blood. 2013;122(6):1062–1071.

68. Novotny VMJ. Prevention and management of platelet transfusion refractoriness. Vox Sanguinis. 1999;76:1–13.

69. Dzik S. How do I: Platelet support for refractory patients. Transfusion. 2007; 47:374–378.

70. Rebulla P. A mini-review on platelet refractoriness. Haematologica. 2005; 90:247–253.

71. Hoffbrand AV, Moss PAH. Blood transfusion. In: Essential haematology, 6 ed. john wiley and sons. West Sussex U.K. 2011;394–423.

72. Mueller-Eckhardt C, Kuenzlen E, Thilo-Korner D, Pralle H. High-dose intravenous

immunoglobulin for post-transfusion purpura. New Engl J. Med. 1983;308:287.

73. Dwyre DM, Holland PV. Transfusion-associated graft-versus-host disease. Vox Sang. 2008;95:85–93.

74. Seghatchian MJ, Ala F. Transfusion-associated graft-versus-host disease: Current concepts and future trends. Transfus Sci. 1995;16:99–105.

75. Rühl H, Bein G, Sachs UJ. Transfusion-associated graft-versus-host disease. Transfus Med Rev. 2009;23:62–71.

76. Schroeder ML. Transfusion-associated graft versus host disease. Br J. Hematol. 2002;117:275–287.

77. Agbaht K, Altintas ND, Topeli A, Gokoz O, Ozcebe O. Transfusion associated graft-versus-host disease in immunocompetent patients: Case series and review of the literature. Transfusion. 2007;47:1405–1411.

78. Treleaven J, Gennery A, Marsh J, Norfolk D, Page L, Parker A, et al. Guidelines on the use of irradiated blood components prepared by the British committee for standards in haematology blood transfusion task force. British Journal of Haematology. 2010;152:35–51.

79. Hoffbrand AV, Hershko C, Camaschella C. Iron metabolism, iron deficiency and disorders of haem synthesis. In: Hoffbrand AV, Catovsky D, et al. (eds.), postgraduate haematology, 6 ed. west sussex. Wiley-Blackwell. 2011;3:26–46.

80. Adewoyin AS, Obieche JC. Hypertransfusion therapy in sickle cell disease in Nigeria. Advances in Hematology; 2014.
Available:http://dx.doi.org/10.1155/2014/923593

81. Vinchinsky EP. Transfusion therapy in sickle cell disease.
Available:http://sickle.bwh.harvard.edu/transfusion.html
(last accessed on 7th February, 2015).

82. Sheth S. SQUID Biosusceptometry in the measurement of hepatic iron. Pediatr. Radiol. 2003;33:373–377.

83. Canavese C, Bergamo D, Ciccone G, Longo F, Fop F, Thea A, et al. Validation of serum ferritin values by magnetic susceptometry in predicting iron overload in dialysis patients. Kidney International. 2004;65:1091–1098.

84. Brittenham GM, Badman DG. Non Invasive measurement of Iron: Report of an NIDDK Workshop. Blood. 2003;101:15–19.

85. Kwiatkowski J. Real World Use of Iron chelators. Hematology. 2011;451–458.

86. Bihl F, Castelli D, Marincola F, Dodd RY, Brander C. Transfusion-transmitted infections. Journal of Translational Medicine. 2007;5:25.
DOI: 10.1186/1479-5876-5-25.

87. Dodd RY, Notari EP, Stramer SL. Current prevalence and incidence of infectious disease markers and estimated window period risk in the American Red Cross blood donor population. Transfusion. 2002;42(8):975–979.

88. Coste J, Reesink HW, Engelfriet CP, Laperche S, Brown S, Busch MP, et al. Implementation of donor screening for infectious agents transmitted by blood by nucleic acid technology: Update to 2003 Vox Sang. 2005;88(4):289–303.

89. Bolton-Maggs PHB, Cohen H. Serious Hazards of Transfusion (SHOT) haemovigilance and progress is improving transfusion safety. British journal of Haematology. 2013;1-12.
DOI: 10.1111/bjh.12547.

90. Brown BJ, Oladokun RE, Ogunbosi BO, Osinusi K. Blood transfusion-associated HIV infection in children in Ibadan, Nigeria. Journal of the International Association of Providers of AIDS Care. 2013;00(0):1–6.
DOI: 10.1177/2325957413500990.

91. Momoh ARM, Okogbo FO, Orhue PO, Aisabokhale FA, Okolo PO. Prevalence of blood pathogens among transfused patients in Ekpoma, Nigeria. International Journal of Community Research. 2013; 2(4):72–76.

92. Ejeliogu EU, Okolo SN, Pam SD, Okpe ES, John CC, Ochoga MO. Is human immunodeficiency virus still transmissible through blood transfusion in children with sickle cell anaemia in jos, Nigeria? British Journal of Medicine and Medical Research. 2014;4(21):3912-3923.

93. Fasola FA, Kotila TR, Akinyemi JO. Trends in transfusion-transmitted viral infections from 2001 to 2006 inIbadan, Nigeria. Intervirology. 2008;51:427–431.
DOI: 10.1159/000209671.

94. Jayaraman S, Chalabi Z, Perel P, Guerriero C, Roberts I. The risk of transfusion-transmitted infections in sub-

Saharan Africa. Transfusion. 2010;50(2): 433–42.

95. Kaur P, Basu S. Transfusion-transmitted infections: Existing and emerging pathogens. J. Post grad Med. 2005; 51:146–151.

96. Llewelyn CA, Hewitt PE, Knight RS, Amar K, Cousens S, Mackenzie J, Will RG. Possible transmission of variant Creutzfeldt-Jakob disease by blood transfusion. Lancet. 2004;363(9407):417–421.

97. Peden AH, Head MW, Ritchie DL, Bell JE, Ironside JW. Preclinical vCJD after blood transfusion in a PRNP codon 129 heterozygous patient. Lancet. 2004; 364(9433):527–9.

98. Khan TH. Transfusion, under-transfusion and over-transfusion. Anaesth Pain & Intensive Care. 2013;17(1):1–3.

99. World Health Organisation. Aide memoire for national blood programmes. Blood safety, WHO, Geneva; 2002.

100. Nurunnabi ASM, Jahan M, Alam MA, Hoque MM. Safe blood transfusion and ethical issues in transfusion medicine. J. Dhaka Med Coll. 2010;19(2):144–149.

5

Cytomegalovirus-induced Pure Red Cell Aplasia Successfully Treated with Ganciclovir: A Case Report

Daisy Ilagan-Tagarda[1], Flordeluna Zapata-Mesina[2*], John S. Delgado[3] and Jomell C. Julian[4]

[1]Department of Medicine, Fellow in Training, University of Santo Tomas Hospital, Section of Infectious Diseases, Philippines.
[2]Department of Medicine, Fellow in Training, University of Santo Tomas Hospital, Section of Adult Clinical Hematology, Philippines.
[3]Department of Medicine, University of Santo Tomas Hospital, Section of Infectious Diseases, Philippines.
[4]Department of Medicine, University of Santo Tomas Hospital, Section of Adult Clinical Hematology, Philippines.

Authors' contributions

This work was carried out in collaboration among all authors. Authors DI-T and FZ-M wrote the initial manuscript, made the critical revisions and managed the literature searches. Authors JSD and JCJ proofread and revised the paper. All authors read and approved the final manuscript.

Editor(s):
(1) Ricardo Forastiero, Department of Hematology, Favaloro University, Argentina.
Reviewers:
(1) Celso Eduardo Olivier, Department of Allergy and Immunology, Instituto Alergoimuno de Americana, Brazil.
(2) Arun Saini, Department of Paediatrics, University of Tennessee Health Science Center, Memphis, TN, USA.

ABSTRACT

Background: Acquired pure red cell aplasia (PRCA) is a rare disease characterized by anemia, severe reticulocytopenia and absent to low bone marrow erythroid precursor cells. There are well-described associations of this disorder with thymomas, lymphoproliferative disorders, autoimmune disorders, certain drugs, and infectious agents. Among the infectious agents, the most common is parvovirus B19, this was rarely reported in association with *Cytomegalovirus* (CMV).
Objective: To describe a rare case of acquired PRCA associated with CMV and its response to antiviral therapy.

Corresponding author: E-mail: plonghema@gmail.com, plonggi@yahoo.com

Methods: We present the clinical and laboratory data of our patient and reviewed the related published literature regarding PRCA, its etiology and response to treatment.

Results: We describe a 64-year-old male who presented with symptomatic anemia. He had a normocytic, normochromic anemia associated with low reticulocyte count. Serum ferritin was elevated. Vitamin B12, folate levels, kidney and liver functions were normal. He was given blood transfusion with packed red cells, hematinics and erythropoietin (EPO) injections for 2 months but there was no response. Bone marrow aspiration and biopsy showed erythroid hypoplasia consistent with PRCA. He was assessed to have PRCA probably EPO-antibody induced. EPO was discontinued and he was started on steroids. After 3 months of steroids there was persistence of anemia and reticulocytopenia. EPO-antibody assay done prior to steroid therapy came out to be negative. He tested negative for Hepatitis A, B and C, Human Immunodeficiency virus, Epstein barr-virus and parvovirus B-19. CMV DNA viral load was elevated. He was started on ganciclovir which resulted to transfusion independence and normalization of hemoglobin.

Conclusion: PRCA may be reversible. High viral load of CMV was detected through PCR. He was treated with antiviral therapy resulting into a favorable response.

Keywords: Pure red cell aplasia; Cytomegalovirus.

1. CASE REPORT

A 64-year-old male, farmer, who presented with symptomatic anemia, weight loss and burning epigastric pain without associated change in character of the stool was admitted in our institution. He was given hematinics and erythropoietin (EPO) injection but no response was seen. Pertinent physical examination showed pallor, absence of lymphadenopathies, non-tender abdomen, absence of hepatosplenomegaly, no palpable abdominal mass and normal rectal exam. He had a normocytic, normochromic anemia associated with low reticulocyte count and reticulocyte production index. His leukocyte and platelet counts were normal. Serum ferritin was elevated. Vitamin B12 and folate levels were normal. Kidney and liver function tests were also normal. Due to the history of epigastric pain and anemia, upper gastrointestinal endoscopy was done, which showed normal findings. He was transfused with packed red cells. Bone marrow aspiration and biopsy showed cellular marrow with erythroid hypoplasia; adequate and intact granulopoiesis; and adequate megakaryocytes consistent with pure red cell aplasia (PRCA). (Figs. 1A-1C) He was initially managed with serial blood transfusions and EPO injection for 2 months but no response was noted. He was then assessed as PRCA probably EPO-antibody induced. Anti-EPO antibody assay was done. Patient was started with prednisone (60 mg/day) and CBC and reticulocyte count was monitored. After three months of steroids, anemia persisted and transfusion requirement was unchanged. Anti-EPO antibody assay came out to be negative. He developed fever and productive

cough and was readmitted as a case of pneumonia, which responded to piperacillin-tazobactam. Further investigation was done for the possible etiology of the disease. Hepatitis A, B, C profile was normal. Epstein Barr Virus (EBV) DNA viral load was not detected but the *Cytomegalovirus* (CMV) DNA viral load was significantly elevated at 382, 000 copies per/ml. Bone marrow aspiration was reviewed for possible parvovirus B19 infection but no characteristic finding of giant pro-erythroblasts with large nuclear inclusions was seen. He was also tested negative for parvovirus B19 IgG. He was treated with intravenous ganciclovir (5 mg/kg twice daily) for two weeks and shifted to oral valganciclovir 900 mg/day. Monitoring of CMV DNA viral load, CBC with platelet count and reticulocyte count during the antiviral treatment was done. CMV DNA was undetected after a month of treatment with maintaining hematocrit at 34-36% and reticulocyte count of 4.0%. He also achieved transfusion independence since the initiation of antiviral. His CMV DNA viral load remained undetected during 2 months follow up after completion of treatment. The patient's diagnostic work-up is shown in Table 1 and course of treatment is summarized in Fig. 2.

2. DISCUSSION

PRCA is characterized by anemia, severe reticulocytopenia, and low to absent bone marrow erythroid precursor cells. It can be classified as congenital or acquired. Acquired PRCA is associated with viral infections most commonly Parvovirus B19 and EBV [1-3] autoimmune diseases such as Systemic Lupus Erythematosus [4] collagen vascular diseases, malignancies [5-8] and medications. Its pathophysiologic mechanism as extensively reviewed by Thompson et al. [9] depends on the primary disease, though heterogeneous, a common finding is an immune-mediated process. Studies showed that there are several factors associated with the primary disease, which inhibit erythropoiesis. It can be due to an antibody against red cell progenitors, [10-11] antibody against EPO, [12] T cell-mediated and the natural killer cells role in hematopoesis.

Table 1. Patient's diagnostic work-up

Laboratory	Results	Normal value
Hemoglobin	48 g/L	120-170 g/L
Hematocrit	13%	37-54%
WBC	6.50×10^9	$4.5\text{-}12 \times 10^9$
Segmenters	75%	40-70%
Lymphocytes	25%	20-40%
Monocytes	0%	0-7%
Eosinophils	0%	0-5%
Platelet count	320×10^9	$150\text{-}450 \times 10^9$
Reticulocyte count	0.02%	0.5-1.5%
Serum ferritin	400 ng/ml	12-300 ng/ml
Serum B12 levels	550 ng/ml	130-700 ng/L
Serum folate	10 ng/mL	3-16 ng/mL
Serum creatinine	0.5 mg/dL	0.5-1.2 mg/dL
Ionized calcium	1.0 mmol/L	1.03-1.23 mmol/L
Hepatitis profile	normal	
EPO-antibody assay	negative	
EBV-DNA viral load	None detected	
CMV viral load	382,000 copies per/ml	

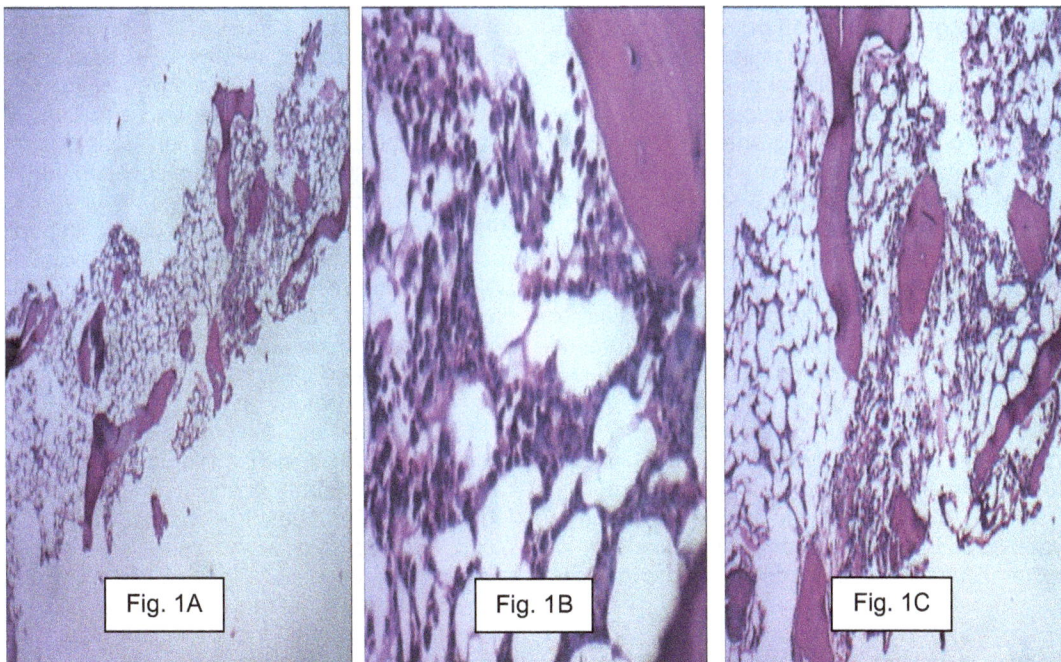

Fig. 1A. Histopathologic finding of the bone marrow aspiration showing erythroid hypoplasia, Fig. 1B. Showing presence of adequate and intact granulopoiesis, Fig. 1C. Low power magnification of bone marrow core showing cellular marrow with erythroid hypoplasia

Hemogram and Clinical Course of Patient's treatment

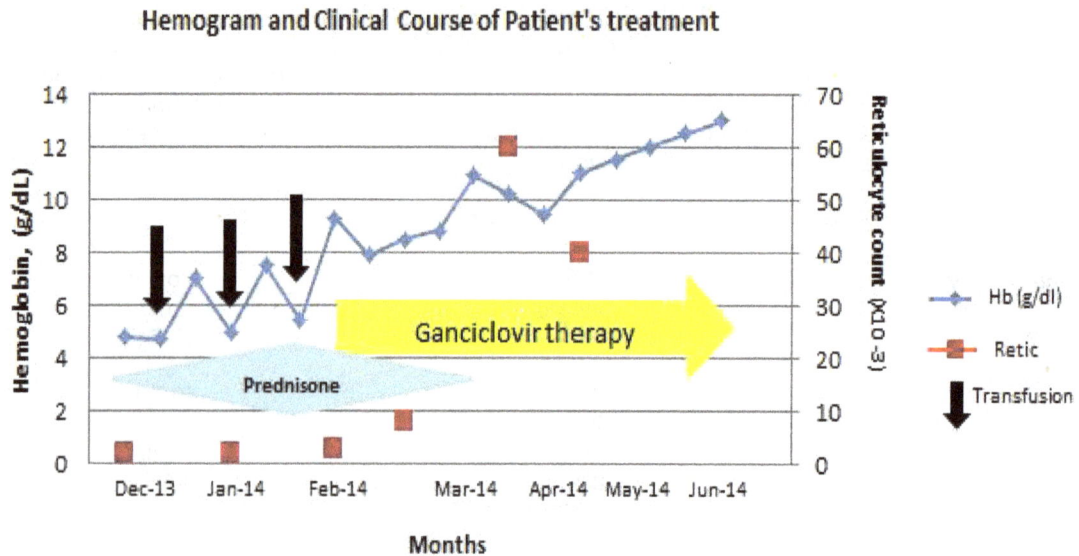

Fig. 2. Clinical course and treatment response of patient. During treatment with prednisone, patient required transfusion with pRBC compared with the increasing hemoglobin level and transfusion independence with treatment of ganciclovir

Acquired PRCA in association with viral infections have been more commonly reported in Parvovirus B19. Other viruses associated with PRCA are hepatitis A and C, HIV, and rarely reported with Human Herpes virus-6, EBV and CMV. Most of the published case reports of CMV primary infection with concomitant PRCA involve pediatric patients. In clinical studies and animal models, Parvovirus B19 induces a block of the erythroid differentiation at the BFU-E/CFU-E level then apoptosis of the infected erythroid progenitors, thus, leading to a sudden cessation of red blood cell production. Parvovirus B19 capsid proteins may play a cytotoxic role either due to accumulation in the nucleus as large inclusions disturbing the nuclear organization, or due a direct toxicity that may potentially related to the recently described phospholipase A2 domain. Due to rarity of CMV induced PRCA, the exact mechanism of erythroid precursor cell destruction remains unclear. An immunologic attack of erythroid precursors or hematopoietic stem cells triggered by the infection has been hypothesized, which causes the inhibition of proliferation of erythroid colony forming units [13].

The task of looking for the primary disease which causes the PRCA is always challenging. In our case, patient has been worked up extensively for other common causes of PRCA such as presence of EPO antibody, parvovirus B19, EBV and viral hepatitis. It was then elucidated that

PRCA was due to CMV. CMV has a double stranded DNA, and a member of Herpesviridae that infects 50 to 80% of the population in United States, and 90% worldwide [14]. This virus, like other members of Herpesviridae, has the ability to become latent, and usually is asymptomatic. The most frequently used tests for the diagnosis of CMV infection are detection of antigen (the pp65 antigenemia assay), DNA, or mRNA. The use of quantitative DNA detection techniques has been increasing in recent years because they are highly sensitive and provide viral load measurements that can give important prognostic information [15]. In the Philippines, DNA quantitative detection by PCR is available. Reactivation of the virus has been associated with several disease entities such as retinitis and pneumonitis, and has been closely associated with different stimuli such as immunosuppression. However, several studies showed that critical illness like sepsis can cause reactivation of latent infection in 30% of case [16]. Associated complications of CMV in the blood, such as thrombocytopenia and hemolytic anemia have been described in several articles. And because of the rarity of cases associated with CMV, no standard of treatment is available. Published case reports and CMV occurring among post-transplant patients have been the basis of treatment of the case presented. Amongpost-transplant patients with CMV disease, treatment recommendation is intravenous ganciclovir 5 mg/kg twice daily with documentation of clearance of virus from the blood as the end point of intravenous therapy. Subsequent administration of oral valganciclovir for 2 to 3 months is also recommended to reduce the relapse of the disease [17]. In a case report of a 3-month-old individual with PRCA secondary to CMV, treatment with ganciclovir 6 mg/kg/dose twice daily showed remarkable improvement after6 weeks [18]. For our patient, he was given a total of 3 months antiviral therapy.

3. CONCLUSION

PRCA is a rare disease with heterogenous etiology. Some cases are reversible and may not require lifetime treatment and/or transfusion such as those induced by CMV. In our patient, we have demonstrated complete response to antiviral therapy.

CONSENT

All authors declare that written informed consent was obtained from the patient for publication of this case report and accompanying images.

ETHICAL APPROVAL

It is not applicable.

COMPETING INTERESTS

Authors have declared that no competing interests exist.

REFERENCES

1.   Frickhofen N, Chen U, Young N, et al. Parvovirus b19 as a cause of acquired chronic pure red cell aplasia. Br J Haematol. 1994;87:818.

2.   Socinski M, Ershler W, Tosato G, et al. Pure red blood cell aplasia associated with chronic Epstein-Barr virus infection: Evidence for T cell-mediated suppression of erythroid colony forming units. J Lab Clin Med. 1984;104:995.

3.   Sung H, Kim S, Lee J, Lee G, et al. Persistent anemia in a patient with diffuse large B cell lymphoma: Pure red cell aplasia associated with latent Epstein-Barr virus infection in bone marrow. J Korean Med Sci. 2007;(22):S167-70.

4.   Cassileth P, Myers A. Erythroid aplasia in systemic lupus erythematosus. Am J Med. 1973;55:706.

5.   Choi J, Oh Y, Park I. Case of pure red cell aplasia associated with angioimmunoblastic T-cell lymphoma. Cancer Res Treat. 2010;42(2):115-7.

6.   Vlachaki E, Tselios K, Charalambidou S, et al. Pure red cell aplasia complicating B cell small lymphocytic lymphoma: A case report. Int J Hematol. 2008;88(3):341-2.

7.   Wong K, Chau K, Chan J, Chu Y, et al. Pure red cell aplasia associated with thymic lymphoid hyperplasia and secondary erythropoietin resistance. Am J Clin Pathol. 1995;103:346.

8.   Suzuki T, Kumagai T, Kitano A, Kubo H, et al. Pure red cell aplasia successfully treated with rituximab in a patient with relapsed diffuse large B-cell lymphoma. Rinsho Ketsueki. 2007;48(1):67-70.

9.   Thompson D, Gales M. Drug-induced pure red cell aplasia. Pharmacotherapy. 1996; 16:1002–1008.

10.   Krantz S, Kao V. Studies on red cell aplasia. I. Demonstration of a plasma inhibitor to heme synthesis and an antibody to erythroblast nuclei. Proceedings of the National Academy of Sciences of the United States of America. 1967;58:493-500.

11.   Alter R, Joshi S, Verdirame J, et al. Pure red cell aplasia associated with B cell lymphoma: Demonstration of bone marrow colony inhibition by serum immunoglobulin. Leuk Res. 1990;14(3):279-86.

12.   Casadevall N, Dupuy E, Molho-Sabatier P, Tobelem G, et al. Autoanti-bodies against erythropoietin in a patient with pure red cell aplasia. New England Journal of Medicine. 2002;334:630-633.

13.   Morinet F, Leruez-Ville M, Pillet S. Anemia caused by viruses Stem cells-Alpha Med Press. 2011;1-7.

14.   Crumpacker Clyde S, Zhang J. Cytomegalovirus. Principles and Practice of Infectious Diseases. 2010;1971-1987.

15.   Hebart H, Lengerke C, Ljungman P, et al. Prospective comparison of PCR-based vs late mRNA-based pre-emptive antiviral therapy for HCMV infection in patients after allo-SCT. Bone Marrow Transplant. 2011;46:408-415.

16.   Cook C. *Cytomegalovirus* Reactivation in "immunocompetent" Patients: A call for scientific prophylaxis. The Journal of Infectious Diseases. 2007;196:1273-1275.

17.   Boeckh M, Ljungman P. How we treat *Cytomegalovirus* in hematopoietic cell transplant recipients. Blood. 2009;113: 5711-5719.

18.   Nandan D, Jahan A, Vivek D, Singh S. et al. Pure red cell aplasia in three months old infant possibly secondary to *Cytomegalovirus*. Indian Journal of Hematology and Blood Transfusion. 2013; 29(1):1-3.

6

Distribution of ABO and Rhesus Blood Groups among Voluntary Blood Donors in Enugu

Ngwu Amauche Martina[1*], Obi Godwin Okorie[1], Anigolu Miriam Obiageli[2] and Eluke Blessing Chekwube[3]

[1]Department of Hematology and Immunology, Enugu State University of Science and Technology, Enugu, Enugu State, Nigeria.
[2]Department of Chemical Pathology, Enugu State University of Science and Technology, Enugu, Enugu State, Nigeria.
[3]Department of Medical Laboratory Science, University of Nigeria, Enugu Campus, Enugu State, Nigeria.

Authors' contributions

This work was carried out in collaboration between all authors. Authors NAM and OGO designed the study, wrote the protocol, managed the analysis of the study and wrote the first draft of the manuscript. Authors AMO and EBC managed the literature searches. All authors read and approved the final manuscript.

Editor(s):
(1) Tadeusz Robak, Medical University of Lodz, Copernicus Memorial Hospital, Poland.
Reviewers:
(1) Celso Eduardo Olivier, Department of Allergy and Immunology, Instituto Alergoimuno de Americana, Brazil.
(2) Liana Maria Tôrres de Araújo Azi, Department of Surgery, Professor Edgard Santos University Hospital – HUPES, Federal University of Bahia, Brazil.

ABSTRACT

Background: ABO and rhesus blood group study is very relevant to the blood transfusion services policy maker and clinicians. ABO and rhesus blood group are the most prevalent blood groups among so many other blood groups discovered.
Aims: The aim of this study was to find out the current distribution of ABO and Rh blood groups among the blood donors in city of Enugu.
Study Design: Two hundred and ninety randomly selected male and female blood donors were grouped according to their ABO and Rh blood group.
Place and Duration of Study: Haematology and Immunology Department, College of Medicine, Enugu State University of Science and Technology, Enugu, Enugu State, Nigeria: April 2012 to

Corresponding author: E-mail: muchyscki@gmail.com

December 2012.

Methodology: Two hundred and ninety voluntary blood donors sample were grouped for ABO and Rhesus 'D' antigen by tile method.

Results: The result showed that blood group O and Rh 'D' positive has the highest frequency, there was no blood group AB in the study.

Conclusion: Blood group AB is completely absent in this study.

Keywords: ABO; rhesus; blood group; antigen.

1. INTRODUCTION

The International Society of Blood Transfusion (ISBT) recently recognized about thirty major blood groups and among the thirty, ABO and Rh blood groups are included [1]. ABO grouping has been shown to be the most common type of grouping. A1, A2, A1B, A2B, A2, A2B, B, B1 & O are subtypes of ABO blood group system, but some of them are very rare [2]. A very important protein plays a great role in the grouping of blood and that protein is Rh factor. If this protein is present on a particular blood type, that blood type is called positive then if absent, it is called negative [3]. In blood transfusion and organ transplant, knowledge of an individual's blood type is required so much. This is because an individual can be exposed to a blood group antigen that is not recognized by self which lead to the sensitization of the person. If somebody is sensitized, the immune system produces a specific antibody which normally binds specifically to a particular blood group antigen and antibodies against that particular antigen will be formed. These formed antibodies do bind to the antigens on the surface of transfused red blood cells which often lead to the destruction of cells [4]. The inheritance of ABO blood type depends on both parents and is controlled by single gene with three alleles; i, IA & IB. Rhesus D antigen is the second most relevant blood group system; this is due to its immunogenicity in Rh D negative individuals during pregnancy and blood transfusion [5]. The higher, the proportions of RhD negative in a population, the higher the incidence of hemolytic disease (HDN) of the new born in that population. Before the introduction of immunoprophylaxis, 1% of HDN was seen in all newborns which accounted for the death of one baby in every 2,200 births. But since the introduction of anti-D prophylaxis, death due to RhD alloimmunisation has reduced from 46 in 100,000 births to 1.6 in 100,000 births [6]. Many studies have been published on ABO blood types link with increase or decrease susceptibility to a particular disease [7,8]. Example, individual of blood group A are at greater risk for some

malignancies [9]. People of blood group O are higher risk of contracting malaria and some infectious diseases, such as cholera [10]. The frequencies of A, B, O, Rh blood group phenotypes are not equal and it has been suggested that environmental factors may be responsible for it. Example, some E. coli has ABO-like antigens on their cell walls. Another one is that H antigen is chemically similar to the capsular antigens of Pneumococcus type XIV. These similarities in antigen make up sometimes confer resistance in individuals that produce the corresponding antibodies, therefore increase the susceptibility of people that their blood group matches the antigen [11]. There is relationship between the blood pH and ABO blood types and these have lead to certain disease conditions. Blood type A&O has an alkaline pH (7.40), blood type B has acidic pH (6.8) and blood type AB has neutral pH (7.00). Study carried out by United States Department of Agriculture (USDA) between 1909 and 2005 showed that population with nearly 95% alkaline blood type A/O and acidic blood type B was as a result of iron poisoning and copper deficiency. The prevalence of blood type B has increased significantly from 1960 until now, and this is observed in diabetes prevalence, which has a high correlation with type B blood [12]. Several researches have been done on relationship between ABO blood group and life span [13,14]. Due to clinical significance of ABO and Rh blood group in transfusion and compatibility, there is need for steady research to discover current status of ABO and rhesus blood group system in our environment. This study was carried out to determine the current distribution of ABO and Rh blood groups among the blood donors in city of Enugu.

2. MATERIALS AND METHODS

2.1 Study Area

The study was carried out in the Department of Haematology and Immunology, Faculty of Medicine, Enugu State University of Science & Technology Enugu, Enugu State. Enugu State euphemistically referred to as the "coal city" is one of the states in the eastern part of Nigeria. The state shares borders with Abia State and Imo State to the south, Ebonyi State to the east, Benue State to the northeast, Kogi State to the northwest and Anambra State to the west. Enugu State has a population of over 3.3 million people. It is also home of the Igbo of southeastern Nigeria. The city is characterized by high level of environmental sanitation, moderate planned housing, portable water supply and proper management of wastes especially in the Enugu urban.

2.2 Study Population

Two hundred and ninety voluntary blood donors are randomly selected during the National blood transfusion blood drive in the higher institutions in Enugu after given informed consent. Before carrying out the research ethical clearance approval was given by the Enugu State University of Science and Technology Teaching Hospital Ethics Committee. Forty of them were selected from Enugu State University of Science & Technology, fifty four blood donors were from Institute of Management and Technology Enugu, one hundred and thirteen blood donors were selected from Federal Cooperative College Oji River, ten of them were selected from Enugu State College of Education Technical, sixty of them were selected from Federal School of Dental Technology Enugu and thirteen blood donors were student of Ebonyi State University. This study was done from April 2012 to December 2012.

2.3 Method

Two milliliters of venous blood was collected into a plain (10 ml) container. ABO and Rhesus 'D' blood group phenotypes were determined using monoclonal anti-A, anti-B and monoclonal anti-D IgG/IgM respectively, according to procedure described by Monica Cheesbrough [15]. The principle of the test was based on the ability of the specific antisera to agglutinate red cell in the presence of the corresponding antigen. One volume of each antisera, anti A, anti B and anti D produced by Carper Laboratories in the UK was placed on a clean white tile and then mixed with a drop of 20% saline suspension of red cells at room temperature; this was then mixed carefully by gentle tilting the tile from side to side for maximum of 2 minutes. Presence of agglutination indicates the presence of the

corresponding blood group. Appropriate controls of known blood groups were applied.

2.4 Statistical Method

Phenotypic frequencies were calculated and expressed as percentage. One Sample T Test was used to compare frequency distribution of ABO and Rh antigen in 20 States in Nigeria.

3. RESULTS

The two hundred and ninety voluntary blood donors selected randomly consist of 223 males and 67 females between ages 18 and 40. Table 1 showed the frequency distribution of ABO according to the sex of the donors in the following order. For male donors O > B > A (59.3% > 14.5% > 3.1%), female donors O > B > A (19.6% > 2.8% > 0.69%). Table 2 showed the distribution of the rhesus factors according to the ABO blood groups. In this study 95.9% of the donors are rhesus D positive while 4.1% are rhesus D negative. The distribution of the rhesus D positive and rhesus D negative in different blood groups occurred in the following order. Rhesus D positive O > B > A (75.9% > 16.2% > 3.8%), rhesus D negative O > B > A (3.1% > 1.0% > 0%). Table 3 showed gender distribution of the rhesus factors. Seventy three point one percent of the male blood donors were rhesus D positive while 3.8% of the males are rhesus D negative. Twenty two point eight percent of the females were rhesus D positive while 0.34% of the females are rhesus D negative. Table 4 showed the donors state of origins, ABO and rhesus blood group distribution according to the states of origins. We observed that 41.38% of the blood donors are indigene of Enugu state. Among the donors from Enugu state, the blood groups were distributed in the following order O+VE > B+VE > A+VE > O-VE > B-VE (82.5% > 7.5% > 5.8% > 2.5% > 1.7%). Table 5 showed that blood group O rhesus D positive and blood group B rhesus D positive were significant in this study ($p = .05$).

Table 1. Distribution of ABO blood group according to sex

	A	B	O
	No (%)	No (%)	No (%)
Male	9 (3.1)	42 (14.5)	172 (59.3)
Female	2 (0.7)	8 (2.8)	57 (19.6)
Total	11 (3.8)	50 (17.3)	229 (79.0)

Table 2. Distribution of rhesus status according to the ABO blood groups

ABO	RhD positive No (%)	RhD negative No (%)
A	11 (3.8)	0 (0)
B	47 (16.2)	3 (1.0)
O	220 (75.9)	9 (3.1)
Total	278 (95.9)	12 (4.1)

Table 3. Distribution of rhesus status according to sex

	RhD positive No (%)	RhD negative No (%)
Male	212 (73.1)	11 (3.8)
Female	66 (22.8)	1 (0.3)
Total	278 (95.9)	12 (4.1)

4. DISCUSSION

ABO and Rh blood groups are known to be very relevant in blood transfusion practice. They are also useful in population genetic studies, researching population migration patterns, as well as resolving certain medico-legal issues, particularly of disputed parentage [15]. It is, therefore, very important to have accurate information on the current distribution of these blood groups in Enugu state. The overall data of this study revealed that percentage frequencies of ABO blood group were 3.79%, 17.24%, 0% & 78.97% for blood group A, B, AB & O while 95.9% and 4.1% for rhesus D positive and negative. We observed that there is deviation between our findings and previous findings on the same subject matter from various parts of the world including Nigeria. For instance in northern part of Nigeria, Kulkarni and Colleagues reported phenotypic frequencies of 23.05%, 29.95%, 4.4% and 46.6% for A, B, AB and O blood groups respectively [16]. Bakare and Colleagues reported phenotypic frequencies of 22.9%, 21.3%, 5.9% and 50% for blood group A, B, AB and O among 7653 individuals in Ogbomoso, South-West Nigeria [17]. Adeyemo and Soboyejo also reported phenotypic frequencies of 25.3%, 16.7%, 2.7% and 55.3% for A, B, AB and O blood groups [18]. A similar study in Hungary reported blood groups phenotypic frequencies of 27.6%, 12.2%, 4.2% and 55.9% for A, B, AB and O blood groups [19]. Also another study in Kuwaiti revealed phenotypic frequencies of 16.1%, 14.0%, 2.7% and 66.8% for A, B, AB and O blood groups [20]. Another study done at Ibadan by Omotade et al. reported phenotypic frequencies of 21.6%, 21.4%, 2.8% and 54.2% for A, B, AB and O blood groups [21]. Again

Iyiola et al. reported phenotypic frequencies of 18.7%, 17.6%, 5.6% and 58.1% for A, B, AB and O blood group in Ilorin, north central Nigeria [22]. In the above previous findings we observed that the pattern of distribution of blood group A, B, AB and O occurred in order of O> A>B>AB which is completely different from our findings. In this work we discovered that the following previous findings were similar to our study in the pattern of O>B>A>AB. For instance a similar study in Adamawa reported blood groups result with phenotypic frequencies of 16.5%, 21.3%,11.7% and 50.6% for blood group A, B, AB and O [23]. Another study in northern Nigeria reported phenotypic frequencies of 23.1%, 29.9%, 4.4% and 46.6% for blood group A, B, AB and O [16]. Another study in Guinea reported blood groups result with phenotypic frequencies of 22.5%, 23.9%, 4.7% and 48.9% for blood group A, B, AB and O [24]. This study also differ from report of research conducted by Yousaf et al. which revealed marginal difference between blood group B and O in Bahawalpur population at Pakistan with phenotypic frequencies of 21%, 36%, 6% and 37% for blood group A, B, AB and O [25]. Another study by Khaliq and Colleagues showed marginal difference between blood group B and O in Hazara population at Pakistan with phenotypic frequencies of 24%, 32%, 11% and 33% for blood group A, B, AB and O [26]. Our data are in line with study conducted among American Indians by Maurant et al, who found no blood group AB in his work with phenotypic frequencies of 3.9%, 1.1%, 0% and 95% for blood group A, B, AB and O [27]. This study was also in consistent with previous study done in northern Nigeria which revealed that phenotypic frequencies of blood group B are on increase in Nigeria population [23].

From our finding, we discovered that percentage phenotypic frequencies of blood group O was predominant in all the parameters used in analyzing the work such as gender and state of origin. The implication of this finding is that blood group O is readily available blood in Nigeria blood banks. The higher proportion of blood group O in this study is an advantage because some research had shown that individual with blood group O had the smallest percentage of severe malaria when compared with other blood groups such as A, B & AB [28,29].The reason for less severe malaria attack seen in blood group O individuals may be due to mechanism of reduced rosettes formation by parasitized RBCs of blood group subjects as shown in the previous study [30].

Table 4. Distribution ABO & Rh according to donor's state of origin

Donor's state of origin	NO of donor according to their state of origin no (%)	A+VE	A-VE	B+VE	B-VE	O+VE	O-VE
Lagos	1 (0.34)	0 (0.0)	0 (0.0)	0 (0.0)	0 (0.0)	1 (100.0)	0 (0.0)
Kaduna	1 (0.34)	0 (0.0)	0 (0.0)	0 (0.0)	0 (0.0)	1 (100.0)	0 (0.0)
River	2 (0.69)	0 (0.0)	0 (0.0)	0 (0.0)	0 (0.0)	2 (100.0)	0 (0.0)
Benue	26 (8.97)	0(0.0)	0 (0.0)	9 (34.6)	0 (0.0)	16 (61.5)	1 (3.8)
Anambra	33 (11.38)	1 (3.0)	0 (0.0)	4 (12.1)	1 (3.0)	23 (69.7)	4 (12.1)
Delta	8 (2.76)	1 (12.5)	0 (0)	0 (0.0)	0 (0.0)	7 (87.7)	0 (0.0)
Imo	36 (12.41)	1 (2.8)	0 (0.0)	12 (33.3)	0 (0.0)	23 (63.9)	0 (0.0)
Akwaibom	1 (0.34)	0 (0.0)	0 (0.0)	1 (100.0)	0 (0.0)	0 (0.0)	0 (0.0)
Ogun	1 (0.34)	0 (0.0)	0 (0.0)	0 (0.0)	0 (0.0)	1 (100.0)	0 (0.0)
Ondo	2 (0.69)	0(0.0)	0 (0.0)	0 (0.0)	0 (0.0)	2 (100.0)	0 (0.0)
Kogi	2 (0.69)	0 (0.0)	0 (0.0)	0 (0.0)	0 (0.0)	2 (100.0)	0 (0.0)
Enugu	120(41.38)	7 (5.8)	0 (0.0)	9(7.5)	2 (1.7)	99(82.5)	3 (2.5)
Edo	4 (1.38)	0(0.0)	0 (0.0)	1 (25.0)	0 (0.0)	3 (75.0)	0 (0.0)
Adamawa	1(0.34)	0 (0.0)	0 (0.0)	1(100.0)	0 (0.0)	0 (0.0)	0 (0.0)
Cross River	13 (4.48)	0 (0.0)	0 (0.0)	2 (15.4)	0 (0.0)	10 (76.9)	1 (7.7)
Abia	11(3.79)	0 (0.0)	0 (0.0)	3 (27.3)	0 (0.0)	8 (72.7)	0 (0.0)
Gombe	1 (0.34)	0 (0.0)	0 (0.0)	1(100.0)	0 (0.0)	0 (0.0)	0 (0.0)
Ebonyi	22 (7.59)	1 (4.5)	0 (0.0)	4 (18.2)	0 (0.0)	17 (77.3)	0 (0.0)
Nassarawa	3 (1.03)	0 (0.0)	0 (0.0)	0 (0.0)	0 (0.0)	3 (100.0)	0 (0.0)
Bayelsa	2 (0.69)	0 (0.0)	0 (0.0)	0 (0.0)	0 (0.0)	2 (100.0)	0 (0.0)
Total	290 (100.0)	11 (3.8)	0 (0.0)	47 (16.2)	3 (1.0)	220 (75.9)	9 (3.1)

Abbreviations: NO: Number: %: percentage, A+ VE: Blood group A rhesus D positive, A-VE: Blood group A rhesus D negative, B+VE: Blood group B rhesus D positive , B-VE: Blood group B rhesus D negative, O+VE: Blood group O rhesus D positive, O-VE: Blood group O rhesus D negative

Table 5. Frequency distribution of A+VE, B+VE, B-VE, O+VE, O-VE within 20 states

N (20)	A+VE	B+VE	B-VE	O+VE	O-VE
Mean±	1.430±	23.670±	0.235±	73.350±	1.305±
STD	3.129	34.975	0.753	34.324	3.182
T value	2.044	3.027	1.395	9.557	1.834
P value	0.055	0.007	0.179	0.000	0.082

P= .05

Also smaller proportion of donors belonging to blood group A in this study is also an advantage because research had shown that frequency of blood group A was significantly higher among people suffering from pancreatic cancer [31]. Reduced blood groups A, B and complete absent of AB in this study may be very advantageous. For instance earlier studies had shown association of oral, pancreatic, ovarian, gastric, leukemia, rectal and cervical cancers among individuals with blood groups A, AB or B [31-35]. Blood group O was highest in both male and female subjects which is consistent with previous study by Adeyemo and Colleagues [18]. This study showed a total percentage of RhD positive distribution of 95.9% and RhD negative distribution of 4.1%. Similar pattern of RhD positive and RhD negative was observed in Nigeria population and other parts of the world.

For instance RhD positive of 91.4% and RhD negative of 8.6% was observed in Mandi Bahanddin (Pakistan) [36], 94% and 6% in Lagos [18], 94.4% and 5.5% in Indian [37], 95% and 5% in Germany [38], 93% and 7% in South Arabia [37], 95% and 4.8% in Ibadan [21], 96.7% and 3.2% in Portharcourt [27], 95.5% and 4.5% in Ilorin [22], 96.7% and 3.3% in Ogbomosho [17]. Study conducted by Yousaf et al. among Bahawal Pur division of Pakistan population differs from ours because the subjects in that study were exclusively RhD positive [25]. Our data on RhD distribution deviated from previous studies in some parts of Nigeria. For instance Adeyemo et al. observed that blood group O RhD positive was highest with percentage frequency of 53.3%, followed by blood group A RhD positive with percentage frequency of 23.3%, followed by blood group B RhD positive of 14.6% and blood group AB RhD positive of 2.6% [18]. Egesie et al. also observed that blood group O RhD positive was highest with a percentage frequency of 48%, followed by group B RhD positive with percentage frequency of 22%, then followed by blood group A RhD positive with percentage frequency of 21% and blood group AB RhD positive with percentage frequency of 7% [39]. Knowledge of the distribution of ABO and Rh blood groups among any population provide useful information for genetic counseling, medical diagnosis, and also help in planning for future health challenges especially in blood transfusion.

5. CONCLUSION

This study showed total absent of blood group AB, which is not common with previous studies in other parts of Nigeria.

ACKNOWLEDGEMENTS

The authors thank the donors and staff of National Blood Transfusion centre Enugu for their permission and assistance during sample collection.

COMPETING INTERESTS

Authors have declared that no competing interests exist.

REFERENCES

1.   Dacie JV, Lewis SM. Practical haematology. In: Lewis SM, Bain BJ, Bates I, editors. 9th edn. London: Churchill Livingstone, Harcourt Publishers Limited. 2001;444–451.

2.   Polesky HF. Blood group, human leukocytes antigens and DNA polymorphism in parenting testing. In: Henry JB, editor. Clinical diagnosis and management by laboratory methods. 19th edn. Philadelphelphia: WB Saunders. 1996;1413–1426.

3.   Reid ME, Mohandas N. "Red blood cell blood group antigens: Structure and function. Seminars in hematology. 2004;41(2):93–117.

4.   Harmening DM. Modern blood banking and transfusion practices. 4th edn. Philadelphia: FA Davis Company. 1915;95–104.

5.   Dennis YM, Hylem NM, Fidler C, Sargent IL, Murphy MF, Chamberlain PF. Prenatal diagnosis of fetal RhD status by molecular analysis of maternal plasma. New Engl. J. Med. 1998;337:1734-1738.

6.   Kumar S, Regan F. Management of pregnancies with RhD alloimmunisation. BMJ. 2005;330(7502):1255-8.

7.   Sharara AI, Abdul-Baki H, ElHajj I, Kreidieh N, Kfoury Baz EM. Association of gastroduodenal disease phenotype with ABO blood group and helicobacter pylori virulence specific serotypes. Digestive and Liver Disease: Official Journal of the Italian Society of Gastroenterology and the Italian Association for the study of the Liver. 2006;38(11):829-833.

8.   Shimazu T, Shimaoka M, Sugimoto H, Taenaka N, Hasegawa T. Does blood type B protect against haemolytic uraemic syndrome? An analysis of the 1996 Sakai outbreak of Escherichia coli 0157: H7 (VTEC 0157) infection. The Osaka Hus critical care study group. The Journal of Infection. 2000;41(1):45-49.

9.   Kay HE, Wallace DM. A and B antigens of tumors arising from urinary epithelium. Journal of the National Cancer Institute. 1961;26:1349-1365.

10. Albert MJ. Epidemiology & molecular biology of Vibrio cholera 0139 bengal. The Indian Journal of Medical Research. 1996;104:14-27.

11. Mourant AE, Kopec AC, Domaniewska-Sobczak K. Blood groups and diseases. Oxford, England: Oxford University Press. 1978.

12. Waltner-Toews D, Lang T.A. New conceptual base for food and agricultural policy: the emerging model of links between agriculture, food, health, environment and society. Glob Change Hum Policy. 2000;1:116-129.

13. Vasto S, Caruso C, Castiglia L, Duro G, Monastero R, Rizzo C. Blood group does not appear to affect longevity a pilot study in centenarians from western Sicily. Biogerontology. 2011;12(5):467-471.

14. Brecher ME, Hay SN. ABO blood type and longevity. American Journal of Clinical Pathology. 2011;135:96-97.

15. Calhoun L, Petz LD. Erythrocyte antigens. In: Beutler E, Lichman MA, Coller BS, Kipps TJ, Selisohn U, editors. Williams hematology. 6th edn. New York: McGraw-

Hill, Inc, Health Professions Division. 2001;1849–1857.

16. Kulkarni AG, Peter B, Ibazebo R, Dash B, Fleming AF. The ABO and Rhesus groups in the North of Nigeria. Ann Trop Med Parasitol. 1985;79:83-88.

17. Bakare AA, Azeez MA, Agbolade JO. Gene frequencies of ABO and rhesus blood groups and haemoglobin variants in Ogbomosho, South-West Nigeria. Afri J Biotechnol. 2006;5(22):224-229.

18. Adeyemo A, Soboyejo OB. Frequency distribution of ABO, RH, blood groups and blood genotypes among the cell biology and genetics students of University of Lagos, Nigeria. Afri J Biotechnol. 2006;5(22):2062-2065.

19. Tuaszik T. Heterogeneity in the distribution of ABO blood groups in Hungary. Gene Geogr. 1995;9:169-176.

20. Al-Bustan S, El-Zawahri M, Al-Azmi D, Al-Bashir AA. Allele frequencies and molecular genotyping of the ABO blood group system in Kuwaiti population. Int J Hematol. 2002;75:147-53.

21. Omotade OO, Adeyemo AA, Kayode CM, Falade SI, Ikpeme S. Gene frequencies of ABO and Rh (D) blood group alleles in a healthy infant population in Ibadan, Nigeria. West Afr J Med. 1999;18(4): 294-7.

22. Iyola OA, Igunnugbemi OO, Anifowoshe AT, Raheem UA. Gene frequencies of ABO and Rh (D) blood group alleles in Ilorin, North-central Nigeria. World J Biol Res. 2011;4(1):6-14.

23. Abdulazeez AA, Alo ED, Rebecca SN. Carriage rate of Human Immunodeficiency Virus (HIV) infection among different ABO and rhesus blood groups in Adamawa State, Nigeria. Biomed Res. 2008;19(1):41-44.

24. Loua A, Lamah MR, Haba NY, Camara M. Frequency of ABO blood group and rhesus D in the Guinean population. Transfus Clin Biol. 2007;14:435-439.

25. Yousaf M, Yousaf N, Zahid A. Pattern of ABO and Rh (D) blood groups distribution in Bahawalpar Division. Pak J Med Res. 1988;27:40-1.

26. Khaliq MA, Khan JA, Shah H, Khan SP. Frequency of ABO and Rh blood groups in Hazara Division (Abbottabad). Pak J Med Res.1984;23:102-3.

27. Jeremiah ZA, Odumody CO. Rh antigens and phenotype frequencies of the Ibibio, Efik and Ibo ethnic nationalities in Calabar, Nigeria. J Blood group Serol Educ Immunohematol. 2005;21:21-24.

28. Hailu T, kebede T. Assessing the association of severe malaria infection and ABO blood groups in northwestern Ethopia. J Vector Borne Dis. 2013;50:292-296.

29. Gupta M, Chowdhuri AN. Relationship between ABO blood groups and malaria. Bull World Health Organ.1980;58(6):913-5.

30. Athreya BH, Coriell L. Relation of blood groups to infection: I A survey and review of data suggesting possible relationship between malaria and blood groups. Am J Epidemiol. 1967;86:292-304

31. Greer JB, Yazer MH, Raval JS, Barmada MM, Brand RE, Whitcomb DC. Significant association between ABO blood group and pancreatic cancer. World J Gastroenterol. 2010;16(44):5588-5591.

32. Wolpin BM, Chan AT, Hartge P, Chanock SJ, Kraft P, Hunter DJ, et al. ABO blood group and the risk of pancreatic cancer. J Natl Cancer Inst. 2009;101(6):424-431.

33. Amundadottir L, Kraft P, Stolzenberge-Solomon RZ, Fuchs CS, Petersen GM, Arslan AA et al. Genome-wide association study identifies variants in the ABO locus associated with susceptibility to pancreatic cancer. Nat Genet. 2009;41(9):986-90.

34. Mortazavi H, Hajian S, Fadavi E, Sabour S, Baharvand M, Bakhtiari S. ABO blood groups in oral cancer: a first case-control study in a defined group of Iranian patients. Asian Pac J Cancer Prev. 2014;15(3):1415-1418.

35. Jaleel BF, Nagarajappa R. Relationship between ABO blood groups and oral cancer. Indian J Dent Res. 2012;23(1):7-10.

36. Anee M, Jawad A, Hashmi I. Distribution of ABO and Rh blood group alleles in Mandi Bahanddin district of Punjab, Pakistan. Proc Pakistan Acad Sci. 2007;44(4):289-294.

37. Khattak ID, Khan TM, Syed P, Shah AM, Khaltak ST, Ali A. Frequency of ABO and Rhesus blood groups in district Swat, Pakistan. J Ayub Med Coll Abbottabad. 2008;20(4):127-129.

38. Akbas F, Aydin M, Cenani A. ABO blood subgroup allele frequencies in the Turkish

population. Anthropol Anz. 2003;61:257-260.

39.   Egesie UG, Egesie OJ, Usar I, Johnbull TO. Distribution of ABO, Rhesus blood groups and hemoglobin electrophoresis among the undergraduate students of Niger Delta University. Nigeria Journal of Physiological Sciences. 2008;23(1-2):5-8.

7

Suitability of Lower K2 EDTA Sample Volumes for Absolute CD4 Count Enumeration by Flow Cytometric Technique

K. A. Fasakin[1*], O. D. Ajayi[2], C. T. Omisakin[1] and A. J. Esan[1]

[1]Department of Haematology, Federal Teaching Hospital, Ido Ekiti, Nigeria.
[2]Department of Pharmacology and Therapeutics, College of Medicine and Health Sciences, University of Afe Babalola, Ado Ekiti, Nigeria.

Authors' contributions

This work was carried out in collaboration between all authors. Author KAF designed the study, wrote the protocol and wrote the first draft of the manuscript and managed the experimental process. Author ODA managed the literature and statistical analysis. Authors CTO and AJE were also involved in experimental process. All authors read and approved the final manuscript.

Editor(s):
(1) Ricardo Forastiero, Department of Hematology, Favaloro University, Argentina.
Reviewers:
(1) Anonymous, India.
(2) Carine Ghem, Instituto de Cardiologia do Rio Grande do, Brazil.
(3) Elizabete Delbuono, Pediatric Oncology Institute, Federal University of São Paulo, Brazil.
(4) José Francisco Zambrano, Autonomous University of Nayarit, Mexico.
(5) Tafireyi Marukutira, Centers for Disease Control and Prevention, Botswana.

ABSTRACT

Background: Incorrect blood sample volume-anticoagulant ratio has been the cause of both haematological and immunological errors especially when K_3 EDTA-containing blood collection tubes were used. Lower whole blood sample volumes collected into 4.0 millilitres spray-dried K_2 EDTA has been shown to overcome incorrect haematology results when analysed on automated haematology analyzers but there is no experimental evidence for the same in the CD4 count enumeration by flow cytometric technique.

Materials and Methods: 9.0 ml of whole blood was collected from each of fifteen retroviral and ten normal volunteers and aliquot into five different 4.0 ml plastic spray-dried K_2 EDTA blood collection tubes containing 4.0, 2.0, 1.5, 1.0 and 0.5 ml respectively. Each well-mixed sample was analysed on Partec Cyflow counter within 4 hours of collection for absolute CD4+T lymphocyte count.

Corresponding author: E-mail: fasakin_kolawole@yahoo.co.uk

Results: Both the reference sample volume 4.0 ml and experimental lower sample volumes (2.0, 1.5, 1.0 and 0.5 mls) of retroviral volunteers in 4.0 ml plastic spray-dried K2 EDTA blood collection tubes gave comparable CD4 count results with percentage mean difference of 1.82%, -1.48%, 2.25% and 0% for 2.0 ml, 1.5 ml 1.0 ml and 0.5 ml respectively. Irrespective of sample volumes, the normal volunteers had higher CD4 count results. There was no statistically and clinically significant difference in the CD4 counts and the percentage mean difference were 0.4%, 0.17%, 1.00% and 0.23% for 2.0 ml, 1.5 ml, 1.0 ml and 0.5 ml respectively. The correlation (slope) and modest logistic regression coefficient (R^2) of experimental lower sample volumes of both retroviral and normal volunteers were between 0.9500 and 1.0000 showing excellent agreement in the CD4 counts of both reference and experimental sample volumes ($p < 0.01$).
Conclusion: Quality CD4 count results can be obtained with a minimum sample volume of 0.5 ml in 4.0 ml spray-dried K2 EDTA vacutainer blood collection tubes both in HIV and healthy individuals with intact immune function.
Funding: This research did not receive any grant from any funding agency in the public, commercial or non-profit sector.

Keywords: CD4 count; K2 EDTA; retroviral volunteers; percentage mean difference; spray-dried cyflow counter.

1. INTRODUCTION

Absolute CD4+ T-lymphocyte count is the diagnostic tool required when considering initiating antiretroviral therapy in newly diagnosed human immunodeficiency virus (HIV) patients as well as for proper monitoring of those already on highly active antiretroviral therapy (HAART). The accuracy and reproducibility of CD4 count results is therefore basic to decision-making in HIV management [1].

Diagnostic medicine like its clinical counterpart is a dynamic scientific world where scientists proffer solution to procedures that pose challenges in the past. One major question that has remained unanswered is whether lower sample volumes collected into spray dried dipotassium ethylene diamine tetra-acetic acid (K2 EDTA) collection tubes are suitable for flow cytometric analysis of CD4 count. The suitability of lower sample volumes collected into spray dried K2 EDTA vacutainer tubes for automated haematologic analysis both in normal and pathologic conditions have been demonstrated by American and Nigerian researchers [2,3]. To the best of our ability, there is virtual lack of data on the suitability of same for CD4 count test given the sensitivity of the test, the cost of the risk of misleading the clinicians, toxicological effects of ART on the recipients of the drugs and overall treatment outcome. However, the challenge of having to collect the standard volumes of 4.5 -5.0 ml into K3 EDTA which is the liquid form of the anticoagulant sometimes pose great challenges to clinicians especially in infants and the elderly as well as highly debilitating patients. Such struggles often times have led to

microclots or fully-clotted, haemolysed, non-homogeneous samples and incorrect blood volume – anticoagulant ratio. These more often than not usually lead to rejection of such samples by clinical laboratory scientists.

Absolute CD4+T- lymphocyte count is the determination of the concentration of CD4+T-lymphocytes in the blood. Depletion of the CD4+ T cell has been proved to be responsible for associated immune deficiency in HIV infection [4,5]. It is one of the hallmarks of the progression of HIV infection and a major indicator of the stage of the disease in HIV infected individuals [6,7]. Clinical and Laboratory Standard Institute, CLSI (formerly, NCCLS) in one of her recent publications, 'Procedures for the Handling of Blood Specimens', stated that the amount of additives placed into a tube is intended for certain volume of blood. If less than the required blood volume is drawn, the excess amount of additives has the potential to adversely affect the accuracy of the test [8] and another publication recommended that the draw volume shall be no more than 10% below the stated volume of the manufacturer [9]. These standards apply to all collection tubes including EDTA.

Several published articles have compared the results of samples collected into glass and plastic K3 EDTA, glass K3 EDTA and plastic K2 EDTA and have obtained comparable results for full blood count carried out by automated analysers [10-12]. In the last two decades, experts have advocated for the use of spray-dried K2 EDTA tubes rather than the usual glass K3 EDTA [13-16,2].

We hypothesized that the spraying of dry K2 EDTA anticoagulant has drastically minimized the immunologic errors due to incorrect anticoagulant – blood volume ratio in just same way it did for haematologic errors.

1.1 The Objective of This Study

We carried out this research to prove our hypothesis that if lower sample volumes collected into spray-dried K2 EDTA gave comparable results with the recommended standard volume (4 ml) in both normal and pathologic samples tested for haematologic parameters, it should do the same for CD4+ T cell count in both normal and pathologic samples; to establish the suitability of analysing absolute CD4 count with flow cytometric method using lower sample volumes, and determine the minimum blood collection volume required for CD4+ T cell count analysis.

2. MATERIALS AND METHODS

2.1 Study Location

This study was carried out at the Haematology department of the Federal Teaching Hospital (FTH), Ido Ekiti, Nigeria. FTH was located in Ido Ekiti, the principal town in Ido Osi local government area of Ekiti state with an estimated population of 107,000. It is geographically located in the northern part of Ekiti state which covers an estimated total area of 6353 km², 2,453 square mile and an estimated population of 2,737,186, where the routes from Kwara and Osun states converge. FTH, Ido Ekiti was upgraded in 2006 to serve as a centre for HIV/AIDS referral, diagnosis and treatment in Ekiti State and serving five contiguous states. The centre since then has been offering free diagnosis and antiretroviral therapy.

2.2 STUDY DESIGN

2.2.1 HIV counselling and testing

All patients newly diagnosed for HIV at our HIV counselling and testing (HCT) site or PEPFAR-supported HIV laboratory (the main laboratory dedicated for confirmation of HIV test results and quality control, and analysis of baseline immunologic, haematologic and other serologic procedures for confirmed HIV/AIDS patients) at the haematology department according to Centre for Disease Control and prevention guideline

serial algorithm II were included in the study [17]. Following pre-test counselling and informed consent, we performed HIV testing using two rapid enzyme immunoassay (EIA) techniques. Whole blood samples obtained by capillary puncture or plasma samples separated from 4 millilitres of whole blood collected into K2 EDTA spray-dried collection tubes were used for the procedures and the tests were performed according to CDC-UMD HIV rapid testing serial algorithm II guideline [17]. Similar results were obtained from Genscreen HIV 1 & 2 ELISA kits (Biorad, France).Diagnostic techniques/algorithm was quality controlled using one world Accuracy HIV samples with already known positive and negative HIV results.

2.2.2 Sample collection

Fifteen (15) newly-diagnosed retroviral volunteers were included in the study with ten (10) normal volunteers serving as research controls. 9.0 ml of whole blood sample was drawn from each of the participating volunteers by venepuncture procedure following due pre-test counselling and informed consent as part of ethical consideration of the Federal Teaching Hospital, Ido Ekiti. Each of the donated 9.0 ml blood volume was aliquoted into five 4.0 ml vacutainer blood collection tubes containing K2 EDTA in the following volumes: 4.0, 2.0, 1.5, 1.0 and 0.5 ml.

2.2.3 Cyflow counter calibration/ research sample analysis

Research samples for CD4 count were prepared and run on the Partec cyflow counter (Partec flow cytometer, GMBH, Munster, Germany) according to the manufacturer's instructions. Partec flow cytometer (Cyflow counter) was first calibrated to ascertain optimal equipment performance by using count check beads of already known concentration following daily cleaning procedure. Samples from normal subjects were tested along with research samples to ensure reagent control and quality of results. A well calibrated cyflow counter must give count check beads reagent control within ±10% of reagent concentration. CD4 monoclonal antibodies were used within the expiry dates. Values within ±10% of known results validated the potency of the CD4 monoclonal antibodies used for our research procedure.

2.2.4 Cyflow counter count check beads calculation

A specific count check bead used during analysis of our research samples had known concentration of 23,470 cells/ml. The equipment displayed absolute CD4 count value of the count check bead as 966 cells/µl, and the pre-set dilution factor is 42, then calculated concentration of the count check beads in cells/ml from the flow cytometer

$$= \frac{(CD4 \text{ count in cells/µl}) \times 1000}{42}$$

$$= \frac{966 \times 1000}{42} = 23,000 \text{cells/ml}.$$

% deviation from the known concentration is calculated from the formula:

% deviation = (23,000-23470)/23470 x 100% = -2.0%.

Since the calculated value of count check beads concentration fell within -10% of known value, the equipment was successfully calibrated.

2.2.5 Principle and procedure of flow cytometry for cd4 count

The cyflow counter operation is based on the simultaneous measurement of multiple physical characteristics of CD4 count in a single file as it flows through the cyflow counter. The counter separated the CD4+ T cell from the monocytes-CD4 bearing cells and noise using a gating system. We prepared the samples and analysed them for CD4 count according to the manufacturer instructions. 20 µl of well-mixed whole blood sample was added to 20 µl of CD4 MAB (monoclonal antibody) in a Rhören tube. This was incubated for 15 minutes in the dark. 800µl of CD4 no-lyse buffer was added (carefully without introducing bubbles) and the mixture was analyzed on Partec cyflow counter and results recorded in cells/µl.

2.3 Statistical Analysis

Data were computed with SPSS statistical software (Statistical Package for Social Sciences Inc, Chicago IL), version 17. The CD4 count results of reference sample volume and lower sample volumes were expressed as means and standards and percentage mean difference using one sample student t-test. The degree of association between the reference CD4 count result (using the standard 4.0 ml sample volume) and the experimental CD4 count results (obtained from lower sample volumes) was further established with Spearman correlation and linear regression analytical tools.

3. RESULTS AND DISCUSSION

9.0 milliliters of blood samples was drawn from each of fifteen (15) retroviral and ten (10) healthy normal volunteers by venepuncture. Each 9.0 ml sample aliquoted into five (5) different 4.0 ml K2 EDTA collection tubes containing 4.0, 2.0, 1.5, 1.0 and 0.5 millilitres samples were analysed on Partec cyflow counter. Mean results, standard deviations and percentage mean difference for absolute CD4 count results of different sample volumes were shown in Tables 1 and 2. The mean CD4 count results for lower sample volumes showed no statistically significant difference from the gold standard 4.0 ml sample volume (p<0.05). For the CD4 count results of lower sample volumes (2.0, 1.5, 1.0 and 0.5 ml) to be diagnostically useful, they must give values within ±10% of the gold standard value. Table 1 showed the means and standard deviations of CD4 count results for lower sample volumes of retroviral volunteers to be 439.2±207.5 cells/µl, 447.2±206.7 cells/µl, 432.7±190.5 cells/µl, 449.1± 210.2 cells/µl and 439.2±203.8 cells/µl respectively. The percentage mean differences obtained for 2.0, 1.5, 1.0 and 0.5 ml sample volumes of retroviral volunteers were 1.82%,-1.48%, 2.25% and 0% respectively. The CD4 count results of normal volunteers were higher than the retroviral volunteers irrespective of the sample volumes. This is expected of persons with intact immune status. Table 2 shows the means, standard deviations and percentage mean differences of CD4 count results obtained from the 4.0 ml and for lower sample volumes of normal volunteers. Comparison of mean with t-test shows no clinically significant difference in CD4 count results of 4.0 ml sample volume and 2.0, 1.5, 1.0 and 0.5ml sample volumes. The percentage mean differences for 2.0, 1.5, 1.0 and 0.5 ml sample volumes were 0.40%, 0.17%, 1.00% and 0.23% respectively. The low percentage mean difference greatly reduces the chance of upward misclassification which can lead to delay in antiretroviral therapy initiation or downward misclassification which can prompt treatment decisions.

To further elucidate the diagnostic usefulness and quality of results of lower sample volumes collected into 4.0 ml K2 EDTA collection tubes, spearman correlation coefficient and modest linear regression R^2 were used to show the degree of association. Both standard volume and lower sample volumes CD4 count results from retroviral and normal volunteers were excellently correlated since the slope and R^2 of all the sample volumes were between 0.9500 and 1.0000 as shown in Tables 3 and 4.

Blood collection tubes containing K2 EDTA have gained popularity in the most clinical laboratories in developed countries but the liquid counterpart (K3 EDTA) is still very much in use in most of our treatment facilities for HIV/AIDS patients in Nigeria. Issues that borders on incorrect blood sample volume – anticoagulant ratio, haemolysis, difficulty in obtaining samples of required volume in exposed babies or geriatric patients and patient assessment requiring that different samples be collected for different tests have all constituted cause of sample rejection by clinical laboratory and the need to collect fresh samples often times based on Clinical and Laboratory Standard Institute guideline [8].

Table 1. Mean ± SD and percentage mean difference of CD4 count values of retroviral samples

Sample volume (millilitre)	Mean±SD (cells/µl)	% Mean difference (%) (Mean CD4 count of GSSV minus mean CD4 count of LSV)/ (Mean CD4 count of GSSV) X 100
4.0	439.2±207.5	-
2.0	447.2±206.7	1.82
1.5	432.7±190.5	-1.48
1.0	449.1±210.2	2.25
0.5	439.2±203.8	-

GSSV: Gold standard sample volume; LSV: Lower sample volume

Table 2. Mean ± SD and percentage mean difference of CD4 count values of normal volunteers (control subjects)

Sample volume (millilitre)	Mean±SD (cells/µl)	% Mean difference (%) (Mean CD4 count of GSSV minus mean CD4 count of LSV)/ (Mean CD4 count of GSSV) X 100
4.0	1193.9±232.7	-
2.0	1198.7±242.2	0.40
1.5	1195.0±244.4	0.17
1.0	1205.8±228.1	1.00
0.5	1196.6±238.4	0.23

GSSV: Gold standard sample volume; LSV: Lower sample volume

Table 3. Correlation and regression analysis comparing the CD4 count results of experimental sample volume of blood collection and 4.0 ml reference sample volume of control (normal volunteers) samples

Sample volume (Milliliter)	Slope of CD4 count values	R^2 of CD4 count values	p-value
2.0	0.9520	0.9940	
1.5	1.0000	0.9830	P = 0.01
1.0	0.9760	0.9830	
0.5	0.9640	0.9690	

Correlation is significant at the 0.01 level (2-tailed)

Table 4. Correlation and regression analysis comparing the CD4 count results of experimental sample volume of blood collection and 4.0 ml reference sample volume of retroviral samples

Sample volume (Milliliter)	Slope of CD4 count values	R^2 of CD4 count values	p-value
2.0	0.9860	0.9910	
1.5	0.9810	0.9900	P = 0.01
1.0	0.9640	0.9890	
0.5	0.9640	0.9920	

Correlation is significant at the 0.01 level (2-tailed)

Our findings based on the use of lower sample volumes in 4.0 millilitres K2 EDTA vacutainer collection tubes revealed the aforementioned problem of incorrect blood sample volume – anticoagulant ratio is not an issue here.

4. CONCLUSION

The study demonstrates that the use of spray-dried K2 EDTA is suitable for CD4 count with a volume of whole blood sample as low as 0.5 millilitre. The statistical analysis shows a high correlation of the small volumes of blood (2.0 millilitres, 1.5 millilitres, 1 millilitre and 0.5 millilitre) with the gold standard volume of 4ml for both abnormal (HIV positive) and normal samples (p=0.01). Standardizing into one 4.0 millilitres spray-dried K2 EDTA tube for vast majority of patients will reduce the need for recollection of samples, simplify pre-analytical testing process, improve staff safety and reduce inventory and supply cost. Where Sysmex KX-21N haematology automated analyser for complete blood analysis and cyflow counter for CD4 count estimation are within the same HIV/AIDS laboratory location, both analyses become highly simplified and patients derive more satisfaction since the minimum sample volume (0.5 millilitre) permits both analyses to be done and gives allowance for repeat of test. Well planned inventory and ordering as well as approval for use is paramount to prevent stock-out and mandatory reverse to old practice. Proper calibration of cyflow cytometer for CD4 count enumeration must also be ensured before analysis for optimal performance and quality results.

INFORMED CONSENT

Pre-test counselling was done and informed consent was obtained from the newly diagnosed HIV individuals before inclusion in the study. Retroviral volunteers already on ART were excluded from the study. No personal bio data was required.

ETHICAL CONSIDERATIONS

CDC guidelines and the ethical guidelines of Federal Teaching Hospital, Ido Ekiti were followed for diagnosis of HIV and inclusion of patients.

ACKNOWLEDGEMENTS

We acknowledge the contributions of the technicians at the department of haematology for their roles in research samples collection and staff of care and support unit especially Mr Ogundana AO for their roles in HIV counselling and testing.

COMPETING INTERESTS

Authors have declared that no competing interests exist.

REFERENCES

1. Hoffman J, van Griensven J, Colebunders R and McKellar M. Role of the CD4 count in HIV management. HIV Ther. 2010;4(1):27-39.

2. Min Xu A, Robbe VA, Jack RM, Ruthledge JC. Under-filled blood collection tubes K2 EDTA as anticoagulant are acceptable for automated complete blood counts, white blood cell differential, and reticulocyte count. International Journal of Laboratory Haematology. 2010;32,491-497.

3. Fasakin KA, Omisakin CT, Esan AJ and Ajayi OD. Lower Sample Volumes Collected Into Spray-Dried K2 EDTA Vacuitaner Bottles Are Suitable For Automated Complete Blood Count. Analysis Including Differential Leukocyte Count. IOSR Journal of Dental and Medical Sciences. 2014;13:1(X),48-53.

4. Shearer WT, Rosenblatt HM, Schluchter MD, Mofenson LM, Denny TN. Immunologic targets of HIV infection: T-cells. Ann. NY Acad. Sci. 1983;693:35-51.

5. Mellors JW, Muñoz A, Giorgi JV, Margolick JB, Tassoni CJ, Gupta P, Kingsley LA, Todd JA, Saah AJ, Detels R, Phair JP, Rinaldo CR. Plasma viral load and CD4+ lymphocytes as prognostic markers of HIV-1 infection. Ann. Intern. Med. 1997;126: 946-954.

6. Hogg RS, Yip B, Chan KJ, Wood E, Craib KJ, O'Shaughnessy MV, Montaner JS. Rates of disease progression by baseline CD4 cell counts and viral load initiating triple drug therapy. JAMA. 2001;286:2568-2577.

7. World Health Organization, WHO. Antiretroviral drugs for the treatment of HIV infection in Adults and Adolescents in resource-limited settings: Recommendations for a public Health Approach (2005 Revision) –Brief meeting Report; 2005.

8. Clinical and laboratory standards institute, CLSI. Procedures for the handling and

processing of blood specimens. Approved guideline- Third edition. 2004;24(21):H18-A3.

9.   Clinical and laboratory Standard Institute, CLSI. Tubes and additives for venous blood specimen collection. Approval guideline-fifth edition. 2003;(16(13),5):HI-A5

10. Brunson DS, Bak A, Przyk E. Sheridan B, Muncer DL. Comparing hematology anticoagulants: K2 EDTA vs K3 EDTA. Lab Hematology. 1995;1:112-119.

11. VS5244 (white paper), BD Vacutainer™ Tube Comparison: Plastic K2 EDTA vs. Glass K3 EDTA Tubes for Blood Counts on the Coulter MAXM™ vol2; 2002.

12. Mamdoor AG. The comparison of Glass EDTA versus Plastic EDTA Blood-drawing tubes for completed Blood Count. Middle East Scientific Research, 2008;3(1):32-35.

13. The International Council for Standardization in Haematology: Expert Panel for Cytometry. Recommendations of the International Council for Standardization in Haematology for ethylene diamine tetra acetic acid anticoagulant of blood for blood cell counting and sizing. Am J Clin Path. 1993; 100:371-372.

14. Lena A. Physical and clinical difference between Glass K3 EDTA and Plastic K2 EDTA. Teck Talk. 2002;8(2).

15. Van Cott EM, Lewandrowski KB, Patel S, Grzybek DY, Kratz A. Comparison of glass K3 EDTA versus plastic K2 EDTA blood drawing tubes for complete blood counts, reticulocyte count, and white blood cell differentials. Laboratory Haematology. 2003;9:10-14. [Pubmed].

16. World Health Organization. Guidance on provider initiated HIV testing and counseling in health facilities. Geneva. World Health Organization; 2007.

17. World Health Organization, WHO. Scaling up antiretroviral health in resource-limited settings. Guidelines for a public health approach. Geneva; 2002.

8

Combined Closed-circuit Acute Normovolemic Hemodilution and Deliberate Hypotension in a Jehovah's Witness: A Case Report

Otu E. Etta[1*] and Emma Etuknwa[1]

[1]*Department of Anaesthesia, University of Uyo Teaching Hospital, Uyo, Akwa Ibom State, Nigeria.*

Authors' contributions

This work was carried out in collaboration between both authors. Author OEE designed the study and wrote the initial draft of the manuscript, while author EE managed the literature search. Both authors read and approved the final manuscript.

Editor(s):
(1) Armel Hervé Nwabo Kamdje, University of Ngaoundere-Cameroon, Ngaoundere, Cameroon.
Reviewers:
(1) Neal Fleming, University of California, Davis, USA.
(2) Anonymous, Federal University of Bahia, Brazil.

ABSTRACT

Aims: To enlighten both clinicians and Jehovah's Witness patients on closed-circuit acute normovolemic hemodilution (ANH) and deliberate hypotension (DH) as safe and acceptable blood conservation strategies.

Case Presentation: A 32 yr old male Jehovah's Witness patient was scheduled for nephrolithotomy on account a right nephrolithiasis (Staghorn calculus). He was fit and young weighing 76 kg with packed cell volume of 34%. The anticipated blood loss during the surgery was 1500 ml or more, hence we decided to use combined closed-circuit ANH and DH. These combined strategies were accepted by the patient; they minimized blood loss to only 400 mls and provided a good operating field visibility.

Discussion: Several blood conservation strategies have been developed and accepted by Jehovah's Witness patients provided the blood circulation circuit is not broken. Our resident doctor and patient were not initially aware of the acceptability of ANH by the Jehovah's witness. Blood conservation strategies could be used either singly or in combination, our patient was suitable for both.

Conclusion: Combined closed-circuit ANH and DH are safe and acceptable to Jehovah's witness patients.

*Corresponding author: E-mail: otuetta@yahoo.com

Keywords: Acute normovolemic hemodilution; deliberate hypotension; Jehovah's Witness.

1. INTRODUCTION

The surgical Jehovah's Witness patients will continue to challenge the clinicians due to their 'no blood transfusion doctrine' even in the presence of life threatening anemia and/or coagulopathy [1]. The Witness's determination that blood transfusion violated God's law was made in 1945 and is based on three biblical passages including Gen 9:3-4: 'Every moving thing that liveth shall be meat for you,… but flesh with life thereof, which is the blood thereof, shall ye not eat' [2]. In a retrospective analysis of Jehovah's Witness patients undergoing non-cardiac surgery, a pre-operative hemoglobin (Hb) concentration <10 g/dl significantly correlated with increased post operative mortality [3]. Several blood conservation strategies have been developed, and are acceptable to many Jehovah's Witness patients [4,5], these include acute normovolemic hemodilution (ANH), intra- and post operative cell salvage (CS), deliberate hypotension (DH), perfluorocarbon emulsion etc, provided the blood circulation circuit in not broken. These are used either in isolation or in combination, however, these techniques are infrequently reported in our environment due to lack of awareness by the clinicians and/or patients, or other factors [4,6]. We describe the successful use of combined closed-circuit ANH and DH in a Jehovah's Witness patient.

2. CASE REPORT

A 32 yrs old male Jehovah's Witness was scheduled for nephrolithotomy on account of right nephrolithiasis (staghorn calculus). He had no previous history of surgery or anaesthesia and no co-morbidities. Medical examination revealed a fit young adult weighing 76 kg, his packed cell volume (PCV) was 34%, other laboratory investigations were within normal limits.

An informed consent for surgery was obtained the previous day during routine preoperative assessment, however, the patient refused consent for any form of blood or blood product transfusion in accordance with his Jehovah's Witness believe. On the morning of surgery, the surgeon alerted that the anticipated blood loss may be up to 1500 ml or more, hence we decided to use a combined closed-circuit ANH and DH to minimize the blood loss.

In the theatre, the patient was counseled on closed-circuit acute normovolemic hemodilution as an acceptable form of blood transfusion by the Jehovah's Witness and consent was eventually obtained for the procedure.

He was attached to a multiparameter monitor and baseline vital signs were as follows: Pulse rate- 90/ m, Blood pressure- 130/70 mmHg, SpO$_2$ – 100% on room air. A tourniquet was applied to the left arm and two intravenous lines were set up with size 18 G canulae, two citrate, potassium, dextrose, adenine (CPDA)– containing blood bags were obtained and blood giving sets were attached to each blood bag. Phlebotomy was performed and blood was collected into the blood bags placed below the arm. At the same time, a size 16 G canula was inserted into the right arm for normal saline infusion. Approximately, a total of 900mls of blood was collected into the two blood bags to roughly reduce the PCV to the estimated 28% before surgery. The blood bags were hung on the drip stand above the patient and the blood giving set connected to the 18 G cannula to establish a closed-circuit after which, the phlebotomy lines were removed (Fig. 1). A total of 3 L of normal saline was infused within 30 minutes to maintain the blood volume.

Anaesthesia was induced with 120 mg of propofol, and halothane at 2%, suxamethonium, 75 mg was given to facilitate endotracheal intubation with size 7.5 mm endotracheal tube, after which pentazocine 30 mg, and atracurium 30 mg were given. Five minutes after intubation, his BP and MAP were 90/68 mmHg and 68 mmHg respectively. He was maintained within a target systolic BP range of 80-90 mmHg, and MAP of 50-70 mmHg using halothane at 1-2%, and controlled manual ventilation (Fig. 3).

The patient was put in the left kidney position and surgery commenced. The kidney stones were removed, the surgery lasted approximately 3 hrs and 50 mins. The estimated blood loss from suction bottle and gauze was 400 ml, and the surgeon was satisfied with the good operating field visibility (Fig. 2).

A total of 2.5 L of normal saline was infused intraoperatively, the two units of blood were reinfused to the patient at the end of surgery. Intravenous paracetamol 1000 mg and intramuscular diclofenac 75 mg were given for immediate post operative analgesia, neuromuscular blockade was reversed with neostigmine/atropine combination. The patient was extubated and transfered to the recovery room. His PCV 48 hrs after surgery was 28%.

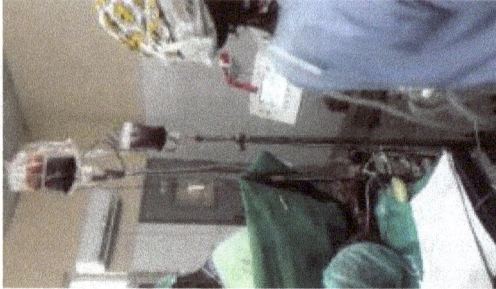

Fig. 1. Patient's blood reinfused

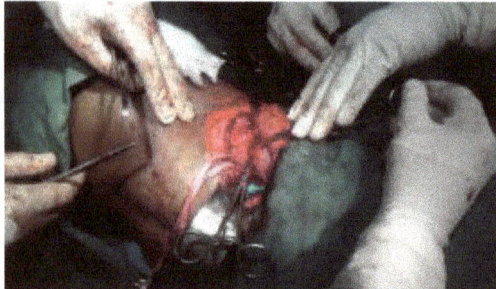

Fig. 2. Good operating field visibility

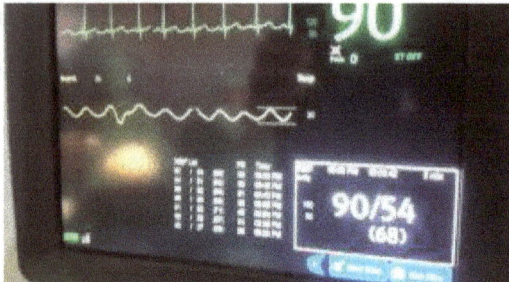

Fig. 3. Hypotension maintained

3. DISCUSSION

The perioperative management of the Jehovah's Witness patient focuses on the prevention of lethal anemia and coagulopathy [7]. Some Jehovah's Witness patients likewise anaesthetists are not familiar with some acceptable blood conservation strategies for Jehovah's Witness [4,6]. Our patient had previously rejected any form of blood transfusion during preoperative assessment the previous day by our resident doctor who was not conversant with closed-

circuit ANH, hence, we counselled the patient in the theatre on closed-circuit ANH and DH as acceptable blood conservation strategies by Jehovah's Witness. To further convince him of the closed-circuit nature of ANH, we performed the phlebotomy before the induction of anaesthesia, against the conventional phlebotomy after induction [5,7].

Blood conservation strategies used either singly or in combnation have been reported by previous researchers [4,5], we opted for combined closed-circuit ANH and DH because the patient was fit for both procedures, also we presumed that outcome of combination technique may be superior to a single measure.

Acute normovolemic hemodilution is based on the concept of removing and storing the patient's Hemoglobin-rich blood before the surgery, replacing the blood with cystalloid or colloid to maintain the blood volume and reinfusing the blood at the end of the surgery. This strategy has been reported to be effective in reducing the total number of units of blood transfused, post operative complications and the overall need for allogenic blood in different types of surgical conditions [4,5,7].

The inclusion criteria for ANH include patients undergoing surgery where greater than 1000 ml of blood loss is anticipated, preoperative hemoglobin concentration is adequate (>9g/dl) and no ischemic heart disease or active bleeding due to coagulopathy are present (8). The American Association of blood banks recommend using the following formula to determine the amount of blood to withdraw for reinfusion [8]: $V = EBV (H_i-H_f)/H_{av}$, where V indicates volume of blood to be withdrawn; EBV, estimated blood volume, typically 70 ml/kg; H_i, initial hematocrit before the procedure; H_f, final desired hematocrit after hemodilution; and H_{av}, average hematocrit during the hemodilution process. Our patient was expected to loose greater than 1500 ml of blood. Although the actual estimated blood loss was only 400mls, this may be attributed to the synergistic effect of combined ANH and DH [9].

Deliberate hypotension or hypotensive anaesthesia entails a controlled lowering of the systolic blood pressure to between 80-90 mmHg or decrease in mean arterial pressure to 50-70 mmHg in a normotensive patient [10]. DH has the risk of hypoperfusion-induced tissue injuries, hence, it is contraindicated in patients with disseminated vascular diseases, ischemic heart disease, carotid artery stenosis and hypertension [11].

DH can be induced by a variety of pharmacological agents and non-pharmacological measures. These include vasodilators such as sodium nitroprusside (SNP), nitroglycerin (NTG); anaesthetic agents such as propofol, halothane and isoflurane; epidural and spinal anaesthesia as well as non-pharmacological techniques such as change in body position and controlled mechanical ventilation [11].

In our patient, only halothane and controlled manual ventilation were used. We maintained the MAP between 50-70 mmHg throughout the procedure, probably the ANH may have augmented the hypotensive strategies.

4. CONCLUSION

Combined closed-circuit ANH and DH are safe and effective in reducing blood loss during surgeries, and are acceptable by Jehovah's Witness patients.

ETHICAL APPROVAL

It is not applicable.

COMPETING INTERESTS

Authors have declared that no competing interests exist.

REFERENCES

1. Dixion JL, Smalley MG. Jehovah's Witness: The Surgical /Ethical challenge. J Am Med Assoc 1981;246:2471-2.

2. Jehovah's Witnesses and the question of blood. New York: Watchtower Bible and Tract Society of New York, Inc; 1977.

3. Carson JL, Duff A, Poses RM, et al. Effect of Anemia and cardiovascular disease on surgical mortality and morbidity. Lancert. 1996;348:1055–60.

4. Nwosu AD. Multimodal approach to blood conservation in the surgical patient. Niger J Clin Pract. 2015;18(3):422-5.

5. Lindstrom E, Johnstone R. Acute normovolemic hemodilution in a jehovah's witness patient: A case report. AANA Journal. 2010;78:326-329.

6. Amucheazi AD, Ajuzeiogu VD,Ezike HA, Odiakosa MC, Nwoke OM, Onyia E. A Survey of blood conservation methods in clinical practice in some urban South-Eastern government hospitals in Nigeria. Asian J Transfus Sci. 2011;5(1):35-38.

7. Habler O, Voss B. Perioperative management of Jehovah's Witness patients: Special consideration of religiously motivated refusal of allogenic blood transfusion. Anaesthetist. 2010;59: 297-311.

8. Brecher M. Ed, for Technical Manual Committee. 14th ed. Bethesda, MD: American Association of Blood Banks. 2002;115-118.

9. Raksamani K, Pongraweewan O, Jirachaipitak S. Anaesthesia for a Jehovah's Witness with Critical Anemia from Ruptured Stomach GIST. Siriraj Med J. 2010;62:215-216.

10. Van Aken H, Van Hemelrijck. Deliberate Hypotension. 1993 Review Course Lectures. 67th Congress of Int'l Anes Res Soc. San Diego. 1993;19-23.

11. Choi WS, Samman N. Risk and benefits of deliberate hypotension in anaesthesia: A systematic review. Int J Oral Maxillofac Surg. 2008;37(8):687-703.

9

A Case of Isolated CNS Relapse in a CML Patient on Chronic Phase

Laurence Adlai B. Morillo[1], Flordeluna Zapata-Mesina[1*]
and Ma Rosario Irene D. Castillo[1]

[1]*Section of Hematology, University of Santo Tomas Hospital, Manila, Philippines.*

Authors' contributions

This work was carried out in collaboration between all authors. Authors FZM and LABM drafted and wrote the manuscript. Author MRIDC reviewed and proofread the manuscript. All authors read and approved the final manuscript.

Editor(s):
(1) Karl-Anton Kreuzer, University Hospital of Cologne, Germany.
(2) Shinichiro Takahashi, Kitasato University School of Allied Health Sciences, Japan.
(3) Tadeusz Robak, Medical University of Lodz, Copernicus Memorial Hospital, Poland.
Reviewers:
(1) Atef Mahmoud Mahmoud Attia, National Research Centre, Egypt.
(2) Golam Hafiz, Bangabandhu Sheikh Mujib Medical University, Bangladesh.

ABSTRACT

We report a patient who achieved hematologic response with Imatinib mesylate and is in chronic phase, but after several years developed neurologic symptoms and was eventually documented to have an isolated CNS relapse. The patient was treated with intrathecal chemotherapy to clear the spinal fluid of the leukemia cells. Imatinib mesylate (STI-571) is a potent and selective inhibitor of BCR-ABL tyrosine kinase and has emerged as a treatment of choice in chronic myeloid leukaemia. However because of poor penetration of the drug to the blood-brain barrier of the central nervous system (CNS), then the CNS acts as a sanctuary site for malignant cells.

Keywords: CNS leukemia; chronic myelogenous leukemia; extramedullary leukemia.

*Corresponding author: E-mail: plonghema@gmail.com

1. INTRODUCTION

Extramedullary leukemia is a well-recognized occurrence and that the central nervous system (CNS) is one of those documented to be affected. In Acute lymphocytic leukemia 6% of patients who were diagnosed with the disease have evidence of CNS involvement; the same number is also noted for those with Chronic myelogenous leukemia with note of involvement of the meninges [1]. Imatinib mesylate (IM) a tyrosine kinase inhibitor used for the treatment of CML allowed patients to achieve hematologic and molecular response. An investigation made by Heike Pfeiffer et al. however showed that 12% of the 103 patient population had relapse with CNS involvement and a portion of which have isolated CNS recurrence without hematologic relapse.

In our case report we are presented with a patient who achieved hematologic response with Imatinib mesylate, however later on developed neurologic symptoms and was eventually documented to have a CNS relapse of CML.

2. CASE

A 42 yr old male was diagnosed with chronic myelogenous leukemia (CML) since 2001 with a cytogenetic finding of hypodiploidy karyotype t (9;22) (q34;q11) Philadelphia chromosome positive. He was started on Imatinib 400 mg/day on 2005, with note of hematologic response during his follow-up. On 2012 his Imatinib dose was adjusted to 600 mg/day and then after a few visits he was lost to follow-up and upon clinical evaluation on 2013 he reported that he was not complaint with Imatinib for almost 10 months.

On August 2013, 7 months prior to admission he was already complaining of frontal headache throbbing in character, unrelieved by intake of pain medications. He then sought consult where a Cranial CT scan image was taken, he was then managed as a case of sub-arachnoid hemorrhage and was treated with medical decompression after which he was discharged stable after a month. He was able to do his usual activity of daily living, and that his Imatinib was reduced to 400 mg/day.

On January 2014, he noted recurrence of the same character of headache severe now accompanied with weakness of extremities, he consulted his physicians and cranial imaging was done once more which showed no change from his previous CT scan imaging, symptoms were persistent, but now with note of blurring of vision. He was admitted for work-up where cervicothoracic MRI was done which showed a suspicious cerebellar enhancement along the cerebellar folla. CNS infection or CNS involvement with leukemia are being considered at this time, hence a lumbar puncture was then performed. Analysis of the CSF collected showed lymphocytosis of 99% in a WBC count of 3660 cells/ul with a protein count of 103 mg/dl, gram stain shows no microorganism, other tests done including special stains and immunologic testing for an infectious cause were performed. The decision then is to treat with Anti-Koch's, based on CSF picture of lymphocytosis. The test however eventually showed negative findings and treatment with anti-Koch's was continued. His symptoms eventually progressed; intermittent headache, progression of blurring of vision and decrease in hearing. A lumbar tap and CSF analysis was done once more still showing only lymphocytosis with WBC count of 1890 cells/ul, 100% of which is lymphocytes no blast cells were reported. Fungal tests were done, results were negative. Ophthalmologic examination was done which revealed a possible nerve pathology of both eyes with note of vitreous infiltrate.

Visual loss was progressive until loss of light perception in a span of 1 month despite initial management. Since all treatment and diagnostic options were explored and still symptom was progressive a reevaluation was then contemplated, a 3rd attempt of lumbar puncture was then decidedly done, this time to start treatment with intrathecal chemotherapy for CNS leukemia, opening pressure at this time was noted to be high at 340 mmH20 and closing pressure of 180. Specimens were still sent for analysis and CSF flow cytometry, intrathecal chemotherapy with hydrocortisone and methotrexate was given. The results of the CSF at this time shows 22% blast cells in a WBC count of 3,103 cells/cu mm and flow cytometry positive for leukemic cells confirming CNS leukemia. He then received 3 doses of Intrathecal Methotrexate (12 mg) given 2x a week (every 5 days) followed by 2 doses of methotrexate, hydrocortisone and cytarabine. CSF analysis was done during every lumbar tap for intrathecal chemotherapy, which showed a decreasing pattern of WBC followed by a decrease in blast cells. The patients visual loss however was noted to be persistent still with no signs of improvement. His headache no longer recurred and hearing loss did not progressed. He continued intrathecal chemotherapy and he was shifted to Nilotinib. During this time his complete blood count was normal. A bone marrow aspiration and biopsy was also done to evaluate the status of his chronic myelogenous leukemia and result was consistent with a chronic phase, CML.

3. DISCUSSION

In the Philippines the annual incidence of CML is at 0.7-0.9 affecting males more than females with a median age of 45-55 [2]. Chronic myelogenous leukemia (CML) is a clonal myeloproliferative disorder of the hematopoeitic stem cell (HSC), associated with an acquired genetic abnormality, the Philadelphia chromosome. Philadelphia chromosome is present in >90% of patients, which is a shortened chromosome 22 resulting from a reciprocal translocation between the long arms of chromosomes 9 and 22 t(9; 22)(q34;q11) this chromosomes causes the formation of BCR-ABL fusion gene which in turn forms the oncogene, p210$^{BCR/ABL}$ [3]. This oncogene then causes an increase in tyrosine kinase activity and the end result is growth factor independence, leukemic cell growth in hematopoietic cell lines and decrease in apoptosis [3]. With the approval and introduction of tyrosine kinase inhibitors such as Imatinib as treatment for Ph+ leukemia (AML and CML) most were able to achieve hematologic and even molecular response. Despite the remarkable therapeutic effect of Imatinib in inducing

remission, some patients still develop refractory disease and some even progress to blastic phase [4]. The progression to blastic phase is influenced by the BCR-ABL gene by which if remained untreated causes genetic instability with impaired DNA repair then DNA damage and eventually leading to blast crisis. [5] Oral tyrosine kinase inhibitors inhibit BCR-ABL-tyrosine kinase. However, the first and second generation tyrosine kinase inhibitors do not penetrate the blood–brain-barrier so that isolated CNS blast crises have been described in several cases [5]. Blastic phase of CML is not limited to peripheral involvement. In a review made by Sohl of 900 patients with CML being treated with Imatinib, they identified 30 patients with extramedullary involvement 15 of which is CNS [6]. Since 1980's reports regarding incidence of CML with extramedullary involvement were documented, most commonly affecting the lymph nodes and a rather small group involving the CNS [7]. CML in accelerated and blastic phase with central nervous system involvement is well known but sporadically reported in literature. Case studies and small series report cerebrospinal fluid with lymphoid or monocytoid blasts as well as parenchymal and dural lesions on patients in blastic phase [8], and more rare are CML in blastic phase presenting as an isolated CNS involvement of leukemia [9-22]. To our knowledge there is no case reported yet in the Philippines regarding CML in blastic phase presenting only in the CSF.

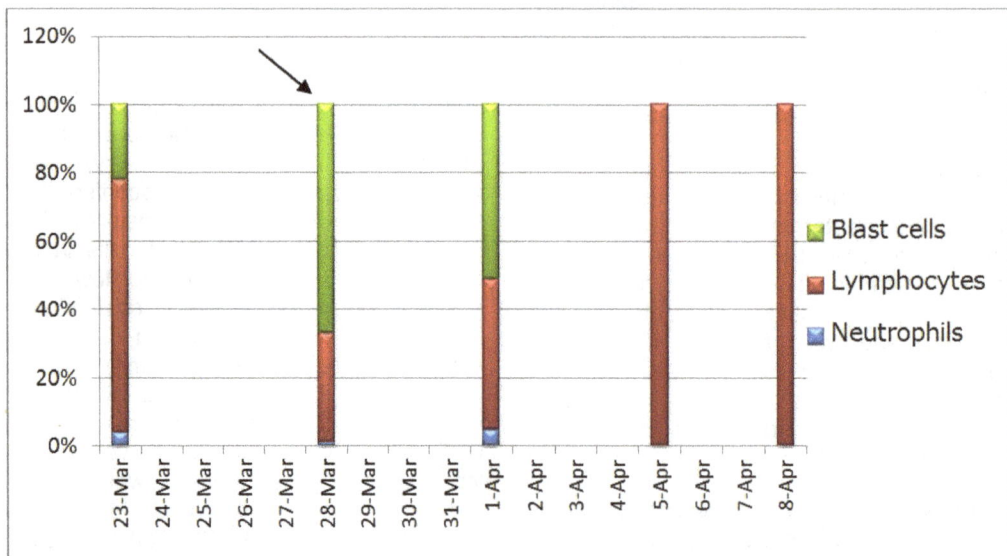

Fig. 1. Spinal cord fluid taken during intrathecal chemotherapy showing a deceasing trend of blast cells upon start of intrathecal chemotherapy, the pointed arrow shows the date of the start of intrathecal chemotherapy

Table 1. Spinal cord fluid analysis showing an overall decrease in total WBC count and a decrease in blast and neutrophil counts, opening and closing pressures was also noted to be decreasing

	Total WBC	Neutrophils	Lymphocytes	Blast cells	Opening pressure	Closing pressure
23-Mar	3,103/mm3	4%	74%	22%	340	180
28-Mar	267/mm3	1%	32%	67%	230	170
1-Apr	843/mm3	5%	44%	51%	270	220
5-Apr	3/mm3	0%	100%	0%	240	190
8-Apr	11/mm3	0%	100%	0%	140	120
28-Apr	19/mm3	0%	100%	0%	120	120
14-May	7/mm3	0%	100%	0%	120	100

The central nervous system is a well-known sanctuary site of leukemic blasts cells. Theoretically, circulating leukemic cells enter the brain or meninges by 5 different routes: 1) passage through the thin walls of the capillaries of the brain and enter the brain tissues directly, 2) migration of leukemic cells through the capillaries and specialized ependymal cells which form the choroid plexus, 3) migration through the walls of vessels which lie in the arachnoid and subarachnoid area, 4) migration through the capillaries of the non-neural areas, and lastly 5) direct migration and growth through perivascular and perineural tissues of vessels and nerves which cross the subdural space. Common to all these routes is the fact that hematogenous spread is the most important vehicle [23].

Leukemia and lymphoma do metastasize to the nervous system but rarely involve brain parenchyma and more characteristically involve the leptomeninges. Leukemic parenchymal tumor also known as chloroma is made up of myeloid leukemic blasts commonly seen in acute myelogenous leukemia and would give mass effect depending on the location of the tumor. While in leptomeningeal metastasis because there is multifocal involvement of the cerebrum, cranial nerves and spinal compartment it may present with symptoms and signs involving one or all of these locations. Headache and mental status changes are the most common cerebral symptoms. Facial weakness, facial numbness, diplopia, visual problems are manifestations of cranial nerve involvement [24]. In our patient, a chronic benign headache was the first manifestation which was attributed to other brain pathology, the clincher to the diagnosis of a possible leptomeningeal metastasis was the development of loss of vision from cranial nerve compression or involvement.

In diagnosis of CNS leptomeningeal leukemia, aside from the patient's clinical presentation of neurologic involvement, a CSF analysis is usually employed to document and strengthen diagnosis. A positive CSF cytology however is just seen in only 50% of patients with documented leptomeningeal metastasis [25]. A repeated spinal tap may sometimes be warranted as it increases the chances of yielding identification of tumor cells and having a positive cytometry test [25]. Neuroimaging may also be used to find diagnostic characteristics of CNS leukemia. Establishing the diagnosis may sometimes be challenging as that said tests may all show negative or equivocal findings, the physician may however deduce the diagnosis by process of elimination and that if all alternative diagnosis has been explored and excluded some clinicians find it acceptable to treat in the absence of diagnostic confirmation [25].

With the introduction of Imatinib more Filipinos are able to achieve hematologic response and even some achieving molecular response [2]. Progression to blastic phase is still documented however, some with CNS involvement or CNS alone despite maintenance of Imatinib. There is no standard of treatment established yet for CML involving the CNS however. Conventional therapy for CNS leukemia, includes intrathecal chemotherapy, high-dose systemic chemotherapy (cytarabine, methotrexate), and radiotherapy. Caution is usually employed in its use however as many patients experience significant toxicity, short-lived responses, and ultimately death resulting from refractory leukemia [26]. Currently tyrosine kinase inhibitor used for CML is Imatinib and though it is effective in controlling CML several studies have shown that the penetration of the drug and its metabolites into the CNS is poor [27].

Table 2. Cases of isolated CNS relapse in CML patients

Case	Year	Author/s	Age	Sex	Presentation	Treatment	Outcome
1	2015	Castillo, Mesina, Morillo (present case)	42yo	Male	Headache, visual loss and hearing loss	IT MTX, Cytarabine and Hydrocortisone Nilotinib	No return of blasts in CSF for a month
2	2015	Gomez J, Dueñas V	33 yo	Male	Headache, Nausea Confusion	Dasatanib 70 mg PO BID Triple Intrathecal chemotherapy	Alive, CCyRwithout signs of systemic and (CNS) relapse
3	2013	Park MJ, Park PW	54 yo	Male	Headache	Dasatinib, intrathecal methotrexate, & cranial irradiation therapy	Alive, Major CyR
4	2013	Nishimoto	22 yo	Male	Headache, Fever Impaired vision	Imatinib+IT+RT+allo-SCT	Alive
5	2012	Fuchs Raenhoffer, Schumm	64 yo	Female	Cognitive and Seizures and polyneuropathy	Triple IT therapy, Cytarabine, MTX, dexamethasone Dasatinib, Allo-PBSCT	Dead
6	2011	Radhika, Minakshi, Rajesh	15 yo	Female	Headache, vomiting and backache	Increased Imatinib to 600 mg/day, with intrathecal and cranial radiotherapy	Not specified
7	2011	Radhika, Minakshi, Rajesh	37 yo	Male	Chills, headache, vomiting and altered sensorium	Increased Imatinib to 600 mg/day, with intrathecal and cranial radiotherapy	Not specified
8	2010	Thomas	33 yo	Male	Back pain and multiple cranial nerve abnormality	IT + RT Dasatanib, Ara-C,Allo-PBSCT	Alive
9	2009	Jeon, Shin et al.	71yo	Male	Dysarthria and R sided weakness with leptomeningeal mass	Imatinib 400 mg/day	Expired
10	2009	Isobe et al.	61 yo	Male	Vomiting and visual disturbances	IT+Auto-PBSCT Imatinib	Alive
11	2009	Lee et al.	39 yo	Male	Headache and diplopia	IT Imatinib	Alive
12	2008	Barlow et al.	68 yo	Male	Headache and cerebellar dysfunction	IT+RT Imatinib	Alive
13	2007	Altintas	39 yo	Male	Headache, vomiting	IT+RT	Alive

	Et al					Imatinib	
14	Aichberger	2007	52 yo	Male	Headache and ataxia	IT+RT Imatinib	Alive
15	Kim et al.	2006	42 yo	Male	Headache and vertigo	IT+craniotomy Imatinib	Dead
16	Johnson et al.	2005	50 yo	Male	Headache, nausea and vomiting	IT+Allo-PBSCT Imatinib	Dead
17	Bujassoum et al.	2004	42 yo	Female	Headache	IT + Allo-PBSCT+RT Imatinib	Alive
18	Bornhauser et al.	2004	56 yo	Female	Ataxia and blurring of vision	IT + Allo-PBSCT+RT Imatinib	Dead
19	Rajappa et al.	2004	39 yo	Male	Headache and vomiting	IT+RT Imatinib	Alive
20	Rytting, Wierda	2004	48yo	Male	Headache, Night sweats and lymphadenopathy	IT therapy with alternating Cytarabine and MTX Craniospinal RT Imatinib	Remission HSCT
21	Meyer and Cuttner	1978	7yo	Male	Frontal headache, vertigo and diplopia	IT Cytosine arabinoside followed by splenectomy and chemoimmunotherapyMylern and methanol extracted residue of BCG	No blastic transformation 42 mos later

Furthermore Robert Ilaria of University of Texas Southwestern Medical Center, USA explains that it does not cross the brain barrier and hence is not effective for CML affecting the CNS. Table 2 shows above different approaches made by different institutions or groups. All of which used Intrathecal therapy with Cytarabine and Methotrexate in combination with Imatinib or Dasatinib. The group of Fuch's however used Dasatinib instead of Imatinib as that it has better penetration to the blood brain barrier and is associated with better survival [27].

4. CONCLUSION

In conclusion an isolated CNS relapse of CML is a rare case, patients on Imatinib with hematologic remission may still progress to blastic phase sometimes presenting as an isolated CNS relapse. CNS leptomeningeal leukemia is challenging to diagnose with a high percentage of the tests to come out negative, however if all other possible disease entities are excluded treatment should already be considered even with the absence of a concrete diagnostic test. Treatment includes Intrathecal therapy with Methotrexate and Cytarabine with Dexamethasone, in combination with a tyrosine kinase inhibitor, among of which Dasatinib as having evidence of blood brain barrier penetration and reduction of mortality. Constant communication with the patient is important especially when diagnosis and treatment is challenging since intrathecal chemotherapy would be frequent, a good rapport with the patient is key and helping them understand their condition better.

CONSENT

All authors declare that 'written informed consent was obtained from the nearest keen for publication of this case report and accompanying images.

ETHICAL APPROVAL

It is not applicable.

COMPETING INTERESTS

Authors have declared that no competing interests exist.

REFERENCES

1. Heike Pfeifer, Barbara Wassmann, Wolf-Karsten Hofmann Martina. Risk and prognosis of central nervous system leukemia in patients with philadelphia Chromosome-Positive acute leukemias treated with Imatinib Mesylate. Clin Cancer Research. 2003;9:4674–4681. Johann Wolfgang Goethe-Universita"t.

2. Wing Y Au, Priscilla B Caguioa, Charles Chuah, Szu Chun Hsu, Saengsuree Jootar, Dong-Wook Kim, Il-Young Kweon, William M O'Neil. Chronic myeloid leukemia in Asia. Int'l Journal of Hematology. 2008;89:14-23.

3. Shet AS, et al. Chronic myelogenous leukemia: Mechanisms underlying disease progression. Leukemia. 2002;16:1402-1411.

4. Richard Meyer, Janet Cuttner. Central nervous system involvement at presentation in the chronic phase of chronic myelogenous leukemia in childhood; 1978.

5. Jerald P Radich. The biology of CML blast crisis, ASH hematology education book; 2007.

6. Solh MM, Kantarjian H, O'Brien S, Giles F, Faderl S, Garcia-Manero G, Rios M, Shan J, Cortes J, Ravandi-Kashani F. Central nervous system (CNS) leukemia after Imatinib Mesylate therapy for chronic myelogenous leukemia (CML). Journal of Clinical Oncology, 2007 ASCO Annual Meeting Proceedings (Post-Meeting Edition). Vol 25, No 18S (June 20 Supplement). 2007;7042.

7. Specchia G, Palumbo G, Pastore D, Mininni D, Mestice A, Liso V. Extramedullary blast crisis in chronic myeloid leukemia. Leukemia Research. 1996;20(11-12):905–908.

8. Rytting ME, Wierda WG. Central nervous system relapse in two patients with chronic myelogenous leukemia in myeloid blastic phase on Imatinib Mesylate therapy. Leukemia & Lymphoma. 2004;45(8):1623–1626.

9. Jeong Shin Bae, et al. Extramedullary B lymphoblastic crisis of CML, presenting as a leptomeningeal tumor. Korean Journal of Pathology. 2005;43(5).

10. Fuchs M, Reinhöfer M, Ragoschke-Schumm A, Sayer HG, Böer K, Witte OW, et al. Isolated central nervous system relapse of chronic myeloid leukemia after allogenic hematopoietic stem cell transplantation. BMC Blood Disord. 2012;12:9.

11. Rajappa S, Uppin SG, Raghunadharao D, Rao IS, Surath A. Isolated central nervous system blast crisis in chronic myeloid leukemia. Hematol Oncol. 2004;22:179-81.

12. Bornhauser M, Jenke A, Freiberg-Richter J, Radke J, Schuler US, Mohr B, et al. CNS blast crisis of chronic myelogenous leukemia in a patient with a major cytogenetic response in bone marrow associated with low levels of imatinib mesylate and its N-desmethylated metabolite in cerebral spinal fluid. Ann Hematol. 2004;83:401-2.

13. Bujassoum S, Rifkind J, Lipton JH. Isolated central nervous system relapse in lymphoid blast crisis chronic myeloid leukemia and acute lymphoblastic leukemia in patients on imatinib therapy. Leuk Lymphoma. 2004;45:401-3.

14. Johnson NA, Fetni R, Caplan SN. Isolated central nervous system relapse in patients with chronic myeloid leukemia on imatinib mesylate. Leuk Lymphoma. 2005;46:629-30.

15. Aichberger KJ, Herndlhofer S, Agis H, Sperr WR, Esterbauer H, Rabitsch W, et al. Liposomal cytarabine for treatment of myeloid central nervous system relapse in chronic myeloid leukaemia occurring during imatinib therapy. Eur J Clin Invest. 2007;37:808-13.

16. Barlow A, Robertson M, Doig A, Stewart W, Drummond MW. Isolated central nervous system lymphoid blast crisis in chronic myeloid leukaemia in major molecular remission. Br J Haematol. 2008;142:327.

17. Altintas A, Cil T, Kilinc I, Kaplan MA, Ayyildiz O. Central nervous system blastic crisis in chronic myeloid leukemia on imatinib mesylate therapy: A case report. J Neurooncol. 2007;84:103-5.

18. Isobe Y, Sugimoto K, Masuda A, Hamano Y, Oshimi K. Central nervous system is a sanctuary site for chronic myelogenous leukaemia treated with imatinib mesylate. Intern Med J. 2009;39:408-11.

19. Thomas A, Stein CK, Gentile TC, Shah CM. Isolated CNS relapse of CML after bone marrow transplantation. Leuk Res. 2010;34:e113-4.

20. Nishimoto M, Nakamae H, Koh KR, Kosaka S, Matsumoto K, Morita K, et al. Dasatinib maintenance therapy after allogeneic hematopoietic stem cell transplantation for an isolated central nervous system blast crisis in chronic myelogenous leukemia. Acta Haematologica. 2013;130:111-4.

21. Kim HJ, Jung CW, Kim K, Ahn JS, Kim WS, Park K, et al. Isolated blast crisis in CNS in a patient with chronic myelogenous leukemia maintaining major cytogenetic response after imatinib. J Clin Oncol. 2006;24:4028-9.

22. Lee KW, Song MK, Seol YM, Choi YJ, Shin HJ, Chung JS, et al. Isolated central nervous system blast crisis in chronic myeloid leukemia. Korean J Med. 2009;77(S2):S441-4.

23. Thomas Louis. Pathology of Leukemia in the Brain and Meninges: Postmortem studies of patients with acute leukemia and of mice given inoculations of L1210 leukemia. Cancer Res. 1965;25:1555-1571

24. Balm M, Hammack J. Leptomeningeal carcinomatosis. Presenting features and prognostic factors. Arch Neurol. 1996;53:626–632.

25. Lisa M Deangelis. Leukemia and lymphoma metastases. Cancer Medicine 6th Ed. Chap 15. 2002;362-374.

26. Kimmo Porkka, Perttu Koskenvesa, TuijaLunda´n. Dasatinib crosses the blood-brain barrier and is an efficient therapy for nervous system Philadelphia chromosome-positive leukemia. Blood Journal. 2008;112(4):1005-1011.

27. Narayan Radhika, Mishra Minakshi, Mohanty Rajesh, Baisakh R. Manas, Mishra Deepak Kumar. Central nervous system blast crisis in chronic myeloid leukemia on imatinib mesylate therapy: Report of two cases. Indian J Hematology Blood Transfusion. 2011;27(1):51–54.

10

Anti-retroviral Treatment Related Haematological Disorders among HIV- Infected Children Attending HIV Clinic at Yekatit 12 Hospital, Addis Ababa, Ethiopia

Mestewat Debasu[1], M. K. C. Menon[2*], Yididya Belayneh[2], Workeabeba Abebe[3], Degu Jerene[4] and Daniel Seifu[2]

[1]Department of Biochemistry, St. Paul's Hospital Millennium Medical College, P.O.Box 1271, Addis Ababa, Ethiopia.
[2]Department of Medical Biochemistry, School of Medicine, Faculty of Health Sciences, Addis Ababa University, P.O.Box 9086, Addis Ababa, Ethiopia.
[3]Department of Pediatrics and Child Health, School of Medicine, Faculty of Health Sciences, Addis Ababa University, P.O.Box 1176, Addis Ababa, Ethiopia.
[4]Department of Preventive Medicine, School of Medicine, Faculty of Health Sciences, Addis Ababa University, P.O.Box 1176, Addis Ababa, Ethiopia.

Authors' contributions

This work was carried out in collaboration between all authors. Authors MD, MKCM, YB, WA, DJ and DS designed the study, wrote the protocol, the first and subsequent drafts of the manuscript. Author MD performed the analytical and experimental process and author DS provided the laboratory facilities and administrative support. All authors read and approved the final manuscript

Editor(s):
(1) Ricardo Forastiero, Department of Hematology, Favaloro University, Argentina.
Reviewers:
(1) Fasakin Kolawole, Federal Teaching Hospital, Nigeria.
(2) Obiako Reginald, Ahmadu Bello University, Nigeria.

ABSTRACT

Background: The Management of drug toxicities is increasingly becoming a crucial component of human immunodeficiency virus infection and improvement of antiretroviral therapy in developing countries like Ethiopia. The severity of hematological abnormalities in children who are taking ART is not known well in Ethiopian Hospitals.

Corresponding author: E-mail: menakathmenon@gmail.com

Objective: The study was undertaken to determine the severity of HAART related hematological disorders in HIV positive children who were on HAART at Yekatit 12 Hospital, Addis Ababa, Ethiopia.

Methods: A cross sectional study was conducted from May 2012 to February 2013 among children who had been on HAART for maximum of twelve months. Data collection using questionnaires and measurement of complete blood count and CD4 + T cell counts were made by using standard methodology. The results were tested using appropriate statistical methods (mean, Standard Deviation, Odd Ratio, p-value and F test value).

Results: A total of 106 patients (<18 years) were enrolled in the study and had a mean age of 6.5±3.4 years, a median age of 7 years and female to male ratio of 1.04:1. The prevalence of anemia was 18.9%, 12.3% and 10.4% at baseline, at six months, and at twelve months post-treatment, respectively. Their mean hemoglobin level increased by 1.0 gm/dl at six months and by 1.7 gm/dl at twelve months of follow up with statistically significant values (p <0.001), and F test value presented 15.87. Patients who were put on AZT based regimen were more likely to develop anemia than those on D4T-based regimen, (OR=4.5, p-value <0.05). The prevalence of thrombocytopenia at baseline was 8.5%, but it was lowered for both at six and twelve months by 5.7%. The thrombocyte count of AZT based regimen showed statistically significant association (p-<0.05) and F test value as 2.98. The prevalence of neutropenia at baseline and at six months was similar with the value of 2.8% while at twelve months it was higher at 5.7%.

Conclusion: Anemia, neutropenia and thrombocytopenia were the hematological abnormalities among HIV infected Ethiopian children taking HAART. Anemia was the most common abnormality, but significantly lesser than in many other hospitals in Ethiopia and among those who were on AZT based regimen. It is recommended that even in limited laboratory monitoring, HAART can be safely used and health professionals may consider other risk factors associated with the development of cytopenia before selection of second line of HAART drug regimen.

Keywords: HAART; anemia; neutropenia; thrombocytopenia; Ethiopian children.

1. INTRODUCTION

In human immunodeficiency virus (HIV) infected individuals hematological abnormalities are common and they increase the risk of morbidity and mortality. In both antiretroviral treated and untreated HIV-individuals, cytopenia is independently associated with an increased risk of disease progression and death. Although highly active anti-retroviral therapy (HAART) is known to profoundly suppress viral replication, by increasing cluster of differentiation 4 (CD4) cell count and delays disease progression; patients on HAART commonly suffer from side effects of the drug. Each antiretroviral drug is associated with specific adverse effects. Among the antiretroviral drugs, Zidovudine (ZDV) formerly Azido thymidine (AZT) remains to be the most widely used drug resulting in myelosuppression [1]. Several studies in developed countries have shown that ZDV alone and ZDV based HAART regimen is associated with significant reduction of hemoglobin (Hgb) level and neutrophil number. Although 25.8 million people are living with HIV/AIDS in Sub Saharan Africa, only few studies tried to assess the safety and efficacy of HAART. In one multicenter study conducted in Uganda, Kenya and Zambia 12% of patients on ZDV based HAART regimen switched drugs because of drug related severe anemia or GI toxicity [1,2].

Globally, there were 3.4 million children living with HIV in 2010, which accounts 390,000 new infections among children, and 250,000 AIDS deaths. By the end of 2008, of the 33.4 million people living with HIV/AIDS worldwide, 15.7 million were women and 2.1 million were children under 15 years of age. In 2009, there were approximately 16.6 million AIDS orphans (children who have lost one or both parents to HIV), most of whom live in sub-Saharan Africa (89%). Additionally, an estimated 2.5 million children were living with HIV at the end of 2009 with 92% in sub-Saharan Africa [3].

In HIV infected infants and children before initiation of ART, many factors need to be considered, including potency of the ART, resistance testing and potential for future sequencing, palatability, available formulations and dosing recommendations, disclosure and adherence issues, and potential drug-drug interactions [4].

Despite the fact, most new HIV infection among children is through vertical transmission (mother to child transmission) (MTCT). HIV positive women pass the virus to the baby during pregnancy, during delivery or by breast feeding. It is estimated that over 90% of children were infected with HIV in utero, during the delivery or breast feeding. Intrapartum transmissions are mediated by direct contact of infant mucosa with HIV-laden maternal blood, amniotic fluid, and cervical/vaginal secretions [5-6]. In Ethiopia, about 1.1 million people are living with HIV, out of which the children constituted about 72000, which is a worrying situation for the Health authorities [7], since most of the infection were vertically transmitted. The roll-out of antiretroviral therapy in Ethiopia has benefited the children, but the spread of the disease vertically through mother-to child transmission, and its control is the major priority in this population.

There are fewer data on ART toxicity in children than in adults, and the full spectrum of ART toxicities observed in adults has also been reported in children. However, some toxicity is less common in children than in adults. For example, hepatotoxicity is rare in children, while others are more commonly reported in children than adult, such as rash or loss of bone density. The most common toxicities include: - Hematological abnormality, mitochondrial dysfunction, lipodystrophy, metabolic abnor-malities, allergic reactions and iron deficiency due to parasitic intestinal infections [8-12].

Anemia was defined as Hgb concentration less than or equal to 10gm/dl for all children less than 18 years and further severity was classified into grades as follows: Hgb level of 8.5–10 gm/dl as Grade 1; 7.5 - <8.5 gm/dl as Grade 2; 6.5 - <7.5 gm/dl as Grade 3; and < 6.5 gm/dl as Grade 4. Grade 3 and 4 are further labelled as severe life threatening anemia [8,1].

The incidence of first severe anemia was assessed among HIV uninfected infants in MTCT prevention trials in Botswana. Severe anemia rates were compared between three groups. The first group was infants exposed to maternal HAART in utero and during breast feeding (BF) and one month of postnatal AZT (HAART-BF). The second group was infants exposed to maternal AZT alone for short term in utero, six months of postnatal AZT, and breastfeeding (AZT-BF) and the third group were infants exposed to maternal short-term AZT alone in utero, one month of postnatal AZT, and formula-feeding (AZT-FF). A total of 1719 infants 691 HAART-BF, 503 AZT-BF, and 525 AZT-FF were analysed Severe anemia was detected in 118 infants (7.4%). By six months, 12.5% of HAART-

BF infants experienced severe anemia, compared with 5.3% of AZT-BF and 2.5% of AZT-FF infants, from this figure, the result obtained for AZT-FF infants were surprisingly low, since AZT has one of the most notorious side effects expressed as anemia. It is important to note that there was no comparison with a group whose mothers were not given any ART during pregnancy [13]. One randomized comparative trial study done to assess the safety and efficacy of AZT and 2',3'-didehydro-2',3'-dideoxythymidine (D4T) or Stavudine in symptomatic HIV infected children showed a prevalence of anemia to be 5% among the AZT group and may occur within 4–6 weeks whereas 2% among the D4T group [14,1]. In a study conducted at Burkina Faso, there was reduction in the frequency of mother-child transmission when mothers received ART. However, mothers CD4+ count cannot be considered as a parameter for setting a ART regimen [5].

In Ethiopia, as a result of rapid expansion of service facilities and improved awareness, the number of patients on ART rose sharply over the years. In 2003, Ethiopia lunched the fee- based ART and free ART in 2005, delivered as part of the comprehensive HIV/AIDS care [15,16]. In 2007, ART was started in many facilities across the country. AZT based HAART is one of the first line regimens in the guideline [1,17,18]. The impact of HAART on the hematological profile of Ethiopian HIV/AIDS patients and children is currently under investigation in many hospitals across Ethiopia. This research was undertaken to fill the gap in the literature about the hematological abnormalities and the associated risk factors and to evaluate it in the HIV infected Ethiopian children admitted to a urbanized hospital.

2. MATERIALS AND METHODS

2.1 Study Design

Cross sectional study design was used to assess the hematological profile among HIV/AIDS infected children who were on HAART at Yekatit 12 Hospital ART clinic, Addis Ababa. Study was conducted from March 2012 to February 2013 in Addis Ababa, ART unit of Yekatit 12 Hospital. This institution is selected based on the availability of patients from all parts of the country as it is referral and urban general specialized teaching hospital in Ethiopia as well as the ease of access and sufficient availability of the data in this unit. As of February 2013, a total of 409 HIV infected children were on ART at Yekatit 12 Hospital. The source population for this study, was HIV positive children age less than 18 years and using ART, and attending follow up at Yekatit 12 Hospital had been considered.

The study population consisted of a total of 409 HIV infected children less than 18 years old who had started HAART (defined as taking two or more antiretroviral drugs for 12 months,), by World Health Organization (WHO) clinical and immunological criteria and who had complete blood count (CBC), CD4 count and thrombocyte counts taken at the time of HAART initiation, and also six and twelve months after initiation of the treatment.

The hospitals in Addis Ababa, Ethiopia provides to HIV- infected children both first line and second line drug regimens. An Etiologic classification on anemia is based on the various conditions that can result from any of the physiologic changes and helps determine direction for planning care [19,20]. First line regimens that children were taking included 4a = d4T/3Tc/NVP (Stavudine, Lamivudine, Nevirapine), 4b = d4T/3Tc/EFV (Stavudine, Lamivudine, Efavirenz), 4c = AZT/3Tc/NVP (Zidovudine, Lamivudine, Nevirapine), and 4d = AZT/3Tc/EFV (Zidovudine, Lamivudine, Efavirenz).

Some children in city hospitals in Addis Ababa, were also on the following second line regimens: ABC/ ddi/LPv/r (Abacavir, Didanosine, retonavir enhanced Lopinavir), AZT/3Tc/LPv/r (Zidovudine, Lamivudine, retonavir enhanced Lopinavir) and D4T/3TC/LPv/r (Stavudine, Lamivudine, retonavir enhanced Lopinavir) [7].

2.2 Study Subjects

All HIV positive children age less than 18 years and using ART for 12 months and attending follow up during the study period, who meet the inclusion criteria and who gave their informed consent and assent.

2.3 Sample Size Determination and Sampling Techniques

2.3.1 Sample size

The required sample size for this study is calculated based on the prevalence rate of 16.19% reported in previous study [21] and the 95% confidence interval and 5% marginal error,

the sample size (n) is determined using the following statistical formula:

$$ n = \frac{Z^2 . P (1 - P)}{d^2} $$

$$ n = \frac{1.96^2 \times 0.1619 (1 - 0.1619)}{0.0025} = 106 $$

d = margin of error between the sample and the population
n = sample size
Z = 95% confident interval
P = prevalence rate of hematological disorders based on the previous study
N = 409

2.3.2 Eligibility criteria

2.3.2.1 Inclusion criteria

(1) All HIV positive Children less than 18 years old at the time of HAART initiation.
(2) Who had started ART and had follow up in Yekatit 12 Hospital, Addis Ababa
(3) Baseline (Pre-HAART), six and twelve months follow up data with complete hematological values (CBC, CD4 cells count and thrombocyte count)
(4) Who were not diagnosed as having hematological diseases of any identified cause (including hemolytic anemia, thrombocytopenia and haemoglobino-pathy) before ART initiation.
(5) Those who volunteered to participate in the study (parents or care givers were consulted, and informed consent obtained)

2.3.2.2 Exclusion criteria

(1) HIV positive children, less than 18 years old who were severely sick due to other medical conditions
(2) Those children on treatment for anemia
(3) Those using medications for either anemia, neutropenia or thrombocytopenia. Those who have any hematological abnormality before initiation of ARTs
(4) Those who were on medication (antibiotics, vitamin supplements and tuberculosis treatment) at the time of sampling.

2.4 Sampling Techniques

Non-probability sampling technique was used. HIV positive children who had enrolled at Yekatit

12 Hospital ART unit from May 2012 to February 2013 and those HIV positive children who were meeting the inclusion criteria during the study period were included in the study.

2.5 Data Collection Procedure

2.5.1 Questionnaires

A structured questionnaire was used for data collection. The questionnaire was developed in English and translated into Amharic language. The questionnaire had three parts, the first part for collecting data about socio-demographic characteristics of the study subjects, the second part for collecting data concerning baseline characteristics of the individuals before initiation of HAART mainly clinical, laboratory and immunological characteristics. The third part for collecting data related to HAART treatment and the change in baseline parameters (adverse effect) after taking HAART. The respondents were parents or immediate care givers of the study children.

2.5.2 Anthropometric measurements

The assessment of growth by objective anthropometric methods such as weight and height in relation to their ages, and weight in relation to height is crucial in child care to assess the nutritional status and for the identification of growth failure. Thus, anthropometric measurement helps to diagnose under nutrition (underweight, stunted and wasting), overweight and obesity and, other growth related conditions by referring WHO growth reference charts [22,10]. Therefore anthropometric measurements were carried out according to the WHO recommendations. Nurses and supportive care givers helped with the collection of data.

2.6 Blood Specimen Examination for Hematological Assay and Immunological Assay

2.6.1 Sample collection and preparation

A volume of 5ml of venous blood was collected from each patient. The blood, 2ml and 3ml was then dispensed into two vacutainer ethylene diamine tetra acetic acid (K_2 EDTA) tubes, respectively. The 2 ml sample was used for immunological analysis (CD4 estimation) and 3ml sample was used for CBC analysis.

2.6.2 Hematological assay

2.6.2.1 Complete blood count

Complete hematological parameters white blood cell (WBC) - Differential, WBC, red blood cell (RBC) and platelet (PLT) were performed using Abbott Hematology Analyzer CELL-DYN 1800 (Abbott, USA). The CELL-DYN 1800 System is a bench-top analyzer consisting of the main analyzer with data module, display station with external printer [23].

2.6.3 Immunological assay

CD4 counts in % were assayed by BD FACS COUNT system analyzer, using % software (Becton Dickenson and Company, California, USA). Standard procedures were used for absolute CD4 T cell count [24,25].

N.B Measurements that were used for data collection procedures such as the anthropometric measurement and the hematological measurements that were done, are part of routine procedure for all patients those attending ART unit in Yekatit 12 Hospital.

2.7 Study Variables

2.7.1 Dependent variable: Status of hematologic disorders

Independent variable: It includes age, sex, nutritional status, CD4 count, opportunistic infection and WHO Clinical stage.

2.8 Ethical Approval

Ethical clearance was obtained from Research and Ethics Review Committee of the Department of Medical Biochemistry, School of Medicine, College of Health Sciences, Addis Ababa, University, Ethiopia with a protocol number of SOM/BCHM/010/2012. Detailed explanations were given about the objectives, risks, and benefits of the study to the study subjects, and parents/caregivers. Strict confidentiality of responses were maintained during the study. Data were collected after obtaining informed consent from the parent/ caregiver, and assent from the children aged 12-18 years.

2.9 Data Analysis

The data was analyzed using SPSS (16th version) and expressed at 95% confidence interval and the p-value were considered significant and very significant at p <0.05 and p ≤0.001, respectively. Then data computed using appropriate statistical methods (mean, standard deviation, p-value, odd ratio, F test statistic value and one-way repeated measures ANOVA) and the results are presented using tables and figures.

3. RESULTS

3.1 Socio-demographic Characteristics, Clinical Staging and Drug Regimen

Of the 409 HIV infected children, 106 who were on HAART for maximum of 12 months were included in the study. Their ages ranged from 3 months to 16 years with a mean for age of 6.5±3.4 years and a median age of 7 years. Majority of age groups were between 5 years to 15 years accounting 61.3%, whereas only 0.9% patient fell in the age group between 14 years to 18 years. Out of the 106 patients, 50.9% were females and 49.1% were males giving a female to male ratio of 1.04:1. The result of children's parent status indicated that in 39.6% both parents were alive and in 22.6% both parents were lost. The majority of educational status of caregivers' at the time of the study was grade 12 and above, which accounts 40.6%, whereas grade 7-12, 25.5% and illiterate, 18.9%. 34.0% of the caregivers were unemployed and 25.5% earned monthly income below ≤ 420 Birr. Among the 106, 54.7% children did not know their HIV status.

According to the duration and type of HAART regimen, all study subjects took treatment for the duration of ≥1 year. The most widely used ART regimen in this study was 4a (d4T-3TC-NVP) 45.3% followed by 4c (AZT-3TC-NVP), 25.5%.Based on WHO clinical staging, majority of the study participants were in stage III 59.4%, stage II was seen in 21.7%, stage IV was seen in 14.2% and stage I was seen, in only 4.7% of the study participants. According WHO clinical classification, stage III and stage IV are considered advanced clinical stages (Table 1).

3.2 Clinical and Immunological Characteristics

As shown in Table 2, 66% of the study children at baseline had severe immune suppression (CD4 percentage below 15%) and only 0.9% participant's had CD4 percentage above 25%. After six months of HAART initiation, 41%

participants had CD4 percentage above 25% while 16% participants were above 25%. The finding was statistically significant as p - value < 0.001 indicated. The value of underweight and stunted children before the initiation of HAART was 27.4% and 36.8%, respectively. However after initiation of HAART, these figures were decreased significantly to 19.8% and 19.8% for both underweight children and stunted children, respectively. The decrements of stunted children

Table 1. Baseline Socio-demographic characteristics, WHO clinical staging and drug regimen of HIV infected children who started HAART at Yekatit 12 Hospital

Demography	N(%), (n = 106)
Sex	
Male	52 (49.1)
Female	54 (50.9)
Age in years	
< 18 months	7 (6.6)
18 – 60 months	33 (31.1)
5 -14 years	65 (61.3)
14 – 18 years	1 (.9)
Parent status	
Both alive	42(39.6)
Father alive	24(22.6)
Mother alive	16(15.1)
Neither alive	24(22.6)
Family income	
≤ 420	27(25.5)
421 - 600	14(13.2)
600⁺	65(61.3)
Educational status of caregivers	
Illiterate	20(18.9)
1 - 6	16(15.1)
7 - 12	27(25.5)
12⁺	43(40.6)
Employment status of care givers	
Unemployed	36(34.0)
Employed	70(66.0)
Child Knows HIV status	
Yes	48(45.3)
No	58(54.7)
*Type of ART	
4a	48(45.3)
4b	16(15.1)
4c	27(25.5)
4d	15(14.2)
WHO Clinical stages	
Stage I	5 (4.7)
Stage II	23(21.7)
Stage III	63(59.4)
Stage IV	15(14.2)

*4a=d4T-3TC-NVP, 4b= d4T-3TC-EFV, 4c= AZT-3TC-NVP, 4d= AZT-3TC-EFV

after HAART were statistically significant (p-value <0.001) but the value of underweight did not significant change. At baseline majority of children were in >70 of weight for height (wasting), which accounts 71.7%, and only 6.6% was in ≥ 90. At six months of HAART initiation, the value of >70 weight for height decreased to 40.6% and the value of ≥ 90 was increased to 17%. The statistic showed significant increments of weight for height, (p-value <0.001). At baseline, the majority of children, 67.9%, had history of Opportunistic Infections (OI), the commonest being recurrent pneumonia seen in 16.1%, and oral thrash was seen in 9.4%, while after the initiation of HAART, majority of children 77.4% did not have history of OI while 22.6% had OI (Table 2).

3.3 Hematological Values before and after Initiation of HAART

As shown in Table 3, the mean Hgb concentration was increased and found to be 12.2 gm/dl on base line and 13.3 gm/dl after six months of HAART. The mean Hgb concentration

based on type of HAART regimen was increased in both AZT and D4T based regimen as compared to baseline, it accounts for 12.7±2.6 and13.6±2.5 respectively after treatment with HAART. The mean CD4 count in % showed increment, 13.2±5.2 at baseline and 24.1±7.8 at six months of HAART. Mean corpuscular volume (MCV), mean cell hemoglobin volume (MCH), mean cell hemoglobin concentration (MCHC) and thrombocyte count also showed increment. Whereas ANC showed some decrement in their mean values at six month, that was 3.2±1.7 but at base line it was 4.0±3.7. The increments of Hgb, MCV, MCH, MCHC and CD4 count in % showed statistically significant with p-value < 0.001 whereas thrombocyte count and ANC showed statistically significant association (p-value <0.05) (Table 3).

3.4 Patterns and Severity of Hematological Abnormalities

In the study subjects hematological abnormalities were observed both before and after treatment with HAART (Fig. 1). The study subject whose

Table 2. Clinical, immunological characteristics and anthropometric measurements of HIV infected children at baseline and after six months with HAART

Variable	Before (n=106) N (%)	After six month (n=106) N (%)	P- value
CD4 lymphocyte %			
Less than 15 %	70 (66.0)	17 (16.0)	0.000
15-24 %	35 (33.0)	45 (42.5)	
Greater than 25 %	1 (0.9)	44 (41.5)	
Weight for age			
< 5th percentile	29 (27.4)	21(19.8)	0.088
> or = 5th percentile	77 (72.6)	85(82.2)	
Height for age			
< 5th percentile	39 (36.8)	21 (19.8)	0.001
>or = 5th percentile	67 (63.2)	85(80.2)	
Weight for Ht			
<70	76 (71.7)	43(40.6)	0.000
70-79	16 (15.1)	23(21.7)	
80-89	7 (6.6)	22(20.8)	
>or= 90	7 (6.6)	18(17)	
Opportunistic Infections			
Chronic GE	3(2.8)	3(2.8)	0.298
Recurrent Pneumonia	27(25.5)	9(8.5)	
*PCP	5(4.7)	1(0.9)	
PCP + pneumonia	6(5.7)	1(0.9)	
Oral thrush	10(9.4)	2(1.9)	
*Chronic GE+ Oral thrush	10(9.4)	1(0.9)	
*Others	11(10.4)	7(6.6)	
No OI	34(32.1)	82(77.4)	

*__GE__ = Gastro enteritis,   *__PCP__ = Pneumocystis carinii pneumonia pneumonia*
__others__= Unexplained persistent fever, Herpes zoster, fungal nail infection, Unexplained persistent parotid enlargement, and Recurrent or chronic upper respiratory tract infections (otitis media, sinusitis, tonsillitis)

Table 3. Mean hematological values and mean hemoglobin values between drug regimens and mean CD4% on HIV infected children before and after six months with HAART

Variables	Hematological values		
	Before HAART Mean ±SD (n=106)	After HAART (six months) Mean± SD (n=106)	p-value
Hemoglobin (Hgb)	12.2±2.2	13.3±2.5	0.000
AZT based	12.5±2.0	12.7±2.6	
D4T based	12±2.3	13.6±2.5	
MCV	80.5±13.5	93±12.5	0.000
MCH	27±5.3	31.7±5.3	0.000
MCHC	33.2±3.7	33.9±2.4	0.000
WBC X 10^3	6.8±3.9	6.6±2.7	0.436
TLC X 10^3	2.6±1.6	2.7±1.4	0.491
ANC X 10^3	4.0±3.7	3.2±1.7	0.034
Thrombocyte X 10^3	317±153	356±136	0.026
CD4 %	13.2±5.2	24.1±7.8	0.000

Hgb concentration > 10 mg/dl had increased their number after taking six months and twelve months of taking ART it accounted 87.7% and 89.6% respectively compared to the number of subjects before HAART 81.1%. Anemia (Hgb ≤10 gm/dl) was found in 18.9% of subjects before and 12.3% at six and 10.4% at twelve months of the subjects after initiation of HAART. Among the anemic cases, the majorities were grade I, 10.4% were at baseline, 6.6% at six

months and 7.5% at twelve months of HAART. This study showed that 2.8%, 0.9 and 1.9% had severe life threatening anemia before, at six and twelve months after initiation of HAART, respectively. Total anemic patients at baseline, among them the number of patients at six months 6.6% and at twelve months 8.5% of post HAART were improved from anemia. The result showed the number of anemic cases decreased.

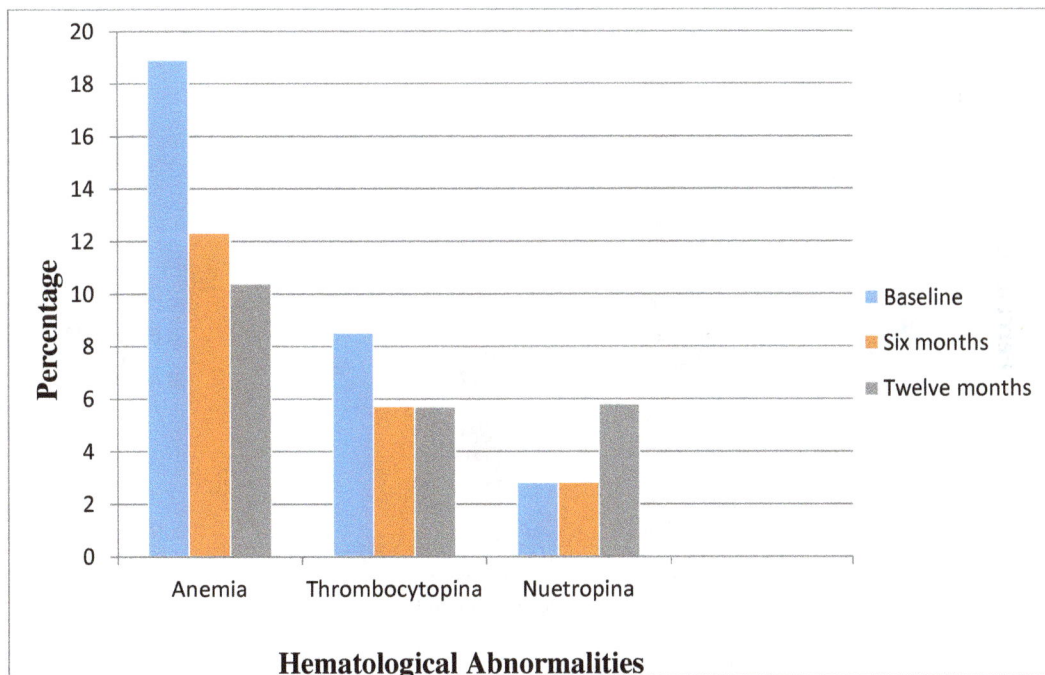

Fig. 1. Comparison of the prevalence of Hematological abnormalities (Anemia, Thrombocytopenia and Neutropenia) and its percentage at baseline, at six months and at twelve months of HAART

Neutropenia was seen in 2.8% before and after six month of HAART but 5.7% was seen at twelve months (Fig. 1). Thrombocytosis was seen for 17%, 22.6% and 19.8% at baseline, at six and twelve months respectively as well as thrombocytopenia was seen in 8.5% at baseline and twelve months where as 5.7% after six month of initiation of HAART.

The type of anemia also assessed in this study. Thus among the total number of cases, before HAART normocytic normochromic anemia was present in 45.3%, whereas after HAART it was increased to 56.6%. It was also found that before HAART, microcytic hypochromic and macrocytic normochromic anemia were present in 46.2% and 7.5%, respectively. After six months of HAART, microcytic hypochromic anemia reduced to 12.3% while macrocytic normochromic anemia was raised to present in 30.2% as shown in Fig. 2.

The result on Table 4 revealed that the study subjects were observed having mean Hgb level, neutrophil and thrombocyte count at baseline, six and twelve months of treatment with HAART. The mean Hgb level increased statistically as very significant (p <0.001) and thrombocyte

count increased statistically significant (p < 0.05), whereas neutrophil count showed decrement. At time of HAART initiation, the mean and standard deviation of Hgb concentration, neutrophil and thrombocyte count were 12.2±2.2, 13.2±2.6 and 13.7±2.2 respectively. After HAART, Hgb concentration, neutrophil and thrombocyte count were 13.2±2.6, 3.23±1712.5 and 356.3±136.4 and 13.7±2.2, 3.53±2091.7 and 340.3±149.4. Their mean Hgb level showed marked increase by 1.0 gm/dl at six month and by 1.7 gm/dl at twelve month. The observed difference is statistically very significant (p <0.001) using one-way repeated measures ANOVA, F test Statistic value presented with 15.87,where as the thrombocyte count revealed statistically significant values (p <0.05) and F test value was 2.98 after six and twelve month of HAART taking.

3.5 The Probability of Anemia in HIV Infected Children after Six Months of HAART

After controlling confounding effects, the probability of anemia after six months of HAART, multivariate logistic regression (Table 5) demonstrated that, 38 participant who were age

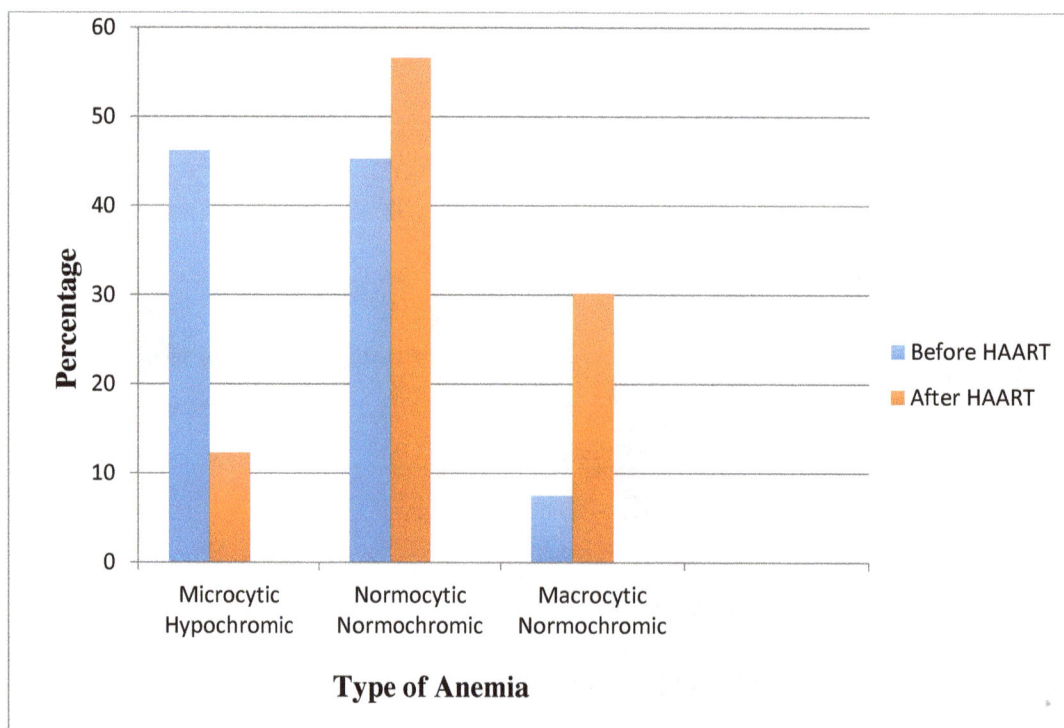

Fig. 2. Summary of type of Anemia (Microcytic Hypochromic, Normocytic Normochromic and Macrocytic Normochromic) and its Percentage of the study subjects before HAART and after HAART

Table 4. Comparison of hematological parameters (Hemoglobin, Neutrophil count and thrombocyte count) between baselines, after six months and after twelvemonths of HAART

Variable	Baseline (n=106) Mean ±SD	After six months (n=106) Mean ±SD	After twelve months (n=106) Mean ±SD	F test statistic value and P - value
Hemoglobin	12.2 ±2.2	13.2±2.6	13.7±2.2	F = 15.87, P = 0.000
Neutrophil Count	3.95±3694.5	3.23±1712.5	3.53±2091.7	F = 2.65, p = 0.09
Thrombocyte count	316.8±153.3	356.3±136.4	340.3±149.4	F= 2.89, p = 0.05

Table 5. Odd Ratio from logistic regression model predicting the probability of anemia in HIV infected children after six months of HAART

Variables	Anemic	Normal	Crude OR (95% CI)	Adjusted OR (95% CI)
Age				
≤ 5 years	7	31	1.88 (0.60-5.82)	3.1 (0.84-11.5)
>5 years	7	61		
Sex				
Female	6	48	0.69 (0.22-2.14)	0.83 (0.25-2.75)
Male	8	44		
Wt for age				
<5 percentile	4	17	1.77 (0.49-6.31)	2.37 (0.41-13.76)
≥ 5percentile	10	75		
Ht for age				
<5 percentile	4	17	1.77 (0.49-6.31)	1.10 (0.19-6.28)
≥ 5 percentile	10	75		
OI				
absent	12	70	1.89 (0.39-9.08)	2.03 (0.38-10.82)
present	2	22		
CD4 % after HAART Rx				
< 25%	9	53	1.33 (0.41-4.26)	3.09 (0.83-11.49)
≥ 25%	5	39		
HAART regimen Based				
AZT	9	33	3.22 (0.99-10.40)	4.54 (1.18-17.43)
D4T	5	59		

below five years, 7 were anemic (OR 3.1,95% CI (0.84-11.5), 52 male participant 8 were anemic (OR 0.83, 95% CI (0.25-2.75) and 21 study participant who were underweight among them 4 were anemic (OR 2.4, 95% CI (0.41-13.76) were independent risk factors to developed anemia. Additionally out of 21 stunted children, 4 were anemic (OR 1.1,95% CI (0.19-6.28), 62 study participant whose CD4 count < 25% among them 9 participant were anemic (OR 3.09, 95% CI (0.83-11.49) and 24 had history of OI among them 2 were anemic (OR 2.03, 95% CI (0.38-10.82) were independent risk factors to developed anemia compared to their each counter parts even if lack of association(with statistical significant) between independent risk factors. This study revealed, 42 participant who were AZT based regimen among them 9 were anemic with statistically significant association (p-value <0.05) compared to D4T based regimen (Table 5).

4. DISCUSSION

Both in infants and children, the use of antiretroviral therapy has been used safely and effectively. Younger children frequently metabolize drugs faster than adults, as food intake varies more in children and may have a greater impact on drug absorption. Growing children need frequent dose adjustments, and altered pharmacokinetic parameters need to be considered when using antiretroviral drugs safely and effectively. Therefore, in children drug dosage recommendations are meant to achieve a targeted drug exposure, usually similar to what is observed in adult patients [4,10].

In Ethiopia, there is lack of baseline data on HIV or HIV treatment related hematological abnormalities in children, in various hospitals. Therefore, the findings of this study in Yekatit 12 Hospital, Addis Ababa, Ethiopia, is an attempt to partially fill this gap. However, the small number of patients in the present study population limits the generalizability of the results.

The main results of this study were that of the 106 HIV infected children developed hematological abnormalities at baseline, at six months and at twelve months of HAART. All study subjects were under first line of antiretroviral therapy. The hematological abnormalities include anemia, thrombocytopenia and neutropenia (Fig. 1). Among these, anemia was the most common observed abnormality in both before-HAART and after-HAART treated children. This is in accordance with studies done in Ethiopia [1,12,26], They described that hematological abnormalities were common problems among the children taking HAART. Another study done elsewhere, macrocytosis, anemia and thrombocytopenia were the commonest hematological adverse events associated with Zidovudine [27]. It is clear that HIV is accompanied by thromboembolic diseases. Supportive evidence from various laboratories indicate that, HIV is cytotonic disregulating β lymphocytes and altered release of cytokines which suppress growth of bone marrow progenitors leading to anemia [28]. Since HAART is widely available in Ethiopia, a crucial adjustment to therapy of haematological complications and even cessation of the drug regimen can be a suggestion to the medical professionals.

4.1 Prevalence of Anemia in HIV Infected Children before HAART and after HAART Initiation

In this study, anemia is the most commonly encountered hematologic abnormality in HIV patients before ART, which is in accordance with a study reported [29].This study, showed similar result in which an overall prevalence of anemia before ART initiation was 18.9%, this means that before ART initiation anemia was observed due to HIV infection and similar results, 18.9% were reported in Uganda [30]. It has been reported that 22.2% prevalence in a urban hospital in Addis Ababa and said to be much lower than the other studies done elsewhere in Ethiopia. Possibly, low prevalence of intestinal parasites in urban children has been attributed as a causative factor in lower percentage of anemic situation in this report. In a separate study at Bahir Dar at Felege Hiwot referal Hospital involving 506 HIV infected children, reported prevalence rate of anemia at baseline was 19.8% [16]. The work reported that 24.2% of the sample population was anemic at registration, but in sharp contrast with the 80% obtained in Port-Harcourt, Nigeria, amongst untreated HIV patients [31,32].

HIV patients before ART initiation had a significantly higher prevalence of anaemia (86.5%) as compared to HIV patients (80.5%) after ART initiation [29]. This study reported higher prevalence of anemia before ART initiation, whereas, the results were in line with Omoregie and colleague but not in agreement with that of Nadler and colleague in which no significant difference in the prevalence of anaemia was observed between HIV patients on HAART and their HAART naive counter parts [33,34]. The difference in anemia definition between the studies may be responsible for the difference in the results. In addition, drugs may cause myelosuppression in HIV infected patients such as antifungal agents, antiviral agents, antiretroviral, anti-Pneumocystis carinii agents and antineoplastic agents [35]. Recently, anemia was correlated with the presence of intestinal parasites/Helminths in HAART naïve patients and it was recommended that a regular check-up of the pharmokinetic data are necessary to prevent the occurrence of anemia in urban children [12].

HAART has been working as the gold standard in the management of HIV patients. This was reported to improve hemoglobin content [34]. However, it was observed that HAART did not improve Hgb content of HIV patients and [33] reports that HIV patients on HAART still develop mild to moderate anemia.

In this study the prevalence of anemia, obtained after ART initiation was 12.3% at six and 10.4% at twelve months. However, earlier reports from Ethiopia [1] states that 21.9% after six months of ART. In separate study, reported AZT based therapy was initiated in 1256 adult patients, among them 16.2% developed AZT induced anemia while 6.8% developed anemia due to D4T regimen [36] Majority of patients had anemia within six months of starting therapy in hospitals located in various regions of Ethiopia [37-41]. Anemia could be caused by the nutrient deficiencies like iron, folic acid and vitamin B12 in patients who are on HAART.

It is reported that the three commonest hematological adverse events after HAART initiation was anemia, macrocytosis and thrombocytopenia, among these anemia was present in 8.3%, of the patients [27].

It is important to note that the lower prevalence of anemia among HIV patients receiving HAART, may indicate the effectiveness of the HAART therapy in reducing viral load and improving Hgb values and it has been reported that HAART increase Hgb concentration and decreases the prevalence of anemia [42,44]. A number of mechanisms have been suggested to explain the prevalence of anemia among HIV patient on HAART. For example they include the presence of antibodies to HAART agents [34] the presence of AZT among the HAART regimen and CD4 counts [43,44,35].

4.1.1 Mean hemoglobin assessment in HIV infected children before HAART and after HAART initiation

In this study after six months and twelve months of HAART initiation the mean Hgb level increased by 1.1 mg/dl at six months and 1.5 mg/dl at twelve months of treatment from baseline. In another study conducted in Jimma, Ethiopia showed mean Hgb increment at six months by 0.7 g/dl from baseline. On further analysis, the increment in the mean Hgb concentration was higher in those patients who had been taking D4T than AZT based HAART (3.5 gm/dl Vs 0.6 gm/dl) [1]. This study revealed by further analysis, the increment in the mean Hgb concentration was higher in those patients who have been taking D4T than AZT based HAART (1.6 g/dl Vs 0.2 g/dl.).

It was also reported that by comparing the mean change of hemoglobin with the meta-analysis of the six prospective, randomized controlled trials which showed a decrement by 0.4 g/dl at six months and 0.2 g/dl at twelve months in AZT group but an increment by 0.45 g/dl at six months and 0.58 g/dl at twelve months in D4T group, our finding showed some increment in both AZT based and D4T based regimen [45].

The different results from the above study is explained due to relatively low baseline prevalence of anemia in the study which is conducted in a developed country and partly due to the difference in study design and size of study populations [46], and also due to the definition of anemia <13 g/dl for males while the females <12 gm/dl and anemia was defined as Hgb ≤ 12.5 gm/dl both for males and females and <10 gm/dl for children [47,43,1]. It is important that a unified definition of anemia, such as WHO definition, be used. The findings in some reports also state that, not all patients on

HAART had AZT in their regimen as was the case in this study. This is important as AZT has been reported by several authors to cause anemia by inhibition of Hbg synthesis and toxicity to bone marrow cells, particularly, erythroid lines [33,43,44].

4.1.2 Risk factors for the development of anemia in HIV infected children both before HAART and after HAART initiation

The risk factors for anemia in HIV infected children are multifactorial. Among those AZT related anemia reported in various studies, include age, gender, advanced HIV stage (WHO stage III and stage IV), low baseline CD4 counts, opportunistic infections, low body weight and low body height. In this study, it was found that only descriptive association of these factors exist, but did not find any statistical significant association with, age, gender, advanced HIV stage, low baseline CD4 count, opportunistic infections, low body weight, low body height, which may be attributed by the small sample size. Our results support the data presented in [36], that anemia did not show any statistically significant association with low body weight, low CD4 count, WHO clinical staging.

In Some studies done elsewhere described that the prevalence of AZT associated anemia is about 10% at six months of ART; the pathophysiologic mechanism being bone marrow toxicity [47]. Similarly study done in Ethiopia, the prevalence of AZT associated anemia was found to be 36.2%. This indicates that AZT associated anemia is a significant problem causing morbidity and increasing treatment cost. The risk of developing AZT associated anemia is found to be higher in children started ART at WHO clinical stage III [48]. These differences can be attributed to different study design and use of different methodologies pertaining to inclusion and exclusion criteria.

A number of reports illustrated that the independent CD4 count is related to viral load, and it has been stated that CD4 count is a predictor of anemia [43,33,35]. However, the value for CD4 count differs and that CD4 count < 50 cells/µl is a significant predictor of anemia. A CD4 count of < 200 cells/µl was the value associated with anemia. Further studies are needed to resolve the effect of CD4 count on the prevalence of anemia.

This study shows post HAART treated male was more in possibility for the development of anemia than females. However, there was no statistical significance associated between them. However, among HAART naive HIV patients, males had significantly higher prevalence of anemia than their female counterparts. In another study reported by female gender had been reported as a risk factor for anemia among HIV patients [33,43]. The findings in this study differ most probably due to the difference in the modes of defining of anemia. Also, as the study subjects were adults, it might be due to large attribution of menstrual blood loss and drains on iron stores that occur with pregnancy and delivery [35].

4.1.3 Type of anemia before HAART and after HAART initiation

When assessed the type of anemia among the total number of cases, before HAART normocytic normochromic anemia was present 45.3%, whereas after HAART it was 56.6%. The high risk of developing the other types of anemia (normocytic hypochromic, normocytic normochromic and macrocytic normochromic) in pre-HAART patients, in this study, can be attributed to the multifactorial etiology of anemia as related to the study conducted earlier [49] where causes of anemia were associated to blood loss or decreased RBC production, increased RBC destruction and ineffective RBC production. The relatively high risk of developing microcytic hypochromic anemia found in before HAART patients as compared to those on HAART. This may reflect the overall nutritional deficiencies (malnutrition and malabsorption) associated with HIV patients. In another cross sectional study done in Ghana, the likelihood of developing microcytic hypochromic anemia in HAART-naive patients was five times more compared to those on HAART [20].

In this study as shown in Fig. 2, it was found that before HAART macrocytic normochromic anemia was present in 7.5% and after HAART macrocytic normochromic anemia present in 30.2% in before HAART and after treatment respectively. This showed that the average MCV for patients on HAART were significantly higher compared to their before HAART. Similar results were reported on macrocytosis anemia which was found in 20.6% of the patients and was one of the three commonest hematological adverse events observed after HAART initiation [27].

Elevated macrocytosis (MCV) is typically associated with vitamin B_{12} or folate deficiency

and in the setting of HIV treatment reflects the use of AZT or D4T [43]. The elevated MCV observed in patients on HAART in this study could therefore be attributed to drug usage since most of them had a combination therapy of either AZT or D4T with lamivudine (3TC). Therefore, other factors will come into play considering the fact that those who were on before HAART had a similar likelihood of developing macrocytosis compared to the patients on HAART. It was also reported that low levels of vitamin B_{12} in HIV positive patients and folate deficiency was also described, in HIV infected patients [50]. Conversely, it was reported that HAART may increase serum B_{12} levels, and patients did not display characteristic findings of vitamin B_{12} deficiency, namely macrocytic anemia [51]. In another retrospective study conducted in Nigeria, the prevalence of 30.6% for macrocytic anemia associated with AZT was reported and is common in HIV-infected children [27]. Similar results (30-40%) were reported in a study done with Jamaican children [52].

It was suggested that low serum B_{12} levels are reflective of low levels of B_{12} transport proteins (transcobalamin I or haptocorrin) which are produced by neutrophil and not a tissue deficiency of B_{12}. A high percentage of neutropenia was observed in the study population with the percentages in patients on HAART being slightly higher than those who were on pre - HAART although the difference was statistically significant. Low levels of transport proteins associated with neutropenia could therefore be indirectly implicated in elevated MCV observed in both before HAART and those on HAART (AZT induced). In this study In this study however, estimations could not be conducted on serum B_{12}. vitamin levels. Therefore, HAART usage and its relationship to B_{12} vitamin levels could not be ascertained [53].

When other types of anemia were assessed amongst the total number of cases as Fig. 2 reveled that, before HAART normocytic normochromic anemia was present in 45.3%, whereas after HAART it was 56.6%. The high risk of developing the other types of anemia (normocytic hypochromic, normocytic normochromic and macrocytic hypochromic) in pre-HAART patients in this study can be attributed to the multifactorial etiology of anemia were associated to blood loss or decreased RBC production, increased RBC destruction and ineffective RBC production. However, reports concerning the relationship between CD4 count and anemia are conflicting. In this study CD4 count and anemia were descriptively associated but not statistically significant [49].

4.2 Prevalence of Thrombocytopenia before HAART and after HAART Initiation

Thrombocytopenia was found to be present before and after treatment with HAART. This study revealed that at baseline the prevalence of thrombocytopenia was 8.5%, similar to that of 10% reported in an earlier study [32]. Whereas both after six and twelve months of ART initiation were 5.7%. [27], Thrombocytopenia was reported to be 2.8%. It was one of the three commonest hematological adverse events observed after HAART initiation. In another study [15], the prevalence of thrombocytopenia before ART initiation was 15.8% of the total 379 patients, similar to the 16.1% reported in another study [31]. Both were higher than the present study. While similar result showed after six month initiation of ART, thrombocytopenia was only in 6.6% of the patients. Yet another study reported that thrombocytopenia can occur in 20% to 33% of pediatric patients with HIV at some time during the course of their disease. HIV directly causes thrombocytopenia in most patients. In other retrospective studies [2] the prevalence of thrombocytopenia before ART initiation was 2.4%. Another cross sectional study, which was done for 64 children in Jimma University Specialized Hospital, Ethiopia, [1] the prevalence of thrombocytopenia at six months of ART initiation was 7.8% and in other study reported which also showed similar finding of the randomized comparative trial of AZT and D4T in children were 7% after treatments [46].

The difference in results seen from the present study is probably due to the difference in the study design and size of the study population. Prevalence of thrombocytopenia after HAART was 14.9% and these findings were correlated with their respective CD4 counts (Immune status). In this study, thrombocytosis was also assessed and found that in 17% at baseline, 22.6% at six months and 19.8% at twelve months of HAART initiation. In another study conducted [1], thrombocytosis was 4.7% at baseline and 14.1% at six months of ART initiation.

But in the present investigation, the results could not be correlated with the immune status of the patients. Since HIV is a prothrombotic condition, disruption of normal balance of coagulation

factors, with an increase of prothrombotic proteins, that fail to normalize the disturbances, can be predicted from the present study [54].

4.3 Prevalence of Neutropenia before HAART and after HAART Initiation

Neutropenia was also observed both at baseline, at six months and at twelve months of initiation of HAART. This study revealed the prevalence of neutropenia for both at baseline and at six months of HAART was same, it accounts 2.8% whereas 5.7% at twelve months of HAART. The prevalence of neutropenia before treatment was 7.8% and after six months of treatment was 4.7% in the first reported case. [1]. Our finding differs from the above report, as it is lower before treatment and higher after treatment. As compared to the meta-analysis which reported 26-46% neutropenia in AZT recipients and the prospective randomized comparative trial of D4T and AZT in children which found neutropenia of 20% over one year among AZT recipients [43]. Our observation shows that it is lower at twelve months of treatment that was 5.7 %. However these differences are explained by the differences in the study population and the study design. A valid comparison is not warranted from these findings [55].

In addition to the hematological abnormalities, this study has also given us some insight about the efficacy of HAART and to ensure the maximum level of safety when delivering ART. This was demonstrated from the anthropometric data collected by improved weight for age, height for age, weight for height from the baseline, decreased rate of opportunistic infection and increased mean CD4 percentage [56].

5. CONCLUSION

Anemia, thrombocytopenia, thrombocytosis and neutropenia were the hematological abnormality encountered in children with HIV/AIDS and who are on highly active antiretroviral therapy. Among those a resulted in increment of the mean hemoglobin concentration irrespective of the regimen used. Hemoglobin level showed significant changes at six months for AZT based regimen, while absolute neutrophil count and thrombocyte count showed statically significant change at twelve months. Accordingly, early diagnosis and appropriate treatment of anemia, thrombocytopenia and neutropenia both before initiation and after initiation of HAART improves the quality of life for HIV-infected children.

AZT drug regimen was a risk factor for anemia. While, other risk factors such as children whose age less than five years, male gender, CD4 count < 25%, the presence of opportunistic infections and advanced WHO clinical staging was associated with the development of anaemia. It can be concluded that before HAART microcytic hypochromic anemia was common whereas, after HAART macrocytic normochromic anemia was common. It is suggested that clinical management of these diseases needs to be adjusted delicately to suit the haematinic deficiencies.

ACKNOWLEDGEMENTS

The authors would like to acknowledge those children attending the ART unit of Yekatit 12 Hospital, Addis Ababa, Ethiopia,their families for giving us the permission to use their medical data and for their cooperation during this work. We extend our appreciation to the staff of Yekatit 12 Hospital, especially Sister Ferdose, and Mr Zerihune for help with the laboratory work and technical support. The authors also thank the Addis Ababa University, Ethiopia for financial and administrative support.

COMPETING INTERESTS

Authors have declared that no competing interests exist.

REFERENCES

1. Abebe M, Alemseged F. Hematologic abnormalities among children on HAART, in Jimma University specialized Hospital, Southwestern Ethiopia. Ethiopian Journal of Health Sciences 2009;19(2):83-89.

2. Choi SE, Kim I, Kim NJ, Lee AS, Choi YA, Bae JY, Kwon JH, Choe PG, Park WB, Yoon SS, Park S, Kim BK, Oh MD. Hematological manifestations of human immunodeficiency virus infection and the effect of highly active anti-retroviral therapy on cytopenia. Korean J Hematol. 2011; 46(4):253–257. PMCID: PMC3259517. DOI:10.5045/kjh.2011.46.4.253.

3. USAIDS/WHO. Ethiopia HIV/AIDS Health profile .USAIDS/WHO HIV/AIDS; 2012.

4. Briars LA, Hilao JJ, Kraus DM. Review of Pediatric Human Immunodeficiency Virus Infection. Journal of Pharmacy Practice. 2004;17:407.

5. Sourabie Y, Ouedraogo SM, Bazie WW, Sanodji N, Barro M, Ouattara ABI, Traore Y, Nacro B. Impact of ART mother and child on the HIV status of the child born to HIV-positive mothers in Burkina Faso: Towards the adoption of an effective PMTCT policy. 2015. J. Hematol. Thrombo Dis. 2015;3(2):198-203.

6. Westerlund E, Jerene D, Mulissa Z, Hallström I, LindjØrn B. Pre-ART retention in care and prevalence of tuberculosis among HIV-infected children at a district hospital in Southern Ethiopia. BMC Pediatrics. 2014;14:250-259.

7. Biressaw S, Abegaz W.E, Abebe M, AbebeTaye W, Belay M. Adherence to antiretroviral therapy and associated factors among HIV infected children in Ethiopia; Unannounced home-based pill count versus caregiver report. BMC Pediatrics. 2013;13:132.

8. Gibb DM, Duong T, Tookey PA, Sharland M, Tudor-Williams G, Novelli V, Butler K, Riordan A, Farrelly L, Masters J, Peckham CS, Dunn DT. The national study of hiv in pregnancy and childhood (NSHPC), and the collaborative hiv pediatrics study (CHIPS). Decline in mortality AIDS and hospital admissions in prenatally HIV-1 infected children. BMJ. 2003;327(7422): 1019.

9. Hunt PW, Wools Kaloustian K, Kimaiyo S, Diero L, Tierney WM, Musick BS, Braitstein P, Bwana MB, Geng E, Bangsberg DR, Martin JN, Yiannoutsos CT. Changing characteristics of HIV-infected patients initiating antiretroviral therapy in East African from 2003-2008. 5th International AIDS Society Conference on HIV Pathogenesis, Treatment and Prevention Cape Town; 2009.

10. World Health Organization (WHO), Antiretroviral therapy of HIV infection in infants and children: Towards universal access: Recommendations for a public health approach - 2010 revision.

11. Luma HN, Doualla MS, Choukem SP, Temfack E, AshuntantangG, Joko HA, Koulla-Shiro S. adverse drug reactions of Highly Active Antiretroviral Therapy (HAART) in HIV infected patients. 2012. The Pan African Medical Journal. 12:87ISSN1937-8688.

12. Mihiretie H, Taye B, Tsegaye A. Magnitude of Anemia and associated

factors among pediatric HIV/AIDS patients attending Zewditu Memorial Hospital ART clinic, Addis Ababa, Ethiopia. Anemia 2015;2015. Article ID 479329. Available:http://dx.doi.org/10.1155/2015/479329

13. Dryden-Peterson S, Hughes MD, Powis K, Ogwu A, Moffat C, Moyo S, Makhema J, Essex M, Lockman S. Increased Risk of Severe Infant Anemia Following Exposure to Maternal HAART, Botswana. Journal Acquir Immune Defic Syndr. 2011;56(5): 428-36.

14. Mark W, Russel B, Jane C, et al. A randomized trial of stavudine verses Zidovudine in children with Human Immunodeficiency Virus Infection. Pediatrics. 1998;101: 214-220.

15. Alemu J. Hematologic profile of HIV infected individuals after receiving highly active antiretroviral therapy (HAART) at Black Lion Specialized Hospital, Addis Ababa. MSC Thesis: School of Medicine, Addis Ababa University; 2011.

16. Koye D, Ayele Tand Zeleke B. Predictors of mortality among children on antiretroviral treatment at referral hospital, Northwest Ethiopia: A retrospective follow up study. BMC pediatrics. 2012;12:161.

17. GAP Report, Panos Global AIDS Programme (GAP), Federal Democratic Republic of Ethiopia: Country progress report on HIV/ AIDS response. AND Ethiopian Health and Nutrition Institute, Federal Ministry of Health. Report on the 2012 Round Antenatal Care based Sentinel HIV Surveillance in Ethiopia; 2012:2013.

18. Derbe M, Monga DP, Daka D. Immunological response among HIV/AIDS patients before and after ART therapy at Zewuditu Hospital Addis Ababa, Ethiopia. American Journal of research communication. 2013; 1(1):103-115.

19. Pamela D. Nature's Pharmacy: Evidence based alternatives to drugs. e. book; 2012.

20. Owiredu W, Quaye L, Amidu N, Mensah OA. Prevalence of anemia and immunological markers among Ghanaian HAART naïve HIV-patients and those on HAART. Afr Health Sci. 2011;11(1):2–15. PMCID: PMC3092327.

21. Aurpibul L, Puthanakit T, Sirisanthana T, Sirisanthana V. Hematological changes after switching from Stavudine to Zidovudine in HIV-infected children receiving highly active antiretroviral therapy. HIV Medicine. 2008;9(5):317–321.

22. Khadilkar VV, Khadilkar AV, Cole TJ, Sayyad MG. Cross-sectional Growth Curves for Height, Weight and Body Mass Index for Affluent Indian Children. Indian Pediatrics. 2007;46.

23. Goldman L, Schafer AL, Cecil medicine 24th ed. Philadelphia, Pa: Saunders Elsevier. 2011;161:1.

24. Leslie AJ, Pfafferott KJ, Chetty P, Draenert R, Addo MM, et al. HIV evolution: CTL escape mutation and reversion after transmission. Nature medicine. 2004;10: 282–289 [PubMed].

25. Tshering KP, Lhamo M. Ministry of Health Royal Government of Bhutan: Guideline for management of pediatric HIV/AIDS; 2008.

26. Addis Z, Yitayew G, Tachebele B. Prevalence of some haematological abnormalities among HIV positive patients on their first visit to a tertiary health institution in Ethiopia: A cross sectional study. International Blood Research and Reviews. 2014;2(6): 270-278.

27. Oshikoya KA, Lawal S, Oreagba IA, Awodele O, Olayemi SO, Iroha EO, Ezeaka VC4,5, Temiye EO, AkinsulieAo, Opanuga O, Adeyemo T, Lesi F, Akanmu AS. Adverse Events in HIV- infected Children on Antiretroviral Therapy at a Teaching Hospital in Lagos, Nigeria: A Retrospective Study. Adv Pharmacoepidem Drug Safety. 2012;1:117. DOI: 10.4172/2167-1052.1000117.

28. Opie J. Haematological complications of HIV infection. S.Afr. Med. J. 2012;102(6): 465-468.

29. Daka D, Lelissa D, Amsalu A. Prevalence of anemia before and after the initiation of antiretroviral therapy at ART centre of Hawassa University referral Hospital, Hawassa, South Ethiopia. Scholarly Journal of Medicine. 2013;3(1):1-6.

30. Mugisha Jo, Shafer LA, Vander Paal L, Mayanja BN, Eotu H, Hughes P, Whitworth JA, Grosskurth H.Anaemia in a rural Ugandan HIV cohort: Prevalence at enrolment, incidence, diagnosis and associated factors. Trop Med Int Health; 2008;13(6):788-94. DOI: 10.1111/j.1365-3156.2008.02069.

31. Akinbami A, Oshinaike O, Adeyemo T, Adediran A, Dosunmu O, Dada M,

Durojaiye I, Adebola A, Vincent O. Hematologic abnormalities in treatment naïve HIV patients. Infectious Diseases: Research and Treatment. 2010;3:45–49. DOI: 10.4137/IDRT.S6033.

32. Erhabor O, Ejele OA, Nwauche CA, Buseri FI. Some hematological parameters in human immunodeficiency virus (HIV) infected Africans: The Nigerian perspective. Niger J Med. 2005;14(1):33–8.

33. Nadler JP, Wills TS, Somboonwit C, Vencent A, Leitz G, Marino K, Naik E, Powers S, Khan N, Almyroudis N, Laatz B. Anemia prevalence among HIV patients: ART and other risk factors; Antivir Ther. 2003;8:1. PubMed Abstract.

34. Omoregie R, Omokaro EU, Palmer O, Ogefere HO, Egbeobauwaye A, Adeghe JE, Osakue SI, Ihemeje V. Prevalence of anaemia among HIV-infected patients in Benin City, Nigeria. Tanzania Journal of Health Research. 2009;11(1).

35. Curkendall SM, Richardson JT, Emons MF, Fisher AE, Everhard F. Incidence of anemia among HIV infected patients treated with HAART. HIV Medicine. 2007; 8:483-490.

36. Agrawal RK, Anuja B, Rohith V, Shubha S, Vinay R, Vikas M. Zidovudine induced reversible pure red cell aplasia. 2010;42 (3):189-191.

37. Alem M, Kena T, Baye N, Ahmed R, Tilahun S. Prevalence of Anemia and associated risk factors among adult HIV patients at the anti-retroviral therapy clinic at the University of Gondar Hospital, Gondar, Northwest Ethiopia. Scientific Reports. 2013;2:3.

38. Wondimeneh Y, Muluye D, Ferede G. Prevalence and associated factors of thrombocytopenia among HAART-naïve HIV positive patients at Gondar University Hospital, Northwest Ethiopia. BMC Research Notes. 2014;7:5.

39. Abebe M, Alemseged F. Hematologic abnormalities among children on HAART, in Jimma University specialized Hospital, Southwestern Ethiopia. Ethiopian Journal of Health Sciences. 2009;19(2):2009.

40. Adane A, Desta K, Bezabih A, Gashaye A, and Kassa D. HIV-associated anemia before and after initiation of antiretroviral therapy at Art Centre of Minilik II Hospital, Addis Ababa, Ethiopia. Ethiopian Medical Journal. 2012;50(1):13-21.

41. Gedefaw L, Yemane T, Sahlemariam Z, Yilma D. Anemia and risk factors in HAART Naïve and HAART experienced HIV positive persons in South West Ethiopia: A comparative study. Plos One. 2013;8(8):e72202. Doi:10.1371/journal.pone.0072202.

42. Belperio PS, Rhew DC. Prevalence and outcomes of anemia in individuals with human immunodeficiency virus: A systematic review of the literature. American Jornal of Medicine. 2004;116 (7A):27 S-43

43. Moyle G. Anaemia in persons with HIV infection: Prognostic marker and contributor to morbidity. AIDS Rev. 2002; 4(1):13-20.

44. Omoregie R, Egbeobauwaye A, Ogefere H, Omokaro EU, Ekeh CC. Prevalence of antibodies to HAART agents among HIV patients in Benin City, Nigeria. Afr J of Biomed, Res. 2008;11:33-37.

45. Ludwig H, Strasser K. Symptomatology of Anemia. Semin Oncol. 2001;28:7-14.

46. Sullivan S, Hanson L, Chu Y, Jeffrey J, John W. Epidemiology of anemia in human immunodeficiency virus (HIV) infected persons: Results from multistate Adult and Adolescent Spectrum of HIV Disease Surveillance Project. Blood. 1998;91:301-308.

47. Mildwan, D. Implications of anemia in human-immunodeficiency virus, cancer and hepatitis C virus. Clin. Infect. Dis. 2003;37:293-296.

48. John G, Tshering KP, Mimi Lhamo. Guideline for Management of Pediatric HIV/AIDS. Wiley and Sons; 2008.

49. Yitbarek A. Prevalence of ARV related adverse drug reactions among children taking HAART at Tikur Anbessa Specialized Hospital [M.A. Thesis]. Dept of statistics: Addis Ababa Univeristy; 2010.

50. Volberding P. The impact of anemia on quality of life in HIV infected patients. J of infectious Disease. 2002;185:110-114.

51. Boudes P, Zittoun J, Sobel A. Folate, vitamin B_{12} and HIV infection. Lancet. 1990;335(8702):1401-1402.

52. Hepburn MJ, Dyal K, Runser LA, Barfield RL, Hepburn LM, Fraser SL. Low serum vitamin B12 levels in an outpatient HIV-infected population. IntJ STD AIDS. 2004; 15(2):127–133.

53. Pryce C, Pierre RB, Steel D, Evans G, Palmer P. Safety of anti-retroviral drug therapy in Jamaican Children with HIV/AIDS. West Indian Med J. 2008;57:238-245.

54. Remacha AF, Cadafalch J. Cobalamin deficiency in patients infected with the Human immunodeficiency virus. Semin Hematol. 1999;36(1):75–87. [PubMed]

55. Bibas M, Biava G, Antinori A. HIV-associated venous thromboembolism. Mediterr J Hemato Infect Dis. 2011;3(1): e2011030. Available:http://dx.doi.org/10.4084%2fmjhid.2011.030

56. Calis, Job CJ, Boele van Hensbroek, Michael, de Haan Rob J, Moons Peter, Brabin Bernard, Bates Imelda. HIV-associated anemia in children: A systematic review from a global perspective. AIDS. 2008;22(10):1099-1112.

11

Cord Blood: A Review

Sunitha Dontha[1*], Hemalatha Kamurthy[1] and Nandakishora Chary Madipoju[1]

[1]*Department of Pharmaceutical Chemistry, Malla Reddy College of Pharmacy, Maisammaguda, Secunderabad-14, Telangana, India.*

Authors' contributions

This work was carried out in collaboration between all authors. Author SD designed the study, wrote the protocol and wrote the first draft of the manuscript. Author HK managed the literature searches, analyses of the study performed and author NCM helped in matter collection. All authors read and approved the final manuscript.

<u>Editor(s):</u>
(1) Armel Hervé Nwabo Kamdje, University of Ngaoundere-Cameroon, Ngaoundere, Cameroon.
<u>Reviewers:</u>
(1) Georgios Androutsopoulos, University of Patras, Rion, Greece.
(2) Georgios Tsoulfas, Aristotle University of Thessaloniki, Greece.

ABSTRACT

The blood collected from a new born baby umbilical cord is known as Cord blood. It is a rich source of hemotopoietic stem cells, used in the treatment of over 80 diseases like various cancers and blood, immune and metabolic disorders. Cord blood is collected from umbilical cord vein attached to the placenta after umbilical cord has been detached from new born. The cord blood is composed of all elements, found in whole blood like red blood cells, white blood cells, plasma, platelets and hematopoietic stem cells. Cord blood which is collected is cryopreserved and is stored in cord blood bank for future transplantation.

Keywords: Cord blood; diseases; stem cells; leukemia; autologous.

1. INTRODUCTION

Umbilical cord blood is blood that remains in the placenta and in the attached umbilical cord after childbirth. Cord blood is collected because it contains stem cells, used to treat hematopoietic and genetic disorders.

Cord blood is a rich source of hematopoietic stem cells (HSC), used to treat certain diseases

*Corresponding author: E-mail: basasunitha@gmail.com

of the blood and immune system. HSC are the stem cells that give rise to all the other blood cells through the process of haematopoiesis. They are derived from mesoderm and located in the red bone marrow. Patients with lymphoma, myelodysplasia and severe aplastic anemia are successfully transplanted with cord blood. Cord blood is collected from the umbilical cord vein attached to the placenta after the umbilical cord has been detached from the newborn. The umbilical vein supplies the fetus with oxygenated, nutrient-rich blood from the placenta. Whereas the fetal heart pumps deoxygenated, nutrient-depleted blood through the umbilical arteries back to the placenta. One unit of cord blood generally lacks stem cells in a quantity sufficient to treat an adult patient. The placenta is a much better source of stem cells since it contains ten times more than cord blood [1]. Some placental blood may be returned to the neonatal circulation if the umbilical cord is not prematurely clamped. According to Eileen and Eman, cord clamping should be delayed a minimum of two minutes to prevent anemia over the first three months of life and enriching iron stores and ferritin levels for as long as 6 months [2]. If the umbilical cord is not delayed clamping, a physiological postnatal occlusion occurs upon interaction with cold air, when the internal gelatinous substance, called Wharton's jelly, swells around the umbilical artery and veins. Cord blood stem cells are blood cell progenitors which forms red blood cells, white blood cells, and platelets, hence cord blood cells are currently used to treat blood and immune system related genetic diseases, cancers, and blood disorders.

There are several methods for collecting cord blood. The method most commonly used in clinical practice is the "closed technique", which is similar to standard blood collection techniques. In this method, the technician cannulates the vein of the severed umbilical cord using a needle that is connected to a blood bag, and cord blood flows through the needle into the bag. The umbilical vein catheter is another source for percutaneous peripheral or central venous catheters or intraosseous canulas and employed in resuscitation or intensive care of the newborn. On an average, by closed technique about 75 ml of cord blood [3] can be collected and cryopreserved, then stored in a cord blood bank for future transplantation.

Cryopreservation or cryoconservation is a process where cells, whole tissues, or any other substances susceptible to damage caused by chemical reactivity or time are preserved by cooling to sub-zero temperatures. At low enough temperatures, any enzymatic or chemical activity which might cause damage to the material is effectively stopped.

Stem cells are immature cells that can both reproduce themselves and have the potential to turn into other types of cells. There are several types such as embryonic (Embryos formed during the blastocyst phase of embryological development stem cell) and Adult tissue (adult stem cells). The umbilical cord blood and bone marrow cells are called hematopoietic progenitor cells (HPCs).

1.1 Storage

Cord blood is stored by both public and private cord blood banks.

1) Public cord blood banks store cord blood for the benefit of the general public, and most U.S. banks coordinate matching cord blood to patients through the National Marrow Donor Program (NMDP). Public cord blood is stored and made available for use by unrelated donors and this banking is widely supported. One important obstacle facing public banks is the high cost required to maintain them, this lead to less number of banks. Because public banks do not charge storage fees, medical centers do not always have the funds required to establish and maintain them. There is a general support in the medical community for public cord blood banking.

2) Private cord blood banks are usually for-profit organizations that store cord blood for the exclusive use of the donor or donor's relatives. Banking is generally not recommended unless there is a family history of specific genetic diseases. Private cord blood is stored for and the costs paid by donor families and is controversial in both the medical and parenting community. Private cord blood banks typically charge around $2,000 for the collection and around $200 a year for storage. For private banking objections raised from many governments and nonprofit organizations.

Although umbilical cord blood is well-recognized to be useful for treating hematopoietic and genetic disorders, some controversy surrounds the collection and storage of umbilical cord blood by private banks for the baby's use. Only a small percentage of babies (estimated between 1 in 1,000 to 1 in 200,000) ever use the umbilical cord blood that is stored. The American Academy of Pediatrics 2007 Policy Statement on Cord Blood Banking states that: "Physicians should be aware of the unsubstantiated claims of private cord blood banks made to future parents that promise to insure infants or family members against serious illnesses in the future by use of the stem cells contained in cord blood".

R. Morgan Griffin reported Umbilical cord blood banking as a procedure in which takes blood from the umbilical cord at birth and stores it for a fee in a blood bank. Because this blood is rich in stem cells -- cells that have the ability to transform into just about any human cell -- it could someday be used as treatment if your child ever became ill with certain diseases. It might also be useful for a sick sibling or relative. Banking cord blood is a way of preserving potentially life-saving cells that usually get thrown away after birth. New parents have the option of storing their newborn's cord blood at a private cord blood bank or donating it to a public cord blood bank. The cost of private cord blood banking is approximately $2000 for collection and approximately $125 per year for storage, as of 2007. Donation to a public cord blood bank is not possible everywhere, but availability is increasing. Several local cord blood banks across the United States are now accepting donations from within their own states. The cord blood bank will not charge the donor for the donation; the OB/GYN may still charge a collection fee, although many OB/GYNs choose to donate their time. After the first sibling-donor cord blood transplant was performed in 1988, the National Institute of Health (NIH) awarded a grant to Dr. Pablo Rubinstein to develop the world's first cord blood program at the New York Blood Center (NYBC), in order to establish the inventory of non embryonal stem cell units necessary to provide unrelated, matched grafts for patients.

1.2 Regulation

In the United States, the Food and Drug Administration regulates cord blood under the category of "Human Cells, Tissues, and Cellular and Tissue Based-Products." The Code of Federal Regulations under which the FDA regulates both public and private cord blood banks. Both the banks are also eligible for voluntary accreditation with either the American Association of Blood Banks (AABB) or the Foundation for the Accreditation of Cellular Therapy (FACT). Potential clients can check the current accreditation status of laboratories from the AABB list of accredited cord blood laboratories.

1.3 Research

The uses of cord blood are beyond blood and immunological disorders, hence some research has been done in other areas [4]. Its uses is limited because cord cells are hematopoietic stem cells (which can differentiate only into blood cells), and not pluripotent stem cells (such as embryonic stem cells, which can differentiate into any type of tissue). Cord Blood for Neonatal Hypoxic-Ischemic Encephalopathy [5] is being studied in humans, and earlier stage research is being conducted for treatments of stroke, [6-8]. However, apart from blood disorders, the cord blood is also used for other diseases in clinical modality and remains a major challenge for the stem cell community [4,9,10]. An alternative approach, Stem Cell Educator therapy induces immune balance by using cord blood-derived multipotent stem cells [11]. A closed-loop system that circulates a patient's blood through a blood cell separator, briefly co-cultures the patient's lymphocytes with adherent CB-SCs *in vitro*, and returns the educated lymphocytes [12-15] to the patient's circulation. From the clinical trial, it was known that a single treatment with the Stem Cell Educator provides lasting reversal of autoimmunity which allows the regeneration of islet β cells. An investigation was also conducted to determine whether cord blood cells have any potential use in repairing damages cardiovascular tissue.

Training programs are also adopted for clinicians and researchers throughout the world, in order to coordinate the research efforts. In 2004 Eurocord,[16] an international platform specialized in clinical research on UCB stem cells, was founded by Pr. Gregory Katz and Eliane Gluckman. Eurocord centralizes and analyzes clinical data from 511 transplant centers in 56 countries. Eurocord funded by the European Union, works closely with the European School of Haematology. In 2007, the association was recognized by the *Medicen* network of cell therapy clusters. Eurocord also develops training programs for clinicians and researchers specialized in blood cancer and cell therapy.

The International Society of Cellular Therapy (ISCT) has established criteria for defining Mesenchymal stem cells MSC [17], differentiate to build bone, cartilage and connective tissue, and they can also mediate the body's inflammatory response to damaged or injured cells [18-21]. Clinical trials are not reported in humans using MSCs derived from cord tissue, but some reports are available, as used in treating certain diseases in animals [22-26].

There is no particular standard procedure or accrediting criteria for the storage of MSC from umbilical cord tissue. Many cord blood banks are storing the cord tissue by freezing a segment of the umbilical cord. This procedure has the advantage of waiting for the technology of cell separation to mature, but has the disadvantage of no guarantee to efficiently retrieve viable stem cells from a previously frozen cord. In few cord blood banks stem cells are extracted from the cord tissue before cryogenic storage. This method has the disadvantage of using current separation method, but the advantage is that it yields minimally manipulated cells which are ready for treatment and compels with FDA regulations on cell therapy products.

1.4 Controversy

The policy of the American Academy of Pediatrics states that "private storage of cord blood as 'biological insurance' is unwise" unless there is a family member with a current or potential need to undergo a stem cell transplantation The American Academy of Pediatrics also notes that the odds of using one's own cord blood is 1 in 200,000.

Banking is not worth for most people. The banks opinion is that, it is a form of "insurance" in case their children ever get sick. But, many medical associations -- like the American Academy of Pediatrics and the American College of Obstetricians and Gynecologists – do not support the practice for most people. They say that possible benefits are too remote to justify the costs.

Stephen Feig, Professor of pediatrics, says that the use of stored cord blood is very less and it is a very expensive insurance policy and he also says that he will not object any one to not to store the cord blood. So the important thing is to make an informed choice. The patients should the know the benefits and costs of cord blood banking before tomake any decisions. Saving a

baby's cord blood for a family member who gets -- or already is -- sick? Siblings are more likely to be a genetic match, which is crucial. The use of child's blood siblings is only about 25% and there is a 75% chance that he or she needs a donation from another donor's cells in a bank instead.

Cord blood is used in treating diseases in children. Only 3 to 5 ounces are taken from the cord, and since cord blood has a limited number of stem cells, which is not enough to treat most adults.

The parents also need to understand that cord blood is not the only possible treatment for these diseases. Most of the people who need a transplant of stem cells, can also get them from donated bone marrow, either from a family member or a bone marrow bank.

The current uses of the CB are limited. But many experts hope that stem cells will be a crucial part of future treatments for diabetes, Alzheimer's, spinal cord injuries, heart failure, stroke, etc. If it is really possible to make stem cells develop into any kind of cell, the uses are endless. But this is only theoretical, it is important to distinguish between what doctors can do now with cord blood stem cells and what they *will* be able to do in the future. Some people do not realize the distinction. They have exaggerated ideas of what is possible today.

Caplan says that people think the stem cell therapy is like its alchemy as a stem cell can be turned into anything, just like alchemists hoped to turn base metals into gold. But it is not true.

Even if researchers do have future successes with stem cells, they may not come from cord blood.

The science is moving fast right now, According to Caplan using stem cells from cord blood will be the new approach to take into the future. Caplan is more optimistic about techniques using embryonic stem cells or stem cells derived from adult tissue.

The controversy centers on varying assessments of the current and future likelihood of successful uses of the stored blood [27].

CB stem cells can be used for other purposes, like for regenerative medicine, says the World Marrow Donor Association (WMDA) and European Group on Ethics in Science and New Technologies. Therefore it is highly hypothetical that CB cells kept for autologous use will be of more value in the future. WMDA, says that there are pediatric cancers (ex: neuroblastoma) and acquired conditions (ex: aplastic anemia) which can be treated by autologous transplant example leukemia.

WMDA Policy Statement for the Utility of Autologous or Family Cord Blood Unit Storage [28] stated that:

1. The use of autologous cord blood cells for the treatment of childhood leukemia is contra-indicated because pre-leukemic cells are present at birth. Autologous cord blood carries the same genetic defects as the donor and should not be used to treat genetic diseases.
2. There is at present no known protocol where autologous cord blood stem cells are used in therapy.
3. If autologous stem cell therapies should become reality in the future, these protocols will probably rely on easily accessible stem cells.

There were several known instances where autologous use of cord blood was possible, though other areas of research are more speculative [29,30].

2. VARIOUS REPORTS ON CORD BLOOD

2.1 Umbilical Cord Blood as a Source of Stem Cells [31]

Umbilical cord blood (UCB) is a source of the hematopoietic stem cells (HSC) and progenitor cells that can reconstitute the hematopoietic system in patients with malignant and nonmalignant disorders treated with myeloablative therapy. UCB cells possess an enhanced capacity for progenitor cell proliferation and self-renewal *in vitro*. The blood remaining in the delivered placenta is safely and easily collected and stored. Currently practiced collection procedure is a simple venipuncture, followed by gravity drainage into a standard sterile anti-coagulant-filled blood bag, using a closed system (similar to the one used for whole blood collection). After aliquots are removed for routine testing, the units are cryopreserved and stored in liquid nitrogen.

Children with both malignant and non-malignant hematologic disorders were transplanted with

UCB from a sibling donor, demonstrated comparable or superior survival to children who received BM transplantation. But the use of UCB transplantation in adult patients is less, since the limited number of HSC that harvested from umbilical cord and resulted in a slower time to engraftment and higher transplant related mortality. This is due to the long aplasia period after transplantation and susceptibility to viral and fungal infections. Despite prolonged periods of aplasia, the apparent reduction in the incidence and severity of graft versus host disease (GVHD). UCB lymphocytes has the lower incidence and severity of GVHD encountered in UCB transplantation compared to the allogeneic BM transplant setting. UCB transplantation is not associated with increased rates of disease relapse. From this data, suggested that nucleated cell dose in UK unit should be the primary criterion for donor selection. In 1991, the UCB transplantation program was established at the Zagreb University Hospital Center for related transplants, and until now only four UCB transplantations were performed successfully. To speed up the engraftment rate, several strategies (such as multiple UCB transplants and *ex vivo* expansion of HSC) have been assayed. The current strategies are focused on the development of much more efficient technologies for *ex vivo* production of progenitor cells. UCB is known to contain extremely immature stem cells (such as pluripotent or multipotent) and these are used for cellular therapy and regenerative medicine. Up to date there is no regarding these possibilities but preliminary *in vitro* and animal studies in the field of tissue regeneration suggest some degree of plasticity and/or trans differentiation. UCB cells are showing unique qualities and potential, and consequently UCB banks are dramatically increasing the scope of their clinical application.

2.2 Hematopoietic Stem-cell Transplantation Using Umbilical-cord Blood [32]

UCB is as an alternative source of hematopoietic progenitors (CD34+) for allogeneic stem cell transplantation, mainly who lack an HLA-matched marrow donor. From 1998, only about 2500 patients have received UCB transplants for a variety of malignant and non-malignant diseases. The vast majority of recipients were children with an average weight of 20 kg, however, more than 500 UCB transplantations (UCBT) have already been performed in adults. The "naive" nature of UCB lymphocytes explains the lower incidence and severity of graft vs. host disease (GvHD) encountered in UCBT. UCB is rich in primitive CD16-CD56++ NK cells, which possess significant proliferative and cytotoxic capacities and used for IL-12 or IL-15, so as to mount a substantial graft vs. leukemia (GvL) effect. The major disadvantage of UCB is the low yield of stem cells, resulting in higher rates of engraftment failure. A rational approach thus involves *ex vivo* expansion of UCB derived hematopoietic precursors.

2.3 Cord Blood for Brain Injury [33]

CB is as an effective therapy for patients with brain injuries since cord blood (CB) cells induces repair through mechanisms like trophic or cell-based paracrine effects or cellular integration and differentiation. Recovery from neurological injuries is typically incomplete and often results in significant and permanent disabilities. Currently, most of the available therapies are limited to supportive or palliative measures. Because restorative therapies targeting the underlying cause of most neurological diseases are not existing. Cell therapies targeting anti-inflammatory, neuroprotective and regenerative potential holds great promise. Both are operative CB therapies for neurologic conditions, and there are numerous potential applications of CB-based regenerative therapies in neurological diseases, including genetic diseases of childhood, ischemic events such as stroke and neurodegenerative diseases of adulthood. This Review, mainly describes the state of science and clinical applications of CB therapy for brain injury.

For neonatal brain injury, UCB transplantation is emerging as a promising therapeutic method for treating hypoxic-ischemic brain injury and ischemic stroke. Number of the human clinical trials were conduced to examine the potential therapeutic benefits of undifferentiated CB cells for the treatment of established ischemic brain injury and established cerebral palsy. It is imperative that the timing of the administration of the UCB with respect to the time of the injury (if known) is defined, as well as the optimal dose of UCB for transplantation. Further, the contribution and beneficial effects of the different cell populations in UCB are to be elucidated in order to determine adequate therapies that leads to further improvement in neurological outcome, based on the clinical scenario.

2.4 Umbilical Cord Blood-derived Cellular Products for Cancer Immunotherapy [34]

Although the vast majority of experience with umbilical cord blood (CB) centers on hematopoietic reconstitution, a recent surge in the knowledge of CB cell subpopulations as well as advances in *ex vivo* culture technology have expanded the potential of this rich resource. Because CB has the capacity to generate the entire hematopoietic system, now a new source for natural killer, dendritic and T cells for therapeutic use against malignancies. This Review mainly focuses on the cellular immunotherapies derived from CB. Expansion techniques, ongoing clinical trials and future directions of CB application are also discussed.

2.5 Stem Cell Comparison: What Can We Learn Clinically from Unrelated Cord Blood Transplantation as an Alternative Stem Cell Source? [35]

Allogeneic hematopoietic cell transplantation (HCT) is an important therapeutic option for a variety of malignant and non-malignant disorders (NMD). The use of umbilical cord blood transplantation (UCBT) has made HCT available to many more patients. The increased level of human leukocyte antigen disparity that can be tolerated makes UCBT a very attractive alternative source of hematopoietic stem cells; however, the increased risk of early death observed after UCBT remains an obstacle. Novel strategies such as *ex vivo* stem cell expansion is now becoming a part of the standard clinical approach, and preliminary results are extremely encouraging with suggestion of reduction of early transplant-related mortality. Although there are no randomized studies that compare the risks and benefits of UCBT relative to those observed with related and unrelated donors both for malignant and NMD, several retrospective studies have compared outcomes between UCBT and other stem cell sources. This review, is aimed to describe and summarize the findings of the principal studies in this field. They hoped that what we can learn from these studies and how we can use this information will improve the outcomes of HCT for patients with malignant and NMD.

2.6 Topping it up: Methods to Improve Cord Blood Transplantation Outcomes by Increasing the Number of CD34+ Cells [36]

CB is increasingly recognized for its excellent stem cell potential, lenient matching criteria, instant availability and clinical behavior in transplant. With 1-2 kg fewer total (stem cell) numbers in the graft compared with other cell sources, the infused cell dose per kilogram is critical for engraftment and outcome, which leads to the development of stem cell support platforms. The co-transplant platforms of haplo cord and double unit cord blood (DUCB) transplantation are aimed toward increasing stem cell dose. Together with the optimization of reduced-intensity protocols, long-term sustained engraftment using CB is available to most patients, including elderly patients. Haplo cord has a low incidence of both acute and chronic GvHD but requires anti-thymocyte globulin ATG for effective neutrophil recovery. DUCB is performed without anti-thymocyte globulin with excellent immune reconstitution and disease-free survival, but engraftment is considerably slower, and GvHD incidence significant. Both haplo-cord and DUCB transplantation appears to be valid alternatives to matched unrelated donors in adults.

2.7 Improving the Outcome of Umbilical Cord Blood Transplantation Through *ex vivo* Expansion or Graft Manipulation [37]

UCBT for adult patients with hematologic malignancies now used for matched unrelated donor transplantation. Multiple strategies are studied to overcome the limitations of low lymphocyte and hematopoietic stem and progenitor cell dose, a source of significant morbidity and mortality. One strategy is *ex vivo* expansion of the UCB unit before transplantation, which increases the number of lymphocytes, committed progenitors and long-term repopulating hematopoietic stem cells. Increasing the numbers of lymphocytes and committed progenitor cells leads to delayed hematopoietic recovery after UCBT. Increasing the hematopoietic stem cell content will improve the availability of adequately sized and matched cord blood units for transplantation. The second strategy is exposure of the UCB graft to compounds for improving the homing and engraftment following transplantation. Such a strategy addresses the problem of slow hematopoietic recovery and the increased risk of graft failure. Many of these strategies are tested in late-phase multi-center clinical trials.

2.8 Umbilical Cord Blood Banking for Transplantation in Morocco: Problems and Opportunities [38]

In 1989, the success of the first UCB transplantation in a child (with Fanconi anaemia), lead to the source of stem cells. UCB provides an unlimited source of diverse stem cells and is an alternative for bone marrow (BM) and peripheral blood (PB) HSCT. Thus, UCB and manipulated stem cells are collected and banked according to international accreditation standards. This work was aimed to identify the problems limiting the creation of a Moroccan cord blood bank and to highlight opportunities and issues of a new legislation promoting additional applications of cell therapy.

2.9 Concise Review: Cord Blood Banking, Transplantation and Induced Pluripotent Stem Cell: Success and Opportunities [39]

HCT became a standard practice to treat a number of malignant and nonmalignant hematologic diseases. Bone marrow, mobilized peripheral blood, and UCB served as primary sources of cells for HCT. Currently a large number of CB units are stored, although it represents only a fraction of potential collections. Since much of the collection is sequestered in private banks only for autologous use. In coming years, the demand for public banks increases by using for the treatment of patients with diseases like leukemia and lymphoma. A possible solution for the private banks is to encourage and share their valuable units and to apply recent methodologies to generate induced pluripotent stem cells from cord cells and to optimize techniques to generate hematopoietic lineages from them. This strategy has an advantage of the units already collected under appropriate regulatory guidelines, to access a pristine cell that can be converted to a pluripotent cell at a much higher efficiency in a shorter time period. The cord blood unit with new cells, for additional therapeutic applications, allows banks to develop an appropriate business model for both private and public cord blood banks.

The cord blood stem cell field is progressing rapidly, with extensive developments and accomplishments in recent years.

2.10 Umbilical Cord Blood–derived Cellular Products for Cancer Immunotherapy [40]

Although a majority of UCB centers on hematopoietic reconstitution, a recent surge in the knowledge of CB cell subpopulations as well as advances in *ex vivo* culture technology have expanded the potential of this rich resource. Because CB has the capacity to generate the entire hematopoietic system, we have a new source for natural killer, dendritic and T cells for therapeutic use against malignancies. This Review was focussed on the cellular immunotherapies derived from CB, expansion techniques, ongoing clinical trials and future directions of CB application are also discussed.

2.11 Therapeutic Potential of Umbilical Cord Blood Cells for Type 1 Diabetes Mellitus [41]

UCB is a rich source of regulatory T cells (Tregs) and multiple types of stem cells, with immunomodulating potential. It has the ability to restore peripheral tolerance toward pancreatic islet β cells by remodeling of the immune responses and suppressing the autoreactive T cells. Type 1 diabetes mellitus (T1DM) which is a chronic disorder results from autoimmune-mediated destruction of pancreatic islet β cells. The optimal therapeutic method for T1DM is to control the autoimmunity, restore immune homeostasis, preserve the residual β cells, reverse β-cell destruction, and protecting the regenerated insulin-producing cells against the re-attacking. Reinfusion of autologous UCB or immune cells from CB is a novel therapy for T1DM. The main advantages are no risk to the donors, minimal ethical concerns, low incidence of graft-versus-host disease (GVHD) and easy accessibility. This review, gives a report on the role of autologous UCB or immune cells from cord blood applications for the treatment of T1DM.

2.12 Fetal Endothelial and Mesenchymal Progenitors from the Human Term Placenta: Potency and Clinical Potential [42]

The phenomenon of fetal micro chimerism (FMC) which occurs during pregnancy, through the transfer of fetal stem/progenitor cells to maternal blood and tissues. Microchimeric mesenchymal stem cells and endothelial progenitors of fetal origin have the capacity for tissue repair in the maternal host. The isolation of fetal stem cell populations from perinatal tissues, such as UCB and placenta, interest has been growing in understanding their greater plasticity compared with adult stem cells and exploring their potential in regenerative medicine. The use of similar fetal stem cells in therapy is significantly hampered by the availability of clinically relevant cell numbers and/or contamination with cells of maternal origin, using the chorionic and decidual placenta. In this review, the researchers highlighted the importance of FMC to the field of fetal stem cell biology and issues of maternal contamination from perinatal tissues and discussed specific isolation strategies to overcome these translational obstacles.

2.13 Allogeneic Haematopoietic Stem Cell Transplantation for Primary Myelofibrosis and Myelofibrosis Evolved from Other Myeloproliferative Neoplasms [43]

Allogeneic haematopoietic stem cell transplantation (allo-HSCT) is the only curative treatment for myelofibrosis. Major improvements in this field are the introduction of reduced intensity conditioning regimens, which made transplant a better tolerated treatment that can be offered to older patients and those with comorbidities. The treatment-related toxicities, GvHD, infectious complications and relapse remains the major problems of post transplant. The authors reviewed here the recent published data and outlined the criteria to select patients with myelofibrosis who can benefit the most from this curative treatment.

2.13.1 Recent findings

Data regarding mutations in myelofibrosis have been useful to better define the prognosis of patients and have provided a tool to monitor minimal residual disease after transplantation. New data regarding the use of age and comorbidities has allowed a better selection of patients who can benefit from transplantation. Janus-activated kinase signal (JAK) 1/2 inhibitors pretransplant can improve patient's performance status and potentially improve transplant outcomes.

2.13.2 Summary

Improvements in the field of allo-HSCT, the ability to improve patient's performance status prior to transplant with JAK1/2 inhibitors and a more accurate disease risk stratification based on molecular mutations to select patients who can benefit from allo-HSCT should result in better transplant outcomes. Efforts should be made to transplant patients with myelofibrosis on prospective studies to answer some unresolved questions.

2.14 Adoptive Immunotherapy with the Use of Regulatory T Cells and Virus-specific T Cells Derived from Cord Blood [44]

Cord blood units are a valuable donor source for the development of cellular therapeutics. Virus-specific T cells and regulatory T cells are two cord blood–derived products that have shown promise in early-phase clinical trials to prevent and/or treat viral infections and GVHD, respectively. CBT is an alternative to traditional stem cell transplants (bone marrow or peripheral blood stem cell transplantation) and an attractive option for patients lacking suitable stem cell transplant donors. The researchers described the current strategies and uses of CB–derived regulatory T cells and virus-specific T cells developed to improve the outcomes for CB transplant recipients.

2.15 Transcription Factor -mediated Reprogramming toward Hemato-poietic Stem Cells [45]

HSCs from renewable cell types are used in regenerative medicine. Paralleling efforts was made recently to use pluripotent stem cells substantial progress was made recently towards HSC generation via combinatorial transcription factor (TF)-mediated fate conversion, a paradigm established by Yamanaka's induction of pluripotency in somatic cells by mere four TFs. This review integrated the recently reported strategies to directly convert a variety of starting cell types toward HSCs in the context of hematopoietic transcriptional regulation and discussed how these findings will be further developed toward the ultimate generation of therapeutic human HSCs.

2.16 Characteristics of Hematopoietic Stem Cells of Umbilical Cord Blood [46]

UCB collected from the postpartum placenta is a rich source of HSCs and is an alternative to BMT. The differences (in phenotype, cytokine production, quantity and quality of cells) between stem cells from UCB, bone marrow and peripheral blood were described. HSCs present in cord blood are more primitive than their counterparts in bone marrow or peripheral blood, and have several advantages including high proliferation. With using proper cytokine combination, HSCs can be effectively developed into different cell lines. This process is used in medicine, especially in hematology.

2.17 Concise Review: Umbilical Cord Blood Transplantation: Past, Present, and Future [47]

UCB is an effective alternate source of hematopoietic stem cell support. Transplantation with CB allows for faster availability of frozen sample and avoids invasive procedures for donors. Allogeneic HSCT is an important treatment option for fit patients with poor-risk hematological malignancies. The lack of available fully matched donors limits its use. In addition, this procedure has demonstrated reduced relapse rates and similar overall survival when compared with unrelated allogeneic HSCT. The limited dose of CD34+ stem cells available with single-unit cord transplantation has been addressed by the development of double-unit cord transplantation. In combination with improved conditioning regimens, double-unit cord transplantation has allowed for the treatment of larger children, as well as adult patients with hematological malignancies. The development of safer techniques to improve homing, engraftment, and immune reconstitution is cuurent development after cord blood transplantation. Here the authors reviewed the past, present, and future of cord transplantation.

2.18 Umbilical Cord Blood Transplantation: A Maturing Technology [48]

CB is used increasingly as a source of allogeneic hematopoietic support for patients who need HCT and do not have access to an HLA-matched donor. To overcome the limitation of low cell doses in single CB units, dCBT has been adopted for many patients and is associated with outcomes comparable to those with other donor sources. There are new strategies under development to improve engraftment with *ex vivo* expansion or homing and to enhance immune reconstitution with the infusion of CB-derived NK cells and cytotoxic T lymphocytes with antiviral and antileukemic specificities. Tregs are being evaluated to reduce the incidence of GVHD. Prospective, multicenter clinical trials are needed to determine the efficacy of these promising technologies that are likely to improve outcome for CBT patients.

2.19 Stem Cell Therapy to Protect and Repair, the Developing Brain: A Review of Mechanisms of Action of Cord Blood and Amnion Epithelial Derived Cells [49]

Stem cell therapy is used to protect and repair the developing brain. In the research, clinical, and wider community the use of stem cells, is of great interest- to reduce the progression, or indeed repair brain injury. Perinatal brain injury results from acute or chronic insults sustained during fetal development, during the process of birth, or in the newborn period. The clinical trials are taking place worldwide targeting cerebral

palsy with stem cell therapies. It takes many years for emerge of strong evidence-based results from these trials. With such trials, it is both appropriate and timely to address the physiological basis for the efficacy of stem-like cells in preventing damage and regenerating, the newborn brain. The experimental animal models are best example. Stem cells that are readily and economically obtained from the placenta and umbilical cord discarded at birth. These cells have the potential for transplantation to the newborn where brain injury is diagnosed or even suspected. The novel characteristics of hAECs and undifferentiated UCB cells are explored. The UCB-derived endothelial progenitor cells (EPCs) and mesenchymal stem cells (MSCs), and how immunomodulation and anti-inflammatory properties are principal mechanisms of action that are common to these cells, and ameliorate the cerebral hypoxia and inflammation that are final pathways in the pathogenesis of perinatal brain injury.

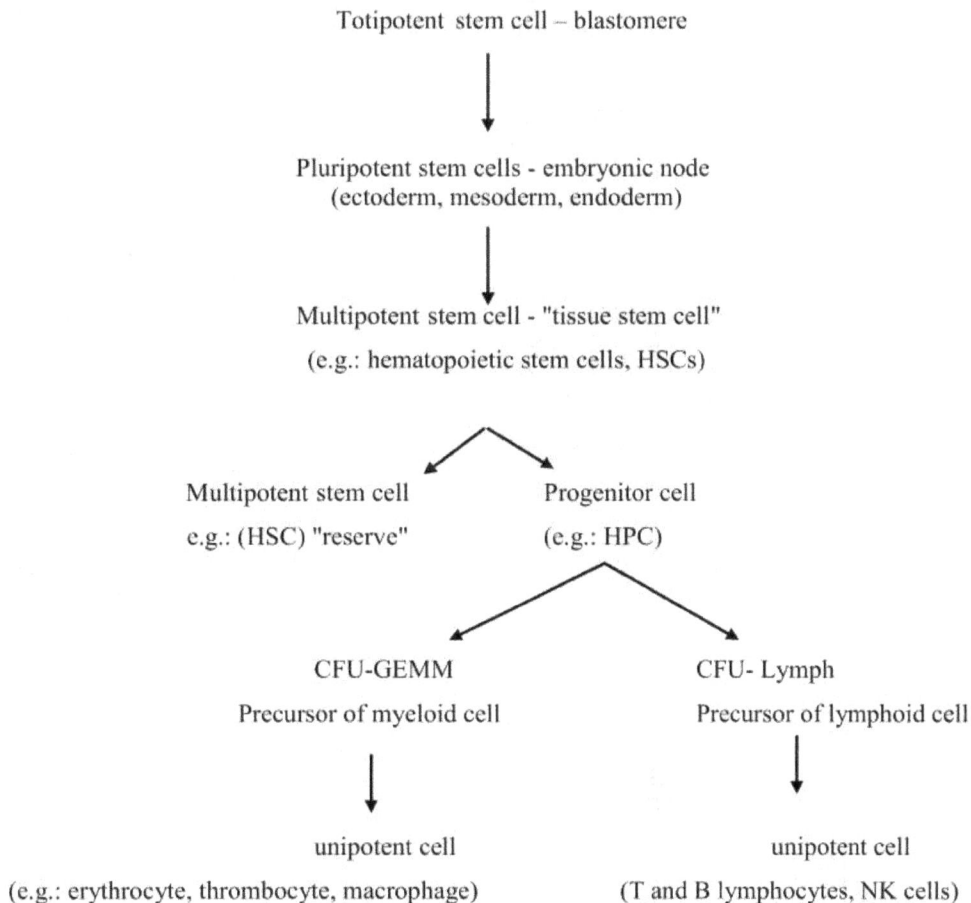

Totipotent stem cell – blastomere

↓

Pluripotent stem cells - embryonic node
(ectoderm, mesoderm, endoderm)

↓

Multipotent stem cell - "tissue stem cell"

(e.g.: hematopoietic stem cells, HSCs)

Multipotent stem cell   Progenitor cell

e.g.: (HSC) "reserve"   (e.g.: HPC)

CFU-GEMM   CFU- Lymph

Precursor of myeloid cell   Precursor of lymphoid cell

↓   ↓

unipotent cell   unipotent cell

(e.g.: erythrocyte, thrombocyte, macrophage)   (T and B lymphocytes, NK cells)

Fig. 1. Functions of stem cells

Table 1. Clinical trials being conducted around the world using umbilical cord blood in regenerative medicine therapies for the management of cerebral palsy and ischemic brain injury in the newborn

Study title	Main objective	Institution	Treatment	Current status	Trial identifier
A randomized study of autologous umbilical cord blood reinfusion in children with cerebral palsy	To determine the efficacy of a single intravenous infusion of autologous umbilical cord blood for the treatment of pediatric patients with spastic cerebral palsy.	Duke University, United States	Intravenous infusion. Autologous umbilical cord blood. Timing: not specified. (Children 12 months–6 years of age enrolled).	Currently recruiting	NCT01147653
Characterization of the cord blood stem cell in situation of neonatal asphyxia (NEOCORD)	To characterize cord blood stem cells of neonates with neonatal asphyxia and to compare them with those from healthy newborn.	Assistance publique Hopitaux de Marseille	*In vitro* characterization of the cord blood stem cell only.	Currently recruiting	NCT01284673
Allogenic umbilical cord blood and erythropoietin combination therapy for cerebral palsy	To determine efficacy of umbilical cord blood and erythropoietin combination therapy for children with cerebral palsy.	Sung Kwang Medical Foundation, Korea	Intravenous allogeneic umbilical cord blood infusion (Total nucleated cells >3 × 10^7/kg) in combination with erythropoietin given twice a week for 4 weeks. Timing: up to 6 months after adverse event.	Completed	NCT01193660
Safety and effectiveness of cord blood stem cell infusion for the treatment of cerebral palsy in children	To test the safety and effectiveness of a cord blood infusion in children who have motor disability due to cerebral palsy. The subjects will be children whose parents have saved their infant's cord blood, who have non-progressive motor disability, and whose parents intend to have a cord blood infusion.	Georgia Health Sciences University, United States	Intravenous infusion of red-cell depleted, mononuclear cell enriched cord blood. Timing: not specified. (Children 1–12 years of age enrolled).	Currently recruiting	NCT01072370

Study title	Main objective	Institution	Treatment	Current status	Trial identifier
Autologous cord blood cells for brain injury in term newborns	To test feasibility and safety of collection, preparation and infusion of autologous umbilical cord blood during the first 3 days of age if the baby is born with signs of brain injury.	National University Hospital, Singapore	Intravenous infusion of autologous cord blood. Timing: 3 days post-birth.	Currently recruiting	NCT01649648
Cord blood for neonatal hypoxic-ischemic encephalopathy	To test feasibility of collection, preparation and infusion of a baby's own umbilical cord blood in the first 14 days after birth if the baby is born with signs of brain injury.	Duke University, United States	Intravenous infusions autologous volume reduced cord blood cells (up to 4 infusions). Timing: first 18 postnatal days.	Currently recruiting	NCT00593242

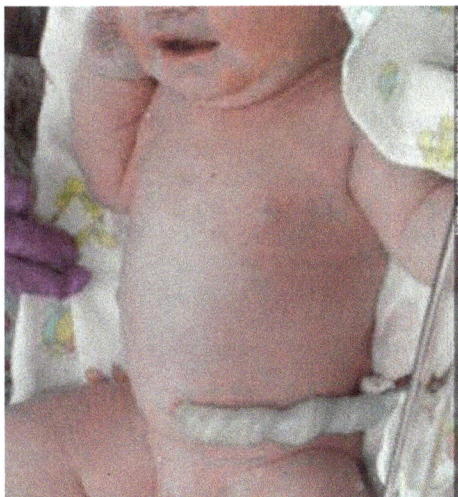

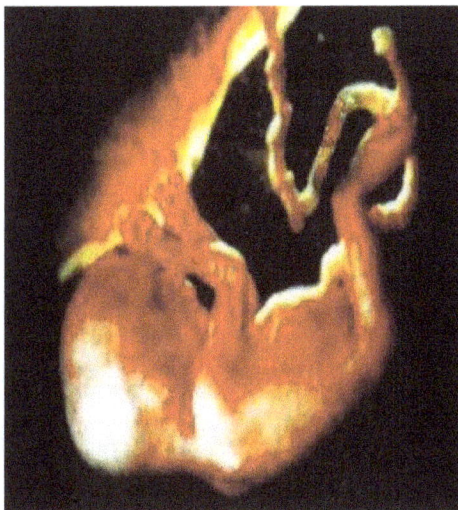

Fig. 2. Umbilical cord stem cells

2.20 Human Umbilical Cord Mesenchymal Stem Cells Transplantation Promotes Cutaneous Wound Healing of Severe Burned Rats [50]

MSC therapy contributes to facilitate wound healing for severe burns (highly lethal trauma) to promote the wound healing as early as possible. In this study, they investigated effect of human umbilical cord MSCs (hUC-MSCs) on wound healing in a rat model of severe burn and its potential mechanism. They concluded that hUC-MSCs transplantation can effectively improve wound healing in severe burned rat model.

3. DISCUSSION

UCB contains a rich and diverse mixture of stem and progenitor cells that have the potential to generate a variety of cell types with neuronal characteristics. It has also been shown that these stem cells have a positive impact on animal models of neural injuries and diseases. UCB stem cells are a potential candidate for clinical therapies for neural injuries and neural degenerative diseases for which current mode of therapy is inadequate [51]. In 1989, Broxmeyer, Gluckman, and colleagues demonstrated the UCB use in clinical settings for stem cell transplantation [52]. Since then, UCB has been used to treat nearly 80 diseases with over 25,000 transplants worldwide. UCB represents an abundant source of non-embryonic stem cells which are easily accessible with non-invasive collection of cells and no risk to the donor. Such cells are more immature than their bone marrow derived counterparts and displays an impressive proliferative potential [53] and have good viability after cells have been cryopreserved for later use.

UCB stem cells have high engraftment rates when used for replacement of haematopoietic stem cell populations, are relatively tolerant of HLA mismatches and thereby show low rates of GVHD, compared to bone marrow derived stem cells. They are rarely contaminated with latent viruses resulting in greater acceptance of UCB stem cells in comparison to bone marrow. UCB is used for the treatment of various hematopoietic disorders but, in the authors reported more recently induced regenerations in the central nervous system [54,55].

UCB is a rich souce of hemapoietic stem/progenitor cells, regulatory T-lymphocytes (Tregs), monocytes, mesenchymal stem cells (MSCs), endothelial progenitor cells (EPCs), and stromal precursor cells and, used for the treatment of neurological disorders. A recent pre-clinical study showed that UCB transplantation resulted in improved sensorimotor ability in a rat model of hypoxic ischemic brain injury. There are only a modest number of animal studies that are examined the effects of UCB transplantation following hypoxic-ischemic injury, predominantly in newborn rats. These experiments using the Rice-Vannuci animal model have reported positive brain results following UCB transplantation including decreased reactive gliosis, increased tissue repair, cognitive improvements amelioration of injury-related effects in the primary somatosensory cortex and enhancement of endogenous neural stem cell proliferation via Hedgehog signalin. These pre-clinical trials have not fully elucidated the mechanism underlying the beneficial effects of UCB transplantation. Nevertheless, autologous intravenous UCB transplantation is shown to be safe and feasible in young children with acquired neurological disorders. The evidence presented suggests that the UCB cells have a great deal of potential as a future treatment for stroke, both ischemic and hemorrhagic, in young and adult alike.

4. CONCLUSION

Collection of cord stem cells is painless and risk free to mother and baby. Cord blood stem cells have a greater ability to differentiate into other cell types. These cells have longer growth potential and have been shown to have a greater rate of engraftment. Cord blood stem cells are much more tolerant to HLA tissue mismatching than bone marrow therefore leading to lower rate of GVHD and are not exposed to the toxins and radiations. Cord blood stem cells are being used in the treatment of 40 medical conditions with over 72 potential disease targets. Research should be oriented towards prolonging their storage and enhancing their expansion.

CONSENT

It is not applicable.

ETHICAL APPROVAL

It is not applicable.

COMPETING INTERESTS

Authors have declared that no competing interests exist.

REFERENCES

1. Cairo MS, Wagner JE. Placental and/or umbilical cord blood: An alternative source of hematopoietic stem cells for transplantation. Blood. 1997;90(12): 4665–4678.

2. Eileen KH, Eman SH. Late vs early clamping of the umbilical cord in full-term neonates. JAMA; 2007.

3. Christopher DH, Ronald GS, Naomi LC Luban. Handbook of pediatric transfusion medicine. Academic Press. 2004;295-296.

4. Hal E Broxmeyer, Franklin OS. Cord blood hematopoietic cell transplantation. Thomas Hematopoietic Cell Transplantation, 4th ed. Wiley-Blackwell, Oxford, UK; 2009.

5. Haller MJ, Viener HL, Wasserfall C, Brusko T, Atkinson MA, Schatz DA. Autologous umbilical cord blood infusion for type 1 diabetes. Exp. Hematol. 2008;36(6): 710–715.

6. Vendrame M, Pennypacker, Keith R, Bickford, Paula C, Davis S, et al. Cord blood rescues stroke-induced changes in splenocyte phenotype and function. Exp. Neurol. 2006;199(1):191–200.

7. Vendrame M, Gemma, Carmelina, Mesquita, Dirson D, Collier, Lisa, Bickford, Paula C, Sanberg CD, Sanberg Paul. Anti-inflammatory effects of human cord blood cells in a rat model of stroke. Stem Cells Dev. 2005;14(5):595–604.

8. Revoltella RP, Papini Sandra, Rosellini Alfredo, Michelini Monica F, et al. Cochlear repair by transplantation of human cord blood CD133+ cells to nod-scid mice made deaf with kanamycin and noise. Cell Transplant. 2008;17(6):665–678.

9. Harris DT, Badowski, Michael Ahmad, Nafees Gaballa, Mohamed A. The potential of cord blood stem cells for use in regenerative medicine. Expert Opin. Biol. Ther. 2012;7(9):1311–1322.

10. Haller MJ, Viener HL, Wasserfall C, Brusko T, Atkinson Mark A, Schatz DA. Autologous umbilical cord blood infusion for type 1 diabetes. Exp. Hematol. 2008;36(6):710–715.

11. Zhao Y, Lin B, Dingeldein M, Guo C, Hwang D, Holterman MJ. New type of human blood stem cell: A double-edged sword for the treatment of type 1 diabetes. Translational Research. 2012;155(5): 211–216.

12. Yong Zhao, Zhaoshun Jiang, Tingbao Z, Mingliang Y, Chengjin H. Reversal of type 1 diabetes via islet β cell regeneration following immune modulation by cord blood-derived multipotent stem cells. BMC Medicine. 2012;10(3):1-11.

13. Yong Zhao, Theodore M. Human cord blood stem cells and the journey to a cure for type 1 diabetes. Autoimmun Rev. Epub. 2010;10(2):103–107.

14. Yong Zhao. Stem cell educator therapy and induction of immune balance. Curr Diab Rep. 2012;12(5):517–523.

15. David Bleich. Diabetes care. 2009;32(11): 2138–2139.

16. Available: http://www.eurocord-ed.org/

17. Dominici M, Le Blanc K, Mueller I, Slaper Cortenbach I, Marini FC, Krause DS. Minimal criteria for defining multipotent mesenchymal stromal cells. The international society for cellular therapy position statement. Cytotherapy. 2006; 8(4): 315–317.

18. Uccelli A, Moretta L, Pistoia V. Mesenchymal stem cells in health and disease. Nature Reviews Immunology. 2008;8(9):726–735.

19. Schugar RC, Chirieleison SM, Wescoe KE, Schmidt BT, Askew Y, Nance JJ, et al. Autologous umbilical cord blood infusion for type 1 diabetes. Journal of Biomedicine and Biotechnology. 2009;1.

20. Sun J, Allison J, Mc Laughlin C, Sledge L, Waters-Pick B, Wease S, Kurtzberg J. Differences in quality between privately and publicly banked umbilical cord blood units: A pilot study of autologous cord blood infusion in children with acquired neurological disorders. Transfusion. 2010; 50(9):1980–1987.

21. Giordano A, Galderisi U, Marino IR. From the laboratory bench to the patient's bedside: An update on clinical trials with mesenchymal stem cells. Exp. Hematol. 2007;211 (1): 27–35.

22. Maurya DK, Chiyo K, Atsushi P, Marla MK, Clay W, Zhihong T, Deryl T, Masaaki. Therapy with un-engineered naive rat umbilical cord matrix stem cells markedly inhibits growth of murine lung adenocarcinoma. BMC Cancer. 2010;10: 590.

23. Fu YS, Cheng YC, Lin MY, Cheng H, Chu PM, Chou SC, Shih YH, Ko MH,Sung MS. Conversion of human umbilical cord mesenchymal stem cells in Wharton's jelly to dopaminergic neurons in vitro: Potential therapeutic application for Parkinsonism. Stem Cells. 2006;24(1):115–124.

24.   Liu Y. Therapeutic potential of human umbilical cord mesenchymal stem cells in the treatment of rheumatoid arthritis. Arthritis Research & Therapy. 2010;12(6): R210.

25.   Limin Wang, Tran I, Seshareddy K, Weiss ML, Detamore MS. A comparison of human bone marrow–derived mesenchymal stem cells and human umbilical cord–derived mesenchymal stromal cells for cartilage tissue engineering. Tissue Engineering Part A. 2009;15 (8):2259–2266.

26.   Rita A Melania LL, Tiziana L, Stefano DA, Giannuzzi P, Farina F, La RG. Wharton's jelly mesenchymal stem cells as candidates for beta cells regeneration: extending the differentiative and immunomodulatory benefits of adult mesenchymal stem cells for the treatment of type 1 diabetes. Stem Cell Reviews and Reports. 2008;7(23):342–363.

27.   Nietfield J, Pasquini MC, Logan BR, Verter F, Horowitz MM. Lifetime probabilities of hematopoietic stem cell transplantation in the U.S. Biology of Blood and Marrow Transplantation. 2008;14(3):316-322.

28.   World Marrow Donor Association. Policy Statement for the Utility of Autologous or Family Cord Blood Unit Storage, World Marrow Donor Association; 2006.

29.   Hayani A, Lampeter E, Viswanatha D, Morgan D, Salvi SN. First report of autologous cord blood transplantation in the treatment of a child with leukemia. Pediatrics. 2007;119(1):296-300.

30.   Haller MJ, Viener HL, Wasserfall C, Brusko T, Atkinson MA, Schatz DA. Autologous umbilical cord blood infusion for type 1 diabetes. Exp. Hematol. 2008;36(6):710–715.

31.   Bojanic I, Golubic Cepulic B. Umbilical cord blood as a source of stem cells. Acta Med Croatica. 2006;60(3):215-25.

32.   Cohena Y, Nagler A. Hematopoietic stem-cell transplantation using umbilical-cord blood. Leuk Lymphoma. 2003;44(8): 1287-99.

33.   Sun JM, Kurtzberg J. Cord blood for brain injury. Cytotherapy; 2015.

34.   Cany J, Dolstra H, Shah N. Umbilical cord blood-derived cellular products for cancer immunotherapy. Cytotherapy; 2015.

35.   Milano F, Boelens JJ. Stem cell comparison: What can we learn clinically from unrelated cord blood transplantation

as an alternative stem cell source? Cytotherapy; 2015.

36.   Lindemans CA, Van Besien K. Topping it up: methods to improve cord blood transplantation outcomes by increasing the number of CD34$^+$ cells. Cytotherapy; 2015.

37.   Horwitz ME, Frassoni F. Improving the outcome of umbilical cord blood transplantation through ex vivo expansion or graft manipulation. Cytotherapy; 2015; 17:4.

38.   Mazini L, Matar N, Bouhya S, Marzouk D, Anwar W, Khyatti M. Umbilical Cord Blood Banking for Transplantation in Morocco: Problems and opportunities. J Stem Cells Regen Med. 2014;10(2):28-37.

39.   Rao M, Ahrlund-Richter L, Kaufman D.S. Concise review: Cord blood banking, transplantation and induced pluripotent stem cell: success and opportunities. Stem Cells. 2012;30(1):55-60.

40.   Jeannette Cany, Harry Dolstra, Nina Shah. Umbilical cord blood–derived cellular products for cancer immunotherapy. Cytotherapy; 2015.

41.   Binbin He, Xia Li, Haibo Yu, Zhiguang Zhou. Therapeutic potential of umbilical cord blood cells for type 1 diabetes mellitus. Journal of Diabetes; 2015.

42.   Abbas Shafiee, Nicholas MF, Dietmar WH, Kiarash K, Jatin Patel. Fetal Endothelial and Mesenchymal Progenitors from the human term placenta: Potency and clinical potential. Stem cells Translational Medicine; 2015.

43.   Tamari Ronia, Castro-Malaspina Hugoa, Allogeneic haematopoietic stem cell transplantation for primary myelofibrosis and myelofibrosis evolved from other myeloproliferative neoplasms. Current Opinion in Hematology. 2015;22(2): 184–190.

44.   Patrick JH, Catherine MB, Claudio GB. Adoptive immunotherapy with the use of regulatory T cells and virus-specific T cells derived from cord blood. Cytptherapy; 2015.

45.   Wataru Ebina, Derrick JR. Transcription factor-mediated reprogramming toward hematopoietic stem cells. EMBO Journal. 2015;34(6):694–709.

46.   Hordyjewska A, Popiołek L, Horecka A. Characteristics of Hematopoietic Stem Cells of Umbilical Cord Blood. Cytotechnology. 2015;67(3):387-96.

47. Munoz J, Shah N, Rezvani K, Hosing C, Bollard CM, Oran B, Olson A, Popat U, Molldrem J, Niece, IK, Shpall EJ. Concise Review: Umbilical cord blood transplantation: Past, present and future. Stem Cells Transl Med. 2014;3(12): 1435-43.

48. Betul Oran, Elizabeth Shpall. Umbilical cord blood transplantation: A maturing technology. Hematology. 2012;1:215-222.

49. Margie Castillo-Melendez, Tamara Yawno, Graham Jenkin, Suzanne LM. Stem cell therapy to protect and repair the developing brain: A review of mechanisms of action of cord blood and amnion epithelial derived cells. Front Neurosci. 2013;7:194.

50. Liu L, Yu Y, Hou Y, Chai J, Duan H. Human umbilical cord mesenchymal stem cells transplantation promotes cutaneous wound healing of severe burned rats. PLOS ONE. 2014;9(2):e88348.

51. Ali H, Bahbahani H. Umbilical cord blood stem cells - potential therapeutic tool for neural injuries and disorders. Acta Neurobiol Exp (Wars). 2010;70(3):316-24.

52. Eliane Gluckman MD, Hal EB. Hematopoietic reconstitution in a patient with Fanconi's anemia by means of umbilical-cord blood from an HLA-identical sibling. N Engl J Med. 1989;321: 1174-1178.

53. Margie Castillo-Melendez, Tamara Yawno, Graham Jenkin, Suzanne LM. Stem cell therapy to protect and repair the developing brain: A review of mechanisms of action of cord blood and amnion epithelial derived cells. Front Neurosci. 2013;7:194.

54. Harris DT, Rogers I. Umblical cord blood: a unique source for regenerative medicine. Curr Stem Cell Res Ther. 2007;2:301-309.

55. Herranz H, Hong X, Pérez L, Ferreira A, Olivieri D, Cohen SM, Milán M. The miRNA machinery targets Mei-P26 and regulates Myc protein levels in the *Drosophila* wing. EMBO. 2010;29(10): 1688-1698.

Anti-HBc and HBV-DNA among Blood Donors in North Africa; Western Libya

Mohamed Kaled A. Shambesh[1*], Ezzadin Areaf Franka[2], Faisal Fathalla Ismail[3], Nagi Meftah Gebril[4], Kamel Ahmed Azabi[4] and Fatma Amar[4]

[1]*Department of Community Medicine, Medical Faculty, University of Tripoli, Libya.*
[2]*Department of Community Medicine, Faculty of Medicine, University of Tripoli, Libya.*
[3]*Department of Medical Science, Faculty of Medical Technology, Omar Al Mukhtar University, Tobruk, Libya.*
[4]*Department of Community Medicine, University of Tripoli, Central Blood Bank, Tripoli, Libya.*

Authors' contributions

This work was carried out in collaboration between all authors. Authors MKAS and FFI designed the study, wrote the protocol and the first draft of the manuscript. Authors FFI and EAF managed the literature searches and helped in discussion writing. Authors MKAS and FFI done the analyses of the study with help of statisticians. Authors NMG, KAA and FA done and supervised the laboratory work. All authors read and approved the final manuscript.

Editor(s):
(1) Armel Hervé Nwabo Kamdje, University of Ngaoundere-Cameroon, Ngaoundere, Cameroon.
Reviewers:
(1) Celso Eduardo Olivier, Department of allergy and immunology, Instituto Alergoimuno de Americana, Brazil.
(2) Krishna Institute of Medical Sciences University, India.
(3) Anonymous, University of Kentucky, USA.
(4) Janaina Luz Narciso Schiavon, Department of Internal Medicine, Federal University of Santa Catarina, Brazil.

ABSTRACT

Background: Post transfusion hepatitis B (PTHB) continues to be an important public health concern with regard to blood transfusion in Libya and in Africa. This concern is related to the screening test which is still used but it is not enough to detect infective cases during window period.
Objectives: To determine the presence of total anti-HBc (hepatitis B core antibodies) and HBV-DNA (hepatitis B viral DNA (in healthy HBsAg (hepatitis B surface antigen) negative blood donors in Tripoli-Libya, North Africa.
Methods: A total of 1256 HBsAg negative blood samples, obtained from healthy blood donors who attended Tripoli's central blood bank, were tested for anti-HBc using the VITROS® 3600

*Corresponding author: E-mail: mkshambesh@yahoo.com

Immunodiagnostic System. The reactive samples were further tested for the presence of HBV-DNA.

Results: From the sample of 1256, 123 (10%) were total anti-HBc positive. Of the 123 anti-HBc positive samples, 13 (10.5%) tested positive for HBV-DNA by PCR (Polymerase chain reaction). The frequency of anti-HBc positive cases among the voluntary donors was 59.2%, and among the replacement donors was 40.7% ($p<0.0001$). The number of anti-HBc positive samples was found to be particularly high in the age group 30-39 years 44).7%) ($p<0.0001$).

All the positive PCR samples were from the age groups 20-39 and 40-59 with highest prevalence among 20-29 ($p<0.0001$). Most occupation who had positivity with anti-HBc and HBV-DNA were civil governmental workers specially militants, free workers and was less in students. Most positive cases were from east of Tripoli the capital (Tagora, SoqAljomaha).

Conclusion: The frequency of anti-HBc among this sample was 10% which is high compared with the international findings. The current study estimated the expected exclusion rate of anti-HBc positive donated blood, as this would be an important factor to consider before adopting anti-HBc testing in addition to HBsAg testing as a mandatory screening test to further enhance transfusion safety.

Keywords: Hepatitis B virus; blood donors; HBsAg; anti-HBc; HBV-DNA; PCR; Libya.

ABBREVIATIONS

HBV-DNA : hepatitis B viral DNA

PTHB : Post transfusion hepatitis B

HBsAg : hepatitis B surface antigen

Anti-HBc : hepatitis B core antibodies

PCR : Polymerase chain reaction

1. INTRODUCTION

Hepatitis B virus infection (HBV) continues to be a major public health problem. More than 240 million people worldwide have chronic hepatitis B infection, leading to the death of more than half a million people each year due to its serious consequences [1]. The prevalence of chronic HBV carriers in Libya is considered to be within the lower limit of the intermediate zone of HBV epidemicity as classified by WHO [2], with a prevalence rate of 2.2% [3].

Considerable efforts have been made by the health authorities in Libya to track and prevent the disease. Perhaps the most important steps have been the adoption of the hepatitis B vaccine for all newborns within the national immunization programe started in the early 1990s, and the screening of blood donors for the presence of HBsAg in the 1980s [4]. However, screening for HBV infection in blood donors in Libya is limited to HBsAg testing, even though several studies have clearly demonstrated that a percentage of donors who are HBsAg negative but anti-HBc positive (which means chronic or acute cases of HBV in the window period) would have been found to be carrying HBV-DNA in their blood when tested using PCR, and thus these donors may be a potential source of PTHB [5-8]. In addition, evidence of PTHB from such donors have been reported by a number of studies, which recommend that the implementation of anti-HBc testing, along with HBsAg testing, of blood donors would help to detect additional HBV-infected donors and improve the safety of blood transfusion specially in countries with high prevalence of HBV [9-12].

Such screening is important especially when considering the lack of an advanced testing system for HBV, such as nucleic acid testing (NAT). The present study has been conducted to determine the seroprevalence of anti-HBc in blood donors in western Libya (Tripoli area), as well as to estimate the presence of HBV-DNA in blood samples that are positive for anti-HBc but negative for HBsAg, and to estimate the exclusion rate of the anti-HBc positive donated blood. This would be an important factor for the health authorities to consider before adopting anti-HBc testing in addition to HBsAg testing as a mandatory screening test to increase transfusion safety.

2. MATERIALS AND METHODS

2.1 Study Design

The study was a Cross sectional study.

2.2 Area

North West of Libya, Tripoli the capital.

2.3 Time

Done in 2014 for one year.

2.4 Ethical Consideration

The study protocol was reviewed and approved by the Ethical Committees of National Authority for Scientific Research (NASR) of Libya. All participants endorsed a written informed consent form.

2.5 Study Population, Design and Sample Size

A total of 1256 blood samples were obtained from healthy blood donors who attended Tripoli's central blood bank during the year 2014. This blood bank serves neighboring cities as well as Tripoli. The donors were interviewed and medically examined before transfusion, as per the blood bank's standard operating protocol; any donors who were anaemic, or who had low body weight or low blood pressure at the time of donation, were excluded. All the donors were counseled and informed about the study, and consent was obtained from each donor to collect an anonymous sample of serum to be used in this study.

Anonymous questionnaires were completed by each donor, which included personal and demographic data. Donors who were donating blood to their relatives or friends were classified as replacement donors, and donors who were donating blood voluntarily were classified as voluntary donors.

2.6 Serological Analysis

All mandatory screening tests for blood-transmitted infections, such as HBsAg, anti-HCV and anti-HIV (anti-HIV-1 and -2), were performed in the central blood bank using the VITROS® 3600 Immunodiagnostic System (France) which is fully automated serologic analyzer. All blood samples which gave a negative result in these tests were simultaneously tested for anti- HBc using the same analyzer in the central blood bank of Tripoli.

2.7 Real-time PCR

All anti-HBc-reactive samples were then further tested by PCR for the presence of HBV-DNA; 500 µL of each sample was extracted, amplified and target HBV DNA fragment detected using the COBAS® AmpliPrep/COBAS® TaqMan® HBV Test, v2.0 system (analysis conducted in France by Taqman Roche, Cerba). The test procedure was carried out according to the manufacturer's instructions. The sensitivity of the real-time PCR used is 20 IU/mL; the conversion factor is 1 IU= 5.82 copies [13,14]. The real-time PCR was performed once.

2.8 Data Statistical Analysis

Was performed using Statistical Package for Social Science (SPSS) computer software (Version 19, SPSS Inc. USA). The contributing blood donors were divided into age groups. Data was calculated and described by using mean, mode, standard deviation, cross tabulations and graphical presentations. A chi-square test was performed to examine and compare the seroprevalence of anti-HBc between age groups.

3. RESULTS

The majority of the donors were males (1248, or 99.4%) and 8 (0.06%) were females. Their age range were from 16 to 93 years old (mean age 34±8.9). Donors occupations were concentrated mainly in civil governmental workers specially militants, free workers and students. The donor population had not previously been screened for anti-HBc.

The donors were from different regions of the Tripoli metropolitan area like Tagora, SoqAljomaha in the east, Alfernag, Almadina Alrithia in the center and Alsrage, Hayalandlas in the west. Of the total 1256, 653 (52%) were voluntary donors who had donated more than once before and have very high risk to transfer hepatitis to others if not diagnosed during the window gap, and 603 (48%) were replacement donors, who were donating only for their relatives or friends for the first time are less dangers because they are not repeaters of blood donation as they may infect their relatives only.

Anti-HBc screening was performed simultaneously with the other mandatory screening tests for blood transmitted infections; 123 samples gave positive results for anti-HBc, giving an overall prevalence 10%.

The frequency of anti-HBc positive cases among the voluntary donors was 59.3% (73 persons), and among the replacement donors it was 40.7% (50 persons) ($p<0.0001$) (Fig.1). The number of anti-HBc positive samples was found to be particularly high in the age group 30-39 years (44.7%) ($p<0.0001$) (Fig. 2 & Table 1).

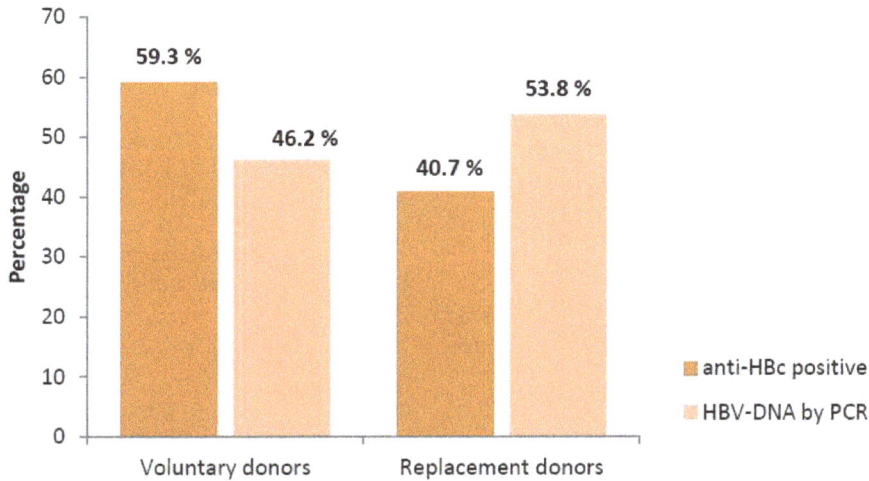

Fig. 1. Frequency of anti-HBc and HBV-DNA in voluntary and replacement donors

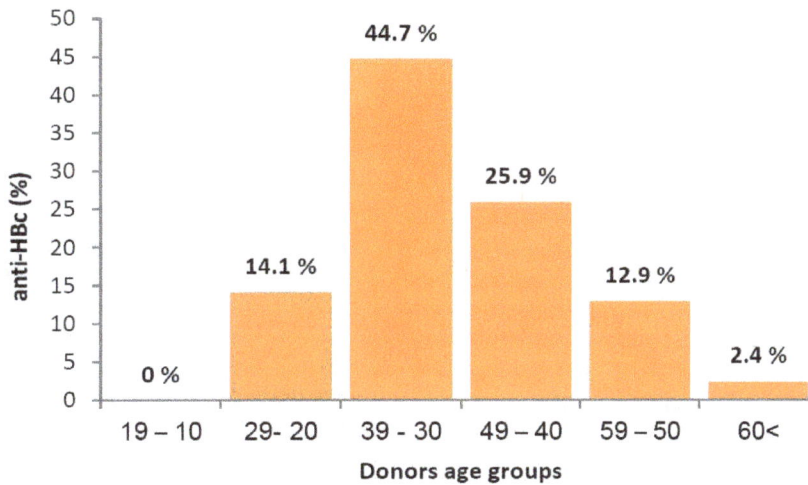

Fig. 2. Percentage of anti-HBc among different age groups

Table 1. Showing age groups screened by total anti-HBc and PCR

Age group	Number of donors screened	Anti-HBc positive cases among whole samples	PCR positive cases (HBV-DNA) among anti-HBc positive cases
10-19	20	0	0
20-29	406	17 (13.8%)	4 (23.5%)
30-39	475	55 (44.7%)	3 (5.5%)
40-49	257	32 (26%)	5 (15.6%)
40-49	80	16 (13%)	1(6.3%)
40-49	18	3 (2.4%)	0
Total	1256	123 (10%)	13 (10.5%)

All anti-HBc positive samples were tested by quantitative real-time PCR. Thirteen samples were found to test positive for HBV-DNA. This figure represents 1% of the whole sample and 10.5% of the anti-HBc positive samples. All the positive PCR samples were from the age groups 20-39 and 40-59 (Fig. 3) with highest prevalence among 20-29 years old ($p<0.0001$) (Table 1). The frequency of HBV-DNA positive cases among the voluntary donors was 46.2%, and among the replacement donors was 53.8%. This confirms that replacement donors in this sample had high positivity rate of HBV-DNA compared to volunteers ($p<0.0001$) (Fig. 1).

Most occupations had positivity with anti-HBc and HBV-DNA were civil governmental workers specially militants and free workers but less in students. Most positive cases were from east of Tripoli the capital (Tagora, Soq Aljomaha).

Exclusion rate for anti-HBc positive donated blood was calculated and estimated that approximately one hundred blood units would be excluded from every thousand donated units if anti-HBc testing were adopted. Moreover, the study estimates that ten donated units per thousand may potentially be infected with HBV.

4. DISCUSSION

Currently, HBsAg is the only serological marker used for the screening of blood donors for HBV infection in most blood transfusion centers in Libya. This study investigated the prevalence of anti-HBc and HBV-DNA in healthy blood donors who had tested negative for HBsAg and other mandatory blood-transmitted infection screening in Libyan transfusion centers. The study examined 1256 healthy blood donors who attended the central blood bank in Tripoli and found that the frequency of anti-HBc among this sample was 123 (10%). This percentage was low in comparison with the findings of a previous pilot study (15.6%) that was conducted by the same authors in the same region, though this difference may be due to the difference in study size [15]. However, the percentage was similar to the results of a preliminary study (9.8%) conducted by the authors in the same place earlier in the same year (2014) [16].

A similar prevalence rate (10.96%) of anti-HBc among HBsAg-negative blood donors was reported in the neighboring country, Egypt [17], although another study in Egypt reported a lower prevalence rate (7.8%) [18]. The reported prevalence of anti-HBc is lower in areas of low endemicity in Europe, where the reported percentages vary between 0.07% in the UK and 1.5% in Germany [19] and are slightly higher (4.85%) in Italy [20].

In contrast, the prevalence has been found to be high in Kuwait (17%) [21], in the Kingdom of Saudi Arabia (15.32%) [22] and Iran (6.5%) [23], and very high (42%) in Sudan. This may be due to the fact that HBV infection is highly endemic in Sudan, as classified by WHO [24].

The prevalence of HBV-DNA in anti-HBc positive donors was 10.5%; this figure was high compared with the previous pilot study (3%) conducted by the authors in the same region [15]. This percentage is similar to that found in Egypt (11.54%) [17]; however, it is higher than that reported (6.25%) in another study in Egypt [18] and higher than the 4.86% reported in Italy [20]. It is broadly similar to the 12.2% found in Iran [23]. These differences could be related to the endemicity of HBV infection among different countries.

The detection of HBV-DNA in anti-HBc positive samples "anti-HBc alone" may be due to chronic unresolved infection with low grade, possibly intermittent virus production and persistent HBV infection, or it may signify the window period in new HBV infection during which anti-HBc is the only detectable marker of recent hepatitis infection. The infection of HBV can be transmitted from HBsAg negative individuals through blood transfusion or organ transplantation [25-27].

As this study estimates that approximately one hundred blood units would be excluded from every thousand donated units if anti-HBc testing were adopted and ten donated units per thousand may potentially be infected with HBV. We recommend that the introduction of anti-HBc screening, at least for first-time donors, would help to detect further infected donors and improve the safety of blood donation. In addition, the introduction of anti-HBc testing would help to identify more chronic HBV carriers; this may allow early access to therapy and thus prevent the serious consequences of HBV infection.

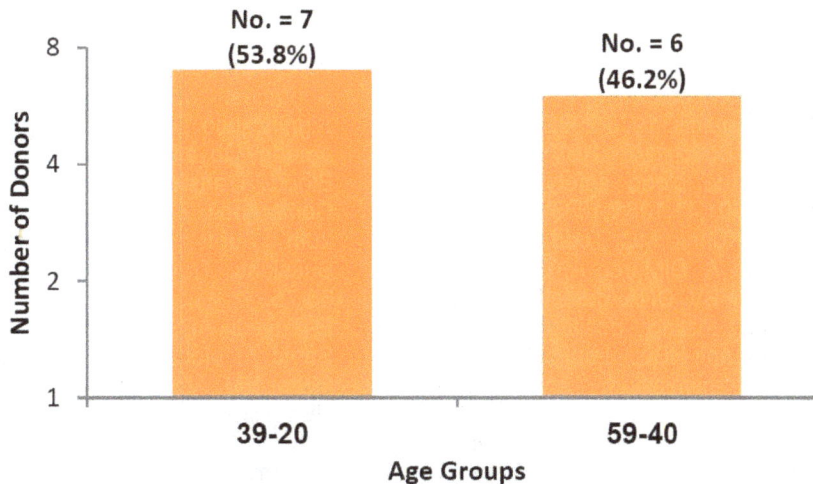

Fig. 3. HBV-DNA positive samples among the age groups

5. CONCLUSION

In conclusion, the prevalence rate of anti-HBc in this study (10%) was low in comparison with a previous study in the region. However, the study emphasizes the importance of implementing anti-HBc in addition to HBsAg testing as mandatory screening tests to further increase transfusion safety. The study also recommends that donated blood from donors who are HBsAg negative but anti-HBc positive should be discarded. In addition, the study has estimated the exclusion rate for anti-HBc positive donated blood, which is an important factor for health authorities to consider before adopting anti-HBc testing as an additional mandatory screening test to enhance the safety of transfusions.

6. STRENGTHS and LIMITATIONS OF THE STUDY

It is the first Libyan big laboratory based study that used anti-HBc and PCR to detect the positivity of hepatitis B disease among blood donors in Libya. Moreover, it uses enough sample size, thus, the result produced from this study reflect the real situation in the Libyan populations living in the capital Tripoli but cannot be generalized among the whole general blood donors of Libya.

7. RECOMMENDATION

To do other studies to measure anti-HBc and PCR in other parts of Libya specially the South

as there is a high level of immigration status in that area.

ACKNOWLEDGEMENTS

The authors would like to thank all staff of the central blood bank of Tripoli. This research is supported by the National Authority for Scientific Research (NASR), Libya.

COMPETING INTERESTS

Authors have declared that no competing interests exist.

REFERENCES

1. World Health Organization. Hepatitis B Virus Infection Fact Sheet. 2013 (No. 204). Available:http://www.who.int/mediacentre/factsheets/fs204/en/
    (Accessed on 23/11/2014)

2. Lavanchy D. Hepatitis B virus epidemiology, disease burden, treatment, and current and emerging prevention and control measures. Journal of Viral Hepatitis. 2004;11:97-107.

3. Daw MA, El-Bouzedi A. In association with Libyan Study Group of hepatitis and HIV prevalence of hepatitis B and hepatitis C infection in Libya: Results from a national population based survey. BMC Infectious Diseases. 2013;14:17-17.

4. Elzouki AN. Hepatitis B infection in Libya: The magnitude of the problem. The Libyan

Journal of Infectious Diseases. 2008;2:20-25.

5.   Lander JJ, Gitnick GL, Gelb LH, Aach RD. Anti-core antibody screening of transfused blood. Vox Sanguinis. 1978;298:77-80.

6.   Kleinman SH, Busch MP. HBV: Amplified and back in the blood safety spotlight. Transfusion. 2001;41:1081-1085.

7.   Kleinman SH, Kuhns MC, Todd DS, Glynn SA, McNamara A, DiMarco A, Busch MP. Frequency of HBV DNA detection in US blood donors testing positive for the presence of anti-HBc: Implications for transfusion transmission and donor screening. Transfusion. 2003;43:696-704.

8.   Dreier J, Krogr M, Diekmann J, Gotting C, Kleesiek K. Low-level viraemia of hepatitis B virus in an anti-HBc and anti-HBs positive blood donors. Transfusion Medicine. 2004; 14 :97-103.

9.   Aach RD, Kahn RA. Post-transfusion Hepatitis: Current perspectives. Annals of Internal Medicine. 1980;92:539-546.

10. Mosley JW, Stevens CE ,Aach RD, Hollinger FB ,Mimms LT, Solomon LR, ET AL. Donor screening for antibody to hepatitis B core antigen and hepatitis B virus infection in transfusion recipients. Transfusion. 1995;35:5-12.

11. Saraswat S, Banerjee K, Chaudhury N, Mahant T, Khandekar P, Gupta RK, Naik, S Post-transfusion hepatitis type B following multiple transfusions of HBsAg negative blood. Journal of Hepatology. 1996;25:639-643.

12. Shastry S, Bhat SS. Prevention of post-transfusion hepatitis by screening of antibody to hepatitis B core antigen in healthy blood donors. Mediterranean Journal of Hematology and Infectious Diseases. 2011;3:e2011-062.

13. Chevaliez S, Bouvier-Alias M, Laperche S, Pawlotsky JM. Performance of the Cobas AmpliPrep/Cobas TaqMan Real-Time PCR Assay for Hepatitis B Virus DNA Quantification. Journal of Clinical Microbiology. 2008;46:1716-1723.

14. Chevaliez S, Bouvier-Alias M, Laperche S, Hézode C, Pawlotsky JM. Performance of Version 2.0 of the Cobas AmpliPrep/Cobas TaqMan Real-Time PCR Assay for Hepatitis B Virus DNA Quantification. Journal of Clinical Microbiology. 2010;48: 3641-3647.

15. Ismail F, Shambesh MK, Aboutwerat A, Elbackush M. Serological and molecular characterization of total hepatitis B core antibodies in blood donors in Tripoli, Libya. The Libyan Journal of Infectious Diseases. 2010;4:24-30.

16. Shambesh MK, Franka EA, Ismail FF. Significance of Screening of anti-HBc among Libyan Blood Donor. The British Blood Transfusion Society 32nd Annual Conference 2014 Harrogate, UK, 24th - 26th September. Abstracts – Poster Sessions. Transfusion Medicine. 2014;24: 33-75.

17. El-Zayadi AR, Ibrahim EH, Badran HM, Saeid A, Moneib NA, Shemis MA, Abdel-Sattar RM, Ahmady AM, El-Nakeeb A. Anti-HBc screening in Egyptian blood donors reduces the risk of hepatitis B virus transmission. Transfusion Medicine. 2008; 18:55-61.

18. Antar W, El-Shokry MH, Abd El Hamid WA , Helmy MF. Significance of detecting anti-HBc among Egyptian male blood donors negative for HBsAg .Transfusion Medicine. 2010;20:409–413.

19. Candotti D, Allain JP. Transfusion-transmitted hepatitis B virus infection. Journal of Hepatology. 2009;51:798-809.

20. Manzini P, Girotto M, Borsotti R, Giachino O, Guaschino O, Lanter M, et al. Italian blood donors with anti-hbc and occult hepatitis B virus infection. Haematologica. 2007;92:1664-1670.

21. Ameen R, Sanad N, Al-Shemmari S, Siddique I, Chowdhury RI, Al-Hamdan S, Al- Bashir A. Prevalence of viral markers among first-time Arab blood donors in Kuwait. Transfusion. 2005;45:1973-1980.

22. Bashawri LA, Fawaz NA, Ahmad MS, Qadi AA, Almawi WY. Prevalence of seromarkers of HBV and HCV among blood donors in eastern Saudi Arabia, 1998-2001. Clinical & Laboratory Haematology. 2004;26:225-228.

23. Behzad-Behbahani A, Mafi-Nejad A, Tabei SZ, Lankarani KB, Torab A, Moaddeb A. Anti-HBc & HBV-DNA detection in blood donors negative for hepatitis B virus surface antigen in reducing risk of transfusion associated HBV infection. The Indian Journal of Medical Research.2006; 123:37-42.

24. Mahmoud OA, Ghazal AA, Metwally DE, Elnour AM, Yousif GE. Detection of occult hepatitis B virus infection among blood donors in Sudan. The Journal of the Egyptian Public Health Association. 2013; 88:14-18.

25. Hoofnagle JH, Seefe LB, Bales ZB, Zimmerman HJ. Type B hepatitis after transfusion with blood containing antibody to hepatitis B core antigen. The New England Journal of Medicine. 1978; 298:1379-1383.

26. Uemoto S, Sugiyama K, Marusawa H, Inomata Y, Asonuma K, Egawa H, Kiuchi T, Miyake Y, Tanaka K, Chiba T. Transmission of hepatitis B virus from hepatitis B core antibody-positive donors in living related liver transplants .Transplantation. 1998;65: 494-499.

27. Antje K, Arndt H, Harald H, Karin W, Wolfgang J. Serological pattern "anti-HBc alone": Characterization of 552 individuals and clinical significance. World J Gastroenterol. 2006;28:12(8): 1255–1260.

13

Microbicidal Activity of Neutrophils Isolated from HIV Patients

J. B. Borges[1], T. Sakurada Jr[1], N. C. S. Santana[2], N. A. Lima[2], S. Lautenschlaugher[1] and A. R. T. Pupulin[1*]

[1]*Department of Basic Health Sciences, State University of Maringa, Maringá, P.R. Brazil.*
[2]*Post Graduate Program in Pharmaceutical Sciences, State University of Maringa, Maringá, P.R. Brazil.*

Authors' contributions

This work was carried out in collaboration between all authors. Authors ARTP and SL designed the study, wrote the protocol, and wrote the first draft of the manuscript. Authors JBB and TSJ managed the literature searches, managed the experimental process. Authors NCSS and NAL performed the spectrophotometry analysis. All authors read and approved the final manuscript.

Editor(s):
(1) Armel Hervé Nwabo Kamdje, University of Ngaoundere, Ngaoundere, Cameroon.
Reviewers:
(1) Nipapan Malisorn, Division of pharmacology, Preclinical Sciences, Faculty of Medicine, Thammasat University, Pathumthani, Thailand.
(2) Anonymous, Brazil.
(3) Anonymous, Italy.
(4) Wagner Loyola, Embrapa Swine and Poultry, Concordia, Brazil.

ABSTRACT

HIV infection is associated with a progressive loss of T cell functional capacity and reduced responsiveness to antigenic stimuli. Neutrophils are crucial cellular components of the innate immune system. Current study evaluates the functional activity of neutrophils isolated from HIV/AIDS patients with similar clinical laboratory parameters differing only in the use of antiretroviral therapy (HAART). Two patients HIV/AIDS patients, a female and a male, were selected for this study, based on clinical history, general physical examination and laboratory tests. Further, two apparently healthy volunteers of the same age and gender former de control group. Neutrophils isolated from human peripheral blood were placed in contact with the yeast in a proportion of 1:10 leukocytes for 1 hour. PMN Fluorescence was detected in FL1 on a flow cytometer and results were recorded as fluorescence intensity and percentage of positive cells in

Corresponding author: E-mail: artpupulin@uem.br

the sample. HOCl formation was monitored by spectrophotometry based on the resulting taurine chloramine-forming reaction of hypochlorous acid with taurine. The experiments revealed that patient I with HAART had a 17.3% lower response activity of neutrophils when compared with the control in the production of hypochlorous acid with PMA stimulation. Patient II, who did not use HAART, was 81% less active than the control in the production of hypochlorous acid. The two patients had similar clinical laboratory parameters differing only in the number of CD4 cells, which was higher in Patient II. Results show that the patient submitted to antiretroviral treatment had a better quality of functional response of neutrophils although with fewer CD4 cells.

Keywords: AIDS; neutrophils; microbicidal activity; HOCl.

1. INTRODUCTION

Despite of 30 years of intensive research, our understanding of how HIV virus undermines the ability of the immune system against common infections is limited. Although we know that T cells, a key cell population that normally invading pathogens lose their function capacity in HIV infected individuals, the reason they do so is unknown. It has been discovered that HIV virus activates another type of cells, called neutrophils, the most common type of white cell in the blood. Activated neutrophils negatively affect the function of T cells and prevent them from producing cytokines, protective proteins that serve as messengers orchestrating the immune response to bacteria and viruses [1].

Neutrophils, the most abundant leukocyte population, are traditionally recognized as essential effector cells of the innate immune system in host defense against invading pathogens [2]. A new appreciation has recently emerged on the role of neutrophils in their interaction with and regulation of the adaptive arm of the immune system [2,3]. Neutrophils co-localize and actively communicate with T cells at sites of infection and migrate to the draining lymph nodes where they are involved in the induction and regulation of cellular and humoral immune responses by exerting a pro-inflammatory or anti-inflammatory function [4]. Accumulated evidence supports the role played by neutrophils in the negative regulation of T cell function via production of reactive oxygen species (ROS) [5-7].

Due to the functional importance of neutrophils in infection by microorganisms particularly with HIV, current study evaluates the microbicide activity of peripheral blood neutrophils of patients with HIV/AIDS when compared to the activity of a control group of healthy volunteer donors.

2. MATERIALS AND METHODS

2.1 Subjects

HIV/AIDS patients treated at the Center for Studies and Support to HIV Patients of the State University of Maringá (Department of Basic Health Sciences) were clinically evaluated and laboratory tests were performed prior to their participation in the projects.

2.2 Inclusion Criteria

Inclusion criteria comprised age between 35 and 45 years and 10 years infection time. After the explanation of the project, patients signed an informed consent approved by the Ethics and Research on Human Experimentation of the State University of Maringá.

Considering their clinical history, general physical examination and laboratory tests, two patients HIV/AIDS, a female and a male were selected for current study. Composite control group of two apparently healthy volunteers of the same age and gender of patients was also selected.

2.3 Clinical and Laboratory Analysis

The clinical history of each patient was obtained by the epidemiological record. The clinical aspects of several other systems (musculoskeletal, neurological, respiratory, cardiovascular, genitourinary and digestive) were evaluated during the general physical examination.

Laboratory evaluation comprised the number of total leukocytes and differential count of neutrophils and lymphocytes obtained by automated cell counter (MINDRAY BC-3000 Plus) coupled to microscopic evaluation. Evaluation of plasma levels of liver enzymes AST, ALT and GGT assessed liver function, total cholesterol, triglycerides and fasting glucose. All biochemical laboratory measurements were performed by specific commercial kits.

2.4 Isolation of Peripheral Neutrophils

2.4.1 Blood collection

Three experiments were performed for each patient, at an interval of at least 30 days. Samples for the HIV/AIDS patients and volunteers (control group) were drawn in experimental day. Samples were collected by anterior-ulnar venipuncture using vacuum collection system. During collection HIV testing was also carried out on patients and volunteers.

2.4.2 Isolation of neutrophils

The blood samples were collected in heparinized tubes (10 U/ml) and then diluted 1: 1 with 10 mM PBS. pH 7.4. The dilution was placed in 10 ml of Histopaque® (BOYUM 1968).

The material was centrifuged at 2500 rpm at room temperature for 20 minutes. An infranatant was added with 15 mL of 5% Dextran diluted in 10 mM PBS pH 7.4 for sterile sedimentation of erythrocytes. The material was kept in an ice bath (with a 45° inclination) for 45 minutes, the supernatant was collected (volume made up to 30 ml of 10 mM PBS) and centrifuged at 2500 rpm at room temperature for 5 minutes. The supernatant was discarded and the infranatant subjected to hemolysis in 10 ml of cold distilled water with constant stirring for one minute. Isotonicity was restored with 5 ml of 2.7% NaCl and 15 mL of sterile 10 mM PBS. The material was centrifuged at 2500 rpm at room temperature for 5 minutes, the supernatant was discarded and the infranatant resuspended in 1 ml RPMI.

2.5 Evaluation of Microbicidal Activity of Neutrophils

2.5.1 Determination of HOCl

HOCl formation was monitored by spectrophotometry based on the resulting taurine chloramine-forming reaction of hypochlorous acid with taurine. Neutrophils ($2x10^6$ cells/mL), activated or not with the standard strain of microorganisms in 10 mM phosphate buffer (pH 7.4) containing 140 mM NaCl, 1 mM CaCl2, 0.5mM $MgCl_2$ and 1 mg/mL glucose were incubated with 15 mM taurine at 37°C under

gentle agitation. The reaction was stopped after 30 minutes by adding of 20 ug/ml catalase (10 minutes, 2000 rpm). The concentration of taurine chloramine-present in the supernatant was estimated by acid oxidation of 5-thio-2-nitrobenzoic acid (TNB) with 5,5'-dithiobis-2-nitrobenzoic acid (DTNB) which measured the decrease in absorbance at 412 nm as described [8].

2.6 Statistical Analysis

Group-comparing statistics were performed with Graph Pad Prism 6.0 (Graph Pad, San Diego, CA, USA) with Student´s t test at p <0.05 considered statistically significant.

3. RESULTS

Two patients were selected for the study after clinical and laboratory examination. Patient I (M.E.D) 45 years old, CD4 cells levels 246 cells/µL, viral load < 50 copies/mL, with no history of liver disease, heart or hypertension. Clinical parameters were within normal levels. He was diagnosed for HIV 10 years ago with levels of CD4 cells 3 cells/µL, once diagnosed treatment began with antiretroviral therapy. Patient II (SRO) 38 years old, 10 years of infection without significant symptoms during the course of the disease, had no history of liver disease, diabetes and hypertension. Viral load 180 cells/µL and the amount of CD4 cells about 400 cells/µL. Post after diagnosis for HIV patient did not use antiretroviral therapy at the moment.

Two healthy volunteers were included in our study after confirmation they had no sign of acute inflammatory and infectious process such as sore throats, fractures, bacterial, fungal, viral and parasitic infections, or suffering from chronic inflammatory diseases.

Table 1 shows clinical laboratory parameters and levels of CD4 + lymphocytes of patients.

Table 2 shows levels of total leucocytes, neutrophils and lymphocytes of HIV patients.

Fig. 1 shows the production of HOCl (hypochlorous acid) of neutrophils (PMN) in healthy patients and HIV-positive patients.

Results show lower activity neutrophils obtained from Patient I in response to the stimulus compared to control, which is 17.3% lower than the control response in the production of hypochlorous acid prior to PMA stimulation.

Table 1. Clinical and laboratory parameters of HIV patients

HIV patient	Gender/Age	Infection time (years)	CD4 cells/mm^3/viral load	HAART	clinical laboratory changes
I	Male/45	10	246 cells /< 50 copies/mL	For 10 years	no
II	Female/38	14	400 cells/180 copies/mL	Not use	no

Table 2. Levels of total leucocytes, neutrophils and lymphocytes of HIV patients

HIV patient	Total leucocytes cells/mm^3	Neutrophils cells/mm^3	Lymphocytes cells/mm^3
I	3,400	1,496	1,394
II	3,500	1,620	1,295

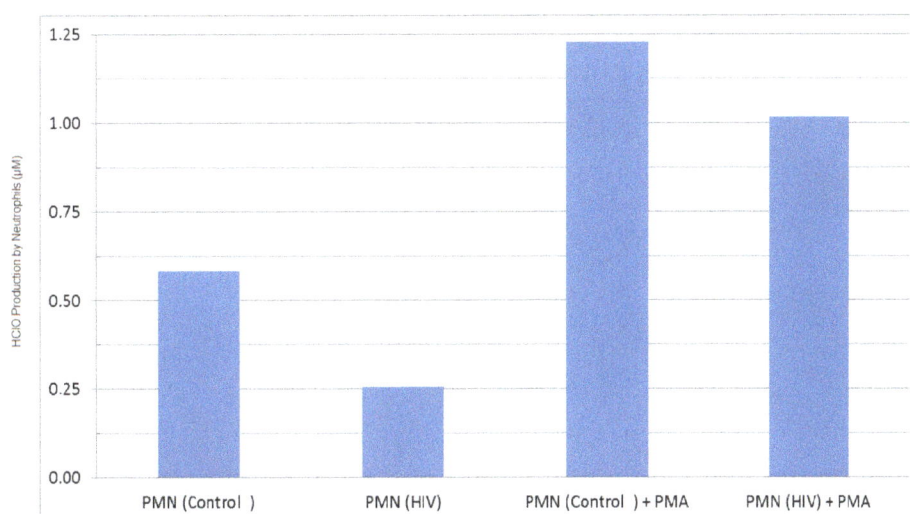

Fig. 1. Determination of the formation of HOCl (hypochlorous acid) accompanied by spectrophotometry of patient I (HIV/AIDS) compared to control, a male without disease
Fig. 1 Production of HOCl (hypochlorous acid) of neutrophils (PMN) in healthy patient and HIV patient I. Comparison of HOCl production of neutrophils (2.0 x 10^6 cells / ml) from healthy patients and in patients with to virus or not stimulated with PMA was determined by spectrophotometry at 655nm

Fig. 2 shows the results of lower activity neutrophils obtained from Patient II in response to stimulus when compared to control, which is 81% lower than the control response in the production of hypochlorous acid prior to PMA stimulation.

Table 3 shows the hypochlorous acid production by neutrophils isolated from the HIV patients compared to healthy controls.

4. DISCUSSION

Neutrophils are crucial cellular components of the innate immune system. They are the first cells recruits to sites of microbial challenges or injury. An essential function of neutrophils include their ability to promptly generate and

release copious amount of reactive oxygen species (ROS) in a process referred to as oxidative burst. The production of ROS is critical to neutrophil antimicrobial activities. A deficiency in oxidative metabolism may result in immune impairment, as may be seen in chronic granulomatous disease [9].

People infected with HIV become progressively immunodeficient, a process that exposes infected individuals to an escalating risk of opportunistic infections. Even though HIV immunodeficiency is generally etiologically likened to CD4 lymphocytes, opportunistic infections organisms observed during HIV disease (i.e. *Pneumocystis carinii*, *Candida albicans* or *Mycobacterium avium)* are suggestive of immunodeficiency in other immune cell type such as neutrophil [10,11]. *Ex vivo* peripheral neutrophils isolated from HIV infected subjects display a dysfunctional phenotype of impaired chemotaxis and deregulated production of ROS [12,13]. ROS production in HIV individuals has been reported to be either exaggerated or reduced when compared to con troll HIV infected subjects. Deregulated responses to stimulation and/or inhibition of neutrophil oxidative metabolism may therefore contribute towards immune dysfunction and oxidative stress in HIV disease [14].

Consequently, repeated microbial challenges and/or inflammatory conditions in the course of HIV disease is likely to result in disproportionate neutrophil oxidative activity, which in turn would aggravate oxidative stress resulting in infections, increased HIV viremia and cardiovascular disease. Consequently, infection and inflammation are a crucial aspect in the management of HIV disease [14].

So that important functions of leukocytes, such as phagocytosis and microbicidal activity, could be maintained, their chemotactic function is preserved [15]. In patients with infections and sepsis to reduce, the neutrophil chemotactic function compared to healthy volunteers. It may be suggested that dysfunction contributes towards the development of infection [16]. In Infectious diseases such as AIDS, the role of neutrophils as a defense cells is well documented In other words, the antiretroviral drugs increase the chemotaxis of neutrophils and monocytes and reduce the incidence of infections [17].

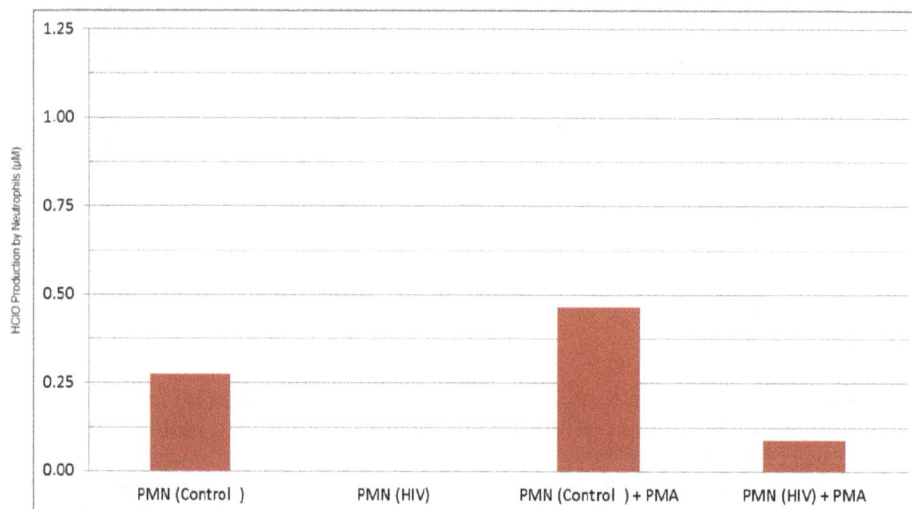

Fig. 2. Determination of the formation of HOCl (hypochlorous acid) accompanied by spectrophotometry of patient II (HIV/AIDS) compared to control, a female did not have the disease

Fig. 2 production of HOCl (hypochlorous acid) of neutrophils (PMN) in healthy patient and HIV patient II. Comparison of HOCl production of neutrophils (2.0 x 10^6 cells / ml) from healthy patients and patients with virus or not stimulated with PMA was determined by spectrophotometry at 655nm

Table 3. Production of hypochlorous acid by neutrophils isolated from HIV patients compared to controls

HIV Patient	PMN	PMN (HIV)	PMN + PMA	PMN(HIV) +PMA
I	4.495±0.37	3.228±0.24	5.268±0.39	4.110±0.13*
II	0.275±0,15	- 0.1±0.001	0.463±0.06	0.088±0.03*

Results were expressed as mean ± SD from at least three independent experiments, with *p≤0.05 considered significant%.PMN (control) = leukocytes isolated from control patient PMN (HIV) = polymorphonuclear leukocytes isolated from HIV-infected patient, PMN (control) + PMA = polymorphonuclear leukocytes isolated from control patients with PMA stimulation to evaluate the production of hypochlorous acid leukocytes PMN (HIV) + PMA = polymorphonuclear leukocytes isolated from HIV patient infected with PMA stimulation to evaluate the hypochlorous acid production by leukocytes

With the evolution of HIV infection, some individuals have physiological and functional changes such as oxidative stress (OS) which enhance the immune dysfunction and promotes an increase in viral replication [18]. In addition, OS may promote apoptosis of T cells and is involved in the mechanism of induction of tumor necrosis factor (TNF) -α [19].

Several studies indicate that human immunodeficiency syndrome is associated with morphological abnormalities in the bone marrow and a decrease of progenitor blood cells. The depletion of these cells could be explained by the same mechanism of apoptosis, including neutrophils, changes in cytokine or other immune factors [20]. Research reveals that progenitor cells from bone marrow of HIV-infected patients undergo apoptosis. Further, the apoptosis of these cells occurs through the Fas-L, cytokine produced by activated T cells, a mechanism by which T cells activated fighting cells infected with HIV [21]. This suggests a mechanism in reducing the chances number of neutrophils and, other cells in HIV-infected patients.

In the late phase of HIV infection, there is a decrease in serum levels of IL-2 and IFN-γ and IL-4 and IL-10 increased with decrease of the adaptive immune response. HAART may lead to an increase in pro inflammatory cytokines such as TNFα. The balance of cytokines such as IL-6, TNFα and IL-10 contributes to the establishment of equilibrium which can be determinant of disease progression.

The above changes may result from the evolution of the infection itself or induced by the use of some drugs of antiretroviral therapy presenting myelosuppressive activity. Results comprise progressive decrease in blood cellularity [22] when compared to healthy patients without HIV.

Although current study presents different results similar the production of HOCl by patients with the same infection period the difference lies in the fact that Patient I uses antiretroviral therapy and patient II does not (Table 3, Figs. 1 and 2). Table 2 also demonstrate that the patients have very similar numbers of total leukocytes, lymphocytes and neutrophils.

On the other hand, as Table 1 shows the number of CD4 cells is higher in Patient II (400 cells/mm^3) when compared to that Patient I (246 cells/mm^3). This fact serves as a laboratory parameter to indicate the non-use of antiretroviral by Patient II.

Results obtained in current study with patients isolated neutrophils indicate that Patient I had a better functional response of neutrophils when compared to Patient II although with a smaller number of CD4 cells. Table 1 shows the number of CD4 cells, or rather, Patient II (400 cells/mm^3) shows highest number with respect to the patient I (246 cells/mm^3). The cells CD4 rate serves as a laboratory parameter to indicate the use of antiretroviral drugs by patients, this patient mode II has no laboratory indication for use of antiretroviral

Results obtained in current study of patients with isolated neutrophils indicate that the Patient I has a better functional response of neutrophils when compared to the Patient II although it has a smaller number of CD4 cells. Thus, the importance of the functional capacity of neutrophils and not merely the number of cells (total leukocytes, lymphocytes, neutrophils and CD4 cells) should be underscored, a fact evidenced in this study.

Despite recent advances in the understanding of HIV infection, major scientific incognita remain and HIV infection is still a global challenge for mankind. Viruses exclusively depend on the host's cellular machinery for their propagation and survival and therefore need to invade the host's cell. HIV infection is associated with a progressive loss of T cells functional capacity and reduced responsiveness to antigenic stimuli. The mechanisms underlying T cell dysfunction in HIV/AIDS are not completely understood. Current author have indicate that HIV virus activates another type of cells, neutrophils, the most common type of white cell in the blood. Activated neutrophils negatively affect the function of the T cells and prevent them from producing cytokines, protective proteins that serve as messengers orchestrating the immune response to bacteria and viruses [1].

HIV establishes persistent infection in human subjects. Although antiretroviral therapy prevents AIDS-related complications and prolongs life expectancy. HIV-1 infected patients have several comorbidities that are usually observed during the human aging process. PMNs are a key component of the early innate response to bacterial and fungal pathogens. In response to pathogens, PMNs rapidly migrate from the blood to inflamed tissues, where their activation triggers microbicidal mechanisms as rapid production of reactive oxygen species (ROS) in oxidative bursts [23]. After they kill microbes, PMNs die spontaneously, mainly through apoptosis. Although they have a very short lifespan their activation by circulating microbial products, as well as by proinflammatory mediators, promotes their survival. In fact, it is a critical mechanism in their effectiveness against pathogens. Nevertheless, inappropriate PMNs survive might lead to a chronic persistent inflammatory mediators and damage associated molecular patters through PMN necrosis [24]. Although PMNs are primarily protective, their inappropriate, excessive or prolonged activation presents the risk of tissue injury and organ dysfunction. It has been involved in various inflammatory diseases, including cardiovascular and osteoarticular disorders [25,26]. The results of this study corroborate these studies, as demonstrated that the patient (II) which is not used HAART showed a neutrophil response less than the patient (I) who used HAART confirming a direct effect of HIV on the quality immunological response of the host even with acceptable number of CD4 cells did.

Finally, further investigation should concentrate the causes for the differences in neutrophil responses observed in HIV disease, at cellular and molecular level. The identification of these causes and the normalization of neutrophil responses may improve the overall immune status and prognosis of HIV infected individuals.

5. CONCLUSION

HOCl is considered the most bactericidal oxidant produced by neutrophils. The production of ROs, as HOCl has a critical role in bactericidal and fungicide activity, and enhances the inflammatory reaction.

During the experiments, which included the isolation of neutrophils and the monitoring the formation of the HOCl isolates, it was possible to compare two HIV/AIDS patients whose antiretroviral treatment was the basic difference. Through experiments, the authors observed that the Patient I with HAART had a response activity of neutrophils 17.3% lower when compared to control in the production of hypochlorous acid before the PMA stimulation. On the other hand, Patient II, who did not use HAART, was active 81% less than control in the production of hypochlorous acid. The two patients had similar clinical laboratory parameters and differed only in

the number of CD4 cells, which were higher in Patient II. Results show that the patient submitted to antiretroviral treatment had a better quality of functional response of neutrophils although with fewer CD4 cells.

ETHICAL APPROVAL

The study was conducted in accordance with the ethical standards set out in Resolution No. 196/96-CNS Ministry of Health on research involving human beings in Brazil, after being approved by the Ethics Committee on Human Research of the State University of Maringa, Maringá PR Brazil. The protocol was approved according to Resolution n° 196/96 and additional CNS/MS in deliberative meeting of COPEP. CAAE n° 10718612.6.0000.0104/2012.

COMPETING INTERESTS

Authors have declared that no competing interests exist.

REFERENCES

1. Bowers NL, Helton ES, Huijbregts RPH, et al. Immune suppression by neutrophils in HIV-1 infection: Role of PD-L1/PD-1 pathway. PLOS/Pathog. 2014;10 (3):572-575.

2. Amulic B, Cazalet C, Haynes GL, et al. Neutrophil function: From mechanisms to disease. Annu Rev Immunol. 2012;30:459-489.

3. Mantovani A, Cassatella MA, Constantini C, Jaillon S. Neutrophils in the activation and regulation of innate and adaptive immunity. Nat Rev Immunol. 2011;11:519-531.

4. Chtanova T, Schaffer M, Han SJ, et al. Dynamics of neutrophil migration in lymph nodes during infection. Immunity. 2008; 29:487-496.

5. Muller L, Munder M, Kropf P, Hansch GM. Polymorphonuclear neutrophils and T lymphocytes: Strange bedfellows or brothers in arms? Trends Immunol. 2009; 30:522-530.

6. Pillay J, Tak T, Kamp VM, Koenderman L. Immune suppression by neutrophils and granulocytic myeloid-derived suppressor cells: Similarities and differences. Cell Mol Life Sci; 2013.

7. Pillay J, Kamp VM, Van Hoffen E, et al. A subset of neutrophils in human systemic

inflammation inhibits T cell responses through Mac -1. J Clin Invest. 2012; 122:327-336.

8. Dypbukt JM, Brooks WM, Thong B, Eriksson H, Kettle AJ. A sensitive and selective assay for chloramine production by myeloperoxidase. Free Radic Biol Med, 2005;39:1468–1477.

9. Kettle AJ, Winterbourn CC. Assays for the chlorination activity of myeloperoxidase. Methods Enzymol. 1994;233:502-512.

10. Eckert JW, Abramson SL, Starke J, Brandt ML. The surgical implications of chronic granulomatosus disease. Am J Surg. 1995; 169(3):320-3.

11. Pitrak DL. Neutrophil deficiency and dysfunction in HIV-infected patients. Am J Health Syst Pharm. 1999;56(5):59-66.

12. Pitrak DL, Mullane KM, Bilek ML, et al. Impaired phagocyte oxidative capacity in patients with human immunodeficiency virus infection. Lab Clin Med. 1998; 132(4):284-93.

13. Valone FH, Paian DG, Abrams DI, Goetz EJ. Defective polymorph nuclear leukocyte chemotaxis on homosexual men with persistent lymph node syndrome. J Infect Dis. 1984;150(2):267-71.

14. Chen TP, Roberts RL, Wu KG, Ank BJ, Stiehm ER. Decreased superoxide anion and hydrogen peroxide production by neutrophils and monocytes in human immunodeficiency virus-infected children and adults. Pedriatr Res. 1993;34(4):544-50.

15. Elbim C, Pillet S, Prevost MH, et al. The role of phagocyte in HIV related oxidative stress. J Clin Virol. 2001;20(3):99-109.

16. MacFadden DK, Saito S, Pruzanski W. The effect of Chemotherapeutic Agents on Chemotaxis and Random Migration of Human Leucocytes. Journal of Clinical Oncology. 1985;3:415-419.

17. Tavares-Murta BM. Failure of neutrophil chemotactic function in septic patients. Critical Care Medicine. 2002;30(5):1056-1061.

18. Mastroianni CM. Improvement in neutrophil and monocyte function during highly active antiretroviral treatment of HIV-1-infected patients. AIDS. 1999;13:883-890.

19. Stehbens WE. Oxidative stress in viral hepatitis and AIDS. Exp Mol Pathol. 2004;77:121-32.

20. Aukrust P, Muller F, Svardal A, et al. Disturbed glutathione metabolism and decreased antioxidants levels in human immunodeficiency virus-infected patients during highly active antiretroviral therapy. J Infect Dis. 2003;2:188-232.

21. Kobari L, Giarratana MC, Poloni A, et al. Flt 3 ligand, MGDF, Epo and G-CSF enhance ex vivo expansion of hematopoietic cell compartments in the presence of SCF, IL-3 and IL-6. Bone Marrow Transplant. 1998;21(8):759-67.

22. Zauli G, Capitani S. HIV-1-related mechanisms of suppression of CD34 + hematopoietic progenitors. Pathobiology. 1996;64(1):53-8).

23. Falguera M., Perez-Mur J., Puig T et al. Study of the role of vitamin B12 and folinic acid supplementation in preventing hematologic toxicity of zidovudine. Eur J Haematol. 1995;55(2):97-102.

24. Borregaard N. Neutrophils, from marrow to microbes. Immunity. 2010;33:657-70.

25. Gabelloni ML, Trevani AS, Saban J, Geffner J. Mechanism regulating neutrophil survival and cell death. Semin Immunopathol. 2013;35:423-37.

26. Cave AC, Brewer AC, Narayanapanicker A et al. NADPH oxidases in cardiovascular health and disease. Antioxid Redox Signal. 2006;8:691-728.

14

Severe Hemolytic Anemia Due to *De novo* Hemoglobin Sabine in an Argentinian Newborn. First Case in South America

Susana Perez[1*], Irma Bragós[1], Mariana Raviola[1], Arianna Pratti[1], Germán Detarsio[1], Sandra Zirone[2], Maria Eda Voss[1], Luciano Verón[2], Irma Acosta[1] and Mara Ojeda[1]

[1]*Departamento de Bioquímica Clínica, Cátedra de Hematología, Facultad de Ciencias Bioquímicas y Farmacéuticas, Universidad Nacional de Rosario. Suipacha 531. Rosario. Santa Fe, Argentina.*
[2]*Departamento de Hematología, Instituto Davoli. Laprida 1061. Rosario. Santa Fe, Argentina.*

Authors' contributions

This work was carried out in collaboration between all authors. Authors SP and IB designed the study, wrote the protocol, wrote the first draft of the manuscript, managed the analyses of the study and managed the literature searches. Authors MR, MO, LV, IA and AP performed laboratory tests. Authors AP, GD, SZ and MEV managed the literature searches.

Editor(s):
(1) Ricardo Forastiero, Department of Hematology, Favaloro University, Argentina.
Reviewers:
(1) Mathew Folaranmi Olaniyan, Department of Medical Laboratory Science, Achievers University, Owo, Nigeria.
(2) Vlachaki Efthymia, Department of Internal Medicine, Aristotle University, Greece.

ABSTRACT

Hemoglobin (Hb) Sabine is an unstable Hb variant that causes hemolytic anemia in heterozygous state, with inclusion bodies in the red blood cells (RBC). This hemoglobin is the result of a point mutation at codon 91(CTG)→(CCG) of the beta-globin gene. We report, for the first time in South America, the identification of Hb Sabine in a nine-month-old female baby, referred to our laboratory bearing a severe hemolytic anemia. We emphasize the need for the correct characterization of this unstable hemoglobin mainly for therapeutic purposes and for genetic counseling.

Keywords: Abnormal hemoglobin (Hb); Hb sabine; unstable hemoglobin.

*Corresponding author: E-mail: perezsusanamabel@gmail.com

1. INTRODUCTION

Up to date, there have been described more than 140 unstable hemoglobins [1], related to hemolytic anemia with different clinical expression. The mutations that cause destabilization of the tetrameric structure are the most frequent cause of hemolytic anemia. Proline introduction in the alpha helix, beyond the third residue, distorts the hemoglobin structure and cause instability. In general, these undergo increased oxidation of the heme with the formation of met Hb and further degradation leading to precipitated Hb and other products within the circulating red cells. [2] In Hb Sabine, as in many of the other unstable hemoglobins, the substitution is a neutral one [β91(F7)Leu-+Pro], so no alteration in charge of the globin chain would be expected. The diminished anodal mobility of these hemoglobins is probably due to loss of heme, an event to which they are peculiarly prone [3]. Hb Sabine is an unstable β chain variant which causes moderately severe hemolytic anemia and has been reported in a few unrelated patients, none of them from South America till date [4-8]. In this paper, we report a new *de novo* case of Hb Sabine in a nine-month-old female baby. The mutation was identified by DNA sequencing following amplification by polymerase chain reaction (PCR). The proband's father is of German origin and her mother is of Spanish descent. The girl has no familial history of anemia. Paternity was confirmed through studies of DNA polymorphism (STRs loci).

1.1 Case Report

The child was admitted to the Service of Pediatrics because of a moderately severe anemia, pallor and a subicteric condition. Her facies indicates expansion of haemopoietic tissue in the skull bones, particularly in the frontal and parietal bones. She had never been transfused. At the age of seven months, she suffered a hemolytic episode in the course of an infection.

Hematological data were obtained with a Sysmex KX21 blood counter. The blood film showed microcytosis, polychromasia, target cells, coarse basophilic stippling, and 2 nucleated erythroid progenitors per 100 white cells. The Hb A2 was measured by elution post electrophoresis at alkaline pH, and Hb F according to the method described by Betke et al. [9].

Isopropanol test (Carrell & Kay) [10] was performed. Cellulose acetate electrophoresis at alkaline pH and globin chains electrophoresis at alkaline pH were carried out using standard methods.

Sickling test was negative. The isopropanol test was positive indicating the presence of an unstable Hb. Cellulose acetate (pH 8.4) electrophoresis detected an additional Hb fraction, between Hb A and Hb A2. (Fig. 1) Globin chains electrophoresis did not show the presence of an abnormal chain.

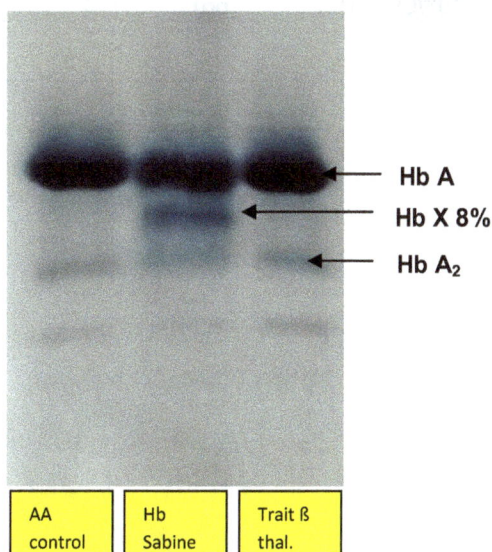

Fig. 1. Hemoglobin electrophoresis at alkaline pH

The patient's hematological and biochemical data are shown in Table 1 and hematological and hemoglobin composition data of parents are shown in Table 2.

DNA was extracted from peripheral blood samples as previously described [11]. Polymerase chain reaction (PCR) was carried out and then the coding regions of the β- and α-globin genes were sequenced. It was performed using a Big Dye Terminators Ready Reaction Kit (Perkin-Elmer Cetus, Norwalk, CT, USA) in an ABI PRISM 310 sequencer (Perkin-Elmer Cetus).

Alpha1 and α2 genes were normal, while sequencing of β gene revealed a CTG→ CCG (Asp→His) substitution at codon 91, corresponding to Hb Sabine (Fig. 2). DNA sequence analysis of the ß-globin gene of both parents showed the absence of the Hb Sabine mutation. Paternity was confirmed by the study of nine short tandem repeats (STRs) and four variable-number tandem repeat (VNTRs) loci.

Table 1. Hematological and biochemical data of the patient

Parameters	Proband
Hb A/X/A2 (%)	8
Hb (g/L)	770
RBC (10^{12}/L)	2.84
MCV (fL)	95.1
MCH (pg)	27.1
Reticulocytes (%)	40
A2 (%)	2.6
Hb F (%)	10
Isopropanol Test	positive
Sickling Test	negative
Total serum bilirrubina (umol/L)	35.2 (NR:5.7-17)
LDH U/l	1075 (NR:360-720)
Ferritina (ug/dl	84 (NR:24-120)
Iron (ug/dl)	114 (80-110)
TIBC (ug/dl)	351 (280-330)

Table 2. Hematological and hemoglobin composition data of parents

Subjet	Hb g/L	RBC (10^{12}/L)	MCV (fL)	MCH (pg)	Reticulocytes (%)	A2 (%)	Hb F (%)	Hb X (%)
Father	152	4.8	91.7	31.7	1.3	2.4	1	0
Mother	134	4.27	88	31.4	1.2	2.6	0.9	0

T G A G C N G C A C

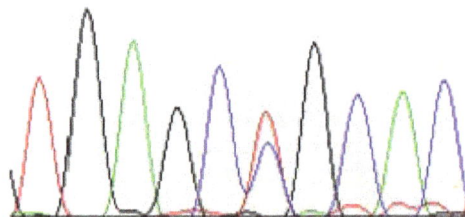

Fig. 2. Sequence of the β-globin gene: CTG→ CCG (Asp→His) substitution at codon 91 corresponding to Hb Sabine

2. DISCUSSION

Numerous cases of hemolytic anemia have been described that are a consequence of the presence in the erythrocyte of unstable hemoglobins.

Most unstable hemoglobin variants in heterozygous state have a variable percentage of the variant. In our case it was 8% of total hemoglobin. This is a much smaller proportion than that found for most Hb variants, presumably because it is precipitated both *in vivo* and *in vitro* during manipulation in the experimental procedures. The erythrocyte containing Hb Sabine, have a markedly shortened survival as a consequence of impaired metabolism, probably due to dissociation and precipitation of abnormal beta polypeptide chains of Hb Sabine. Unstable Hbs are inherited in an autosomal dominant fashion, and virtually all affected individuals are heterozygous. The homozygous state for the unstable variants has not been found.

Our patient, as all Hb Sabine carriers reported so far had significantly increased Hb F levels (HbF:10%) Patients with higher levels of HbF as those refered by Pavlovic S el al. [8] and Panagoula Kollia et al. [12] one had an association with the Xmn I polymorphism at -158 Gγ and the other a compound heterozigocity with non-deletional hereditary persistence of fetal hemoglobin respectively.

Almost all reported patients suffered from severe hemolytic anemia and were splenectomized at early age.

Our patient that now is 17 months is been managed with folic acid and when she was 14 months received one transfusion. Splenectomy cannot be predicted now, it will depend on the transfusion regimen, hypersplenism and how she passes her early childhood. In Pediatrics is ideal to splenectomize after the age of 6.

Even though Hb Sabine is detectable by electrophoresis, its correct characterization requires more sophisticated methods, like high performance liquid chromatography, capillary electrophoresis or molecular analysis.

The so far published cases of Hb Sabine in 1969 [4], 1983 [5], 1992 [6] and 2008 [13] were all de novo presentations. The only inherited case reported in 2004, was the son of a Yugoslavian patient [8].

3. CONCLUSION

We report this case to emphasize the need for the correct identification of this unstable hemoglobin, mainly for therapeutic purposes and for genetic counseling, especially in therapeutic cases [14-15].

These patients present mild to severe chronic hemolytic anemia that may be exacerbated by stress, especially infections, and treatment with oxidizing agents.

CONSENT

All authors declare that written informed consent was obtained from the patient's parents for publication of this case report.

ETHICAL APPROVAL

All authors hereby declare that all laboratoty tests have been examined and approved by the "Comité de Etica de la Facultad de Ciencias Bioquímicas" and have therefore been performed in accordance with the ethical standads laid down in the 1964 Declaration of Helsinki.

COMPETING INTERESTS

Authors have declared that no competing interests exist.

REFERENCES

1. Available:http://globin.bx.psu.edu//hbvar//menu.html Hb Var: a database of human hemoglobin variants and thalassemias (Available:http://globin.cse.psu.edu/hbvar/menu.htm)

2. Beutler E, Lichtman M, Coller B, Kipps T. Hemoglobinopathies associated with unstable hemoglobin, in Wlliams Hemalology (5th ed), edited by. Beutler E, Lichtman MA, Coller BS, Kipps TJ. New York, McGraw-Hill. 1995;650–654.

3. Ueda S, Schneider R. Brief Report: Rapid Differentiation of Polypeptide Chains of Hemoglobin by Cellulose Acetate Electrophoresis of Hemolylsates. Blood. 1969;34:230-235.

4. Schneider RG, Ueda S, Alperin J et al. Hemoglobin Sabine Beta 91 (F 7) Leu → Pro-An Unstable Variant Causing Severe Anemia with Inclusion Bodies. N Engl J Med. 1969;280:739-745.

5. Bogoevski P, Efremov GD, Kezic J, Lam H, Wilson JB, Huisman THJ. Hb Sabine or α2

β2 91(F7) Leu-Pro in a Yugoslavian boy. Hemoglobin. 1983;7:195-200.

6. Gasperini D, Galanello R, Melis MA, et al. Hemoglobin Sabine [β 91(F7) Leu Pro]: occurrence in a Sardinian individual with hemolytic anemia and inclusion bodies. Haematologica. 1992;77:381-3.

7. Hull D, Winter PC, McHale CM et al. Familial hemolytic anemia due to Hb Sabine (beta-91(F7)leu-to-pro) identified by polymerase chain reaction. Hemoglobin. 1998;22:263-266.

8. Pavlovic S, Kuzmanovic M, Urosevic J et al. Severe central nervous system thrombotic events in hemoglobin Sabine patient. Eur J Haematol. 2004;72:67-70.

9. Efremov GD, Huisman THF. Diagnótico de laboratorio de hemoglobinopatías en Hemoglobinas anormales. En: Weatherall DJ. Clínica Hematológica 2/2. Barcelona: Salvat. 1976;A) 319-320 B) 322-323.

10. Carrell RW, Kay R. A simple method for the detection of unstable haemoglobins. Br J Haematol 1972;23:615-9.

11. Noguera N, Tallano C, Bragós I et al. Modified salting-out method for DNA isolation from newborn cord blood nucleated cells. J Clin Lab Analysis. 2000; 14(6);280-283.

12. Panagoula Kollia, Angelos Kalamaras, Christos Chassanidis, Maria Samara, Nikolaos K. Vamvakopoulos. Compound heterozygosity for the Cretan type of non-deletional hereditary persistence of fetal hemoglobin and β-thalassemia or Hb Sabine confirms the functional role of the Aγ −158 C>T mutation in γ-globin gene transcription. Blood Cells, Molecules, and Diseases 41. 2008;263–264.

13. Kollia P, Kalamaras A, Chassanidis C et al. Compound heterozygosity for the Cretan type of non-deletional hereditary persistence of fetal hemoglobin and β-thalassemia or Hb Sabine confirms the functional role of the Aγ−158 C>T mutation in γ-globin gene transcription. Blood Cells, Molecules, and Diseases. 2008;41:263–264.

14. Eandi Eberle S, Noguera N, Calvo K et al. Severe hemolytic anemia due to hemoglobin Hammersmith. Arch Argent Pediatr. 2009;107(4):347-352.

15. Zanotto MI, Calvo K, Schavartzmanb G et al. Hemolytic anemia due to hemoglobin Evans in an Argentinean family. Arch Argent Pediatr. 2010;108(6):e130-e133.

15

Relationship between Glucose Level, Lipid Profiles, and Waist to Height Ratio (WHtR)

Hazizi Abu Saad[1*], Aina Mardiah Basri[1] and Zahratul Nur Kalmi[1]

[1]Department of Nutrition and Dietetics, Faculty of Medicine and Health Sciences, Universiti Putra Malaysia, 43400 UPM Serdang, Selangor, Malaysia.

Authors' contributions

This work was carried out in collaboration between all authors. Author HAS designed the study, wrote the protocol, and wrote the first draft of the manuscript. Authors AMB and ZNK managed the literature searches, data collection, data entry and data analyses. All authors read and approved the final manuscript.

Editor(s):
(1) Tadeusz Robak, Medical University of Lodz, Copernicus Memorial Hospital, Poland.
Reviewers:
(1) Goluch-Koniuszy Zuzanna, Department of Human Nutrition Physiology, West Pomeranian University of Technology, Poland.
(2) Lior Z. Braunstein, Harvard Medical School, USA.
(3) Maciste H Macias Cervantes, Department of Medical Science, Universidad de Guanajuato, Mexico.

ABSTRACT

A cross sectional study was carried out to determine the relationship between glucose level, lipid profiles, and waist to height ratio (WHtR) among adults in a workplace setting. Respondents were recruited from government staff in two ministries, each from the federal territories of Kuala Lumpur and Putrajaya, Malaysia. Socio-demographic information was collected using a set of questionnaire and anthropometric measurement including weight, height, percent body fat, and waist and hip circumference were measured. Antropometric assessments were measured and blood sample was collected in the morning before 10 AM, after the respondents undergone 12 hours of overnight fasting. A fingerpick blood sample was collected to measure blood glucose and lipid profiles. A total of 210 respondents were recruited for this study. The majority of the respondents (81.9%) were aged 34 years and younger. Approximately 16.8% were obese and 25.1% overweight. Based on WHtR, 47.1% of the respondents were classified as having WHtR≥0.5. Based on odds ratio, having a high WHtR (≥0.5) was found to be related to increased risk of having high BMI (OR=18.125; 95% CI 8.583-38.276), high triglyceride (OR=6.202; 95% CI 2.517-15.281), elevated blood pressure (systolic OR=4.351; 95% CI 2.026-9.344, diastolic OR=4.932; 95% CI 1.571-15.484), high blood glucose (OR=3.084; 95% CI 1.186-7.831) and low HDLC (OR=3.506; 95% CI 1.862-6.600). For the

---

*Corresponding author: E-mail: hazizi@upm.edu.my

subjects of this study, WHtR was found to be significantly related to lipid profile and blood glucose level.

Keywords: WHtR; lipid profile; glucose; odds ratio.

1. INTRODUCTION

Obesity is a condition where the body has excessive levels of fat. The relationship between obesity and health risk has been studied by many researchers and it has been established that obesity causes increases in many risk factors. Excess body fat has been shown to be related to several conditions such as diabetes, cardiovascular disease (CVD), dyslipidaemia, hypertension metabolic syndrome, dyslipidaemia, inflammation, thrombosis and certain cancers [1-4].

Several methods can be used to estimate body composition and its relation to disease risk, such as computed tomography, magnetic resonance imaging, dual energy X-ray absorptiometry, and bioelectrical impedance analysis. In large epidemiological studies, Body Mass Index (BMI), waist circumference (WC), waist to hip ratio (WHR) and body fat percentage (%BF) are the most popular indicators used in assessing the relationship between disease risk and body composition. The nature and strength of association between each indicator and risk of disease varies.

Obesity, as measured by BMI, has been reported in many studies to be related to risk of premature death [5], CVD [6], type II diabetes [7] and colon cancer [8]. On the other hand, WC and WHR, indicators of abdominal fat accumulation in the body, are better indicators than BMI for all obesity-related causes of mortality [9]. Among subjects with Coronary Artery Disease, Coutinho et al. [10] reported that WC and WHR is directly associated with mortality, but not BMI.

The relationship between CVD risk and body composition, as represented by BMI, WHR, WC and WHtR classifications, has been described at length in the literature, and the majority of sources suggested central adiposity (WC, WHR & WHtR) to be superior to BMI in predicting CVD risk [11]. A publication by Lee, Huxley, Wildman and Woodward [12] further showed that the best discriminator for hypertension, diabetes, and dyslipidaemia in both sexes is WHtR, as compared to BMI and WC. However, a review paper by Qiao and Nyamdorj [13] surmised that, based on prospective studies, risk of type II diabetes is equally associated with all anthropometric measures of BMI, WC, WHR and the WHtR.

Although there are many comparative studies carried out on the relationship between BMI, WHR, WHtR and WC with the risk of disease, studies reported on WHtR in Malaysia is still limited. Most published studies involving WHtR and its relationship with disease risks were carried out among western populations, and research among people in Asia were focused on populations in Japan, China, Hong Kong, Taiwan, Bangladesh and several Arab countries. Therefore this study was performed to describe waist circumference to height ratio (WHtR) among a sample of government staff in Malaysia, and to assess the relationship between WHtR and health risks, such as lipid profile and glucose level.

2. METHODS AND MATERIALS

2.1 Respondents

The respondents of this study were recruited from one ministry in Putrajaya and another in Kuala Lumpur, Malaysia. Invitation to participate in this study was distributed to all staff in these ministries between 18 to 60 years old, without any physical impairment and not pregnant. All procedures performed were in accordance with the ethical standards and ethical approval to conduct this study was granted from the Medical Research Ethics Committee, Faculty of Medicine and Health Sciences, Universiti Putra Malaysia. All subjects were briefed about the study and signed a consent form to participate in this study.

2.2 Measurements

2.2.1 Questionnaire

A structured questionnaire was used to obtain information on sociodemographic characteristics, such as gender, age, monthly income, education level and work position in the agency. Physical Activity level was measured using the International Physical Activity Questionnaire (IPAQ) Short and Malay version. The IPAQ Scoring Protocol was used to calculate MET/min and classification of physical activity level was made based on IPAQ [14].

2.2.2 Anthropometric measurements and blood pressure

Antropometric assessments were determined and blood sample was collected in the morning (before 10 AM) after the respondents undergone 12 hours of overnight fasting. Anthropometric measurements were carried out, including weight, height, and waist and hip circumference. Height was measured accordingly and followed methods as described by Gibson [15], using a Seca Bodymeter (Model 201, Germany) to the nearest 0.1 cm. Weight and percent body fat were measured using a Tanita Body Fat Analyser (Model 418, Japan) in light clothing and without shoes and socks. To minimize errors in body fat analysis, using a Tanita Body Fat Analyser and via the 8-electrode segmented BIA technique, all measurement procedures as well as subject preparation instructions described in the Tanita Body Composition Analyser BC418 manual, were followed. BMI was calculated automatically by the Tanita Body Fat Analyser and classified based on standards suggested by the World Health Organization [16]. Body fat percentage was classified according to the classifications suggested by the American College of Sports Medicine [17]. Waist (midpoint between the lower margin of the last rib and the top of the iliac crest) and hip (widest portion of the buttocks) circumference were measured to the nearest 0.1 cm with non-stretchable measuring tape. Classification of WC was based on WHO/IASO/IOTF [18] and WHR was calculated as ratio of waist circumference to hip circumference; individuals were classified as having central obesity if WHR≥0.9 for males and ≥0.8 for females, respectively (World Health Organization, 1999 [19]). WHtR was determined from waist circumference (cm) divided by height (cm) and classified according to Ashwell & Hsieh [20], proposing the boundary value of WHtR≥0.5 to indicate increased risk for adult males and females. Blood pressure was measured after 5 minutes of sitting and resting, using an Omron blood pressure monitors (Model HEM-780, Japan).

2.2.3 Biochemical assessments

A capillary blood sample was collected by using a finger prick technique. A total of 30 μl of blood sample was collected using capillary tubes for measurement of blood glucose level. Micro blood collection tubes- K2EDTA were used to collect 0.5 ml of blood from the respondent. The blood sample was centrifuged at 3000 rpm and the resulting plasma sample was used to determine the level of triglyceride (TG) and high density lipoprotein cholesterol (HDLC). Reflotron Test Reagent Strips was used to measure the level of total cholesterol, TG, and HDLC using the Reflotron plus Clinical Chemistry Analyzer (Germany). Low density lipoprotein cholesterol (LDLC) was calculated automatically by the Reflotron plus Chemistry Analyzer based on the Friedewald formula. One of the respondents had a TG concentration >4.5 mmol/l.A standard LDL analysis was performed with an automatic chemical analyser. Blood glucose, lipid profile and blood pressure were classified based on the American Diabetes Association [21], the National Cholesterol Education Program [22] and Ministry of Health Malaysia [23] respectively.

2.3 Statistical Analysis

Data was analyzed using IBM SPSS Statistics version 19. Univariate analysis, including frequency, percentage, mean, and standard deviation, were applied to the sociodemographic, anthropometric, and blood profiles. A t-test was performed to determine the mean difference between two groups, specifically WHtR<0.5 and WHtR≥0.5. The association between variables studies was determined by using Pearson's correlation and odds ratio. An alpha level of 0.05 was set as significant level.

3. RESULTS

A total of 210 respondents were recruited in this study and almost 70% were female respondents. Table 1 showed the distribution of respondents according to sociodemographic characteristics, anthropometric characteristics, blood pressure glucose level, lipid profile and physical activity level. About 60% of the respondents were between 25-35 years of age and about the same proportion had received up to tertiary education (college/university).Mean age of the respondents was 31.18±8.43 years. About one in four respondents was classified as overweight and another 16.8% as obese. Percentages of overweight and obese individuals were higher among males, as compared to females. More than 70% of the respondents were classified as having high body fat percentage and high risk, as classified by waist to hip classification. About one in four respondents had elevated blood pressure (classified as systolic blood pressure ≥135 mmHg and/or diastolic blood pressure ≥85 mmHg).

Approximately 11.8% of the respondents exhibited elevated blood glucose and the percentage was higher among males as compared to females. Similar trends were observed for total cholesterol, triglyceride and LDLC, but with different percentages. The percentage of respondents classified as having high total cholesterol was almost the same for males (7.4%) and females (8.3%) in this study. Low HDLC was more prevalent among females (39%), as compared to males (3.8%). About one third of the respondents were sedentary, more so among females than males. Central obesity, as classified as WHtR≥0.5, was more prevalent among males (67.2%) than females (38.2%).

Table 2 showed distribution, mean, and standard deviation of WHtR, according to socio-demographic and anthropometric characteristics, blood pressure, blood glucose level, lipid profile and physical activity level. Mean WHtR was significantly higher among males compared to females, as well as among older compared to younger, but not significantly different in terms of occupational status. Mean WHtR was also significantly higher among respondents with elevated blood pressure and significantly higher among respondents with elevated total cholesterol, triglyceride and LDLC. WHtR was significant lower among respondents with HDLC ≥1.03 mmol/l as compared to groups with HDLC <1.03 mmol/l. There was no significant difference in mean WHtR between sedentary and non-sedentary respondents (p>0.05).

WHtR and BMI were moderately correlated with percent body fat and blood pressure. Correlation between WHtR and BMI with lipid profiles and blood glucose were weak but significant. WHtR and BMI were not significantly correlated with physical activity level of the respondent. Based on odds ratio, having high WHtR was found to be related to increased risk of having high blood glucose, triglyceride, blood pressure, and low HDLC. For lipid profile and blood glucose, odds ratio of having high blood glucose and low HDLC were three times higher among respondent with WHtR≥0.5, compared to respondent with WHtR <0.5. The highest odds ratio among lipid profiles was odds of having high triglyceride, which was equal to 6.2 among respondents with WHtR≥0.5 as compared to respondents with WHtR<0.5. Odds of having elevated systolic and diastolic blood pressure were 4 times higher among respondents with WHtR≥0.5 compared to respondents with WHtR<0.5. Based on calculated odds ratio, percent body fat was not significantly related to WHtR.

4. DISCUSSION

Ashwell and Hsieh [20] suggested that the waist-to-height ratio (WHtR) is more useful for assessing health risk than BMI for several reasons, such as WHtR is more sensitive, cheaper, and easier to measure and calculate than BMI. Further, a cut off value of WHtR≥0.5 indicates increased risk for both males and females across ethnic and population groups. WHtR may also allow the same cut off values for children, adolescents and adults.

In this study, the mean WHtR was significantly higher among male respondents, and the percentage of respondent with WHtR≥0.5 was higher among males as compared to females. This is in line with BMI results that showed that the percentages of overweight and obesity (BMI ≥25 kg/m^2) were higher among males as compared to females. The mean WHtR was significantly higher among older respondents as compared to younger ones, but not significantly different between work positions (professional vs. non-professional). These results contradict those of a study conducted by Flora et al. [24] in Bangladesh, which found that females had a higher risk of having a WHtR greater than males (OR = 7.898; 95% CI 7.110-8.774). However, our study was in agreement with this study in terms of the risk of having high WHtR was higher among the older than the young. However, in terms of employment, Flora et al. [24] showed that the risk was higher among the professional and business people compared to other fields of work.

The prevalence of overweight and obesity among adults in Malaysia, based on the latest National Health and Morbidity Survey of 2011, was 44.5% (females 45.4% vs. males 43.6%), and abdominal obesity was also higher among females (54.1%) than males (37.4%) [25]. A study among 1,530 respondents in one state in Malaysia showed that WHR also followed a similar trend (females 76.3% vs. males 49.5%) [26]. In this study, based on BMI, obesity and overweight occurred more frequently in males than in females. Whereas, based on waist circumference, the prevalence of abdominal obesity also showed similar trend. In contrast, based on fat percentages, prevalence of high body fat was lower (17.2%) among males compared to females (93.9%). Each of the indices of obesity projected differences in prevalence, even though all are clustered as obesity indices. Differences in prevalence, as shown above, indicated that each indicator used in assessing obesity and its relationship with disease risk is unique and may differ in terms of its role and association in the prediction of disease. This requires researchers to conduct further studies to identify the most sensitive and accurate indicators related to risk of chronic diseases, such as diabetes and CVD.

Table 1. Distribution of respondents according to sociodemographic and anthropometric characteristics, blood pressure, blood glucose level, lipid profile and physical activity level

	Male n (%)	Female n (%)	Total n (%)
Sex	64 (30.5)	146 (69.5)	210 (100)
Age (years)			
<25	13 (20.3)	37 (25.3)	52 (23.8)
25-34	37 (57.8)	85 (58.2)	122 (58.1)
35-44	7 (10.9)	8 (5.5)	15 (7.1)
>44	7 (10.9)	16 (11.0)	23 (11.0)
Education level			
Primary school	3 (4.7)	18 (12.3)	21 (10.0)
Secondary school	12 (18.8)	23 (15.8)	35 (16.6)
Upper Secondary School	7 (10.9)	15 (10.3)	22 (10.5)
Collage/ University	42 (65.6)	90 (61.6)	132 (62.9)
Occupation			
Non-professional	44 (68.8%)	99 (67.8%)	143 (68.1%)
Professional	20 (31.3%)	47 (32.2%)	67 (31.9%)
BMI (kg/m^2)			
Underweight (<18.5)	1 (1.7)	11 (8.3)	12 (6.3)
Normal Weight (18.5-24.9)	24 (41.4)	75 (56.4)	99 (51.8)
Overweight (25-29.9)	19 (32.8)	29 (21.8)	48 (25.1)
Obese (≥30)	14 (24.1)	18 (13.5)	32 (16.8)
Fat Percentage			
Normal (male<25%/ female <32%)	48 (82.8)	8 (6.1)	56 (29.6)
High (male ≥25%/ female ≥32%)	10 (17.2)	123 (93.9)	133 (70.4)
Waist circumference (cm)			
Normal (<90 for male or <80 for female)	31 (53.4)	88 (67.2)	119 (63.0)
High risk (≥ 90 for male or ≥80 for female)	27 (46.6)	43 (32.8)	70 (37.0)
WHR			
Normal (<0.9 form male and <0.80 for female)	36 (62.1)	109 (83.2)	145 (76.7)
High risk (≥0.9 form male and ≥0.80 for female)	22 (37.9)	22 (16.8)	44 (23.3)
Systolic blood pressure (mmHg)			
Normal (<135)	32 (55.2)	114 (87.7)	146 (77.7)
Elevated (≥135)	26 (44.8)	16 (12.3)	42 (22.3)
Diastolic blood pressure (mmHg)			
Normal (<85)	50 (86.2)	120 (91.6)	170 (89.9)
Elevated (≥85)	8 (13.8)	11 (8.4)	19 (10.1)
Systolic blood pressure ≥135 mmHg and/or diastolic blood pressure ≥85mmHg			
Normal blood pressure	32 (58.2%)	110 (84.6%)	142 (76.8%)
Elevated blood pressure	23 (41.8%)	20 (15.4%)	43 (23.2%)
Total glucose (mmol/l)			
<5.6	44 (80.0)	113 (91.9)	157 (88.2)
5.6-6.9	8 (14.5)	8 (6.5)	16 (9.0)
>6.9	3 (5.5)	2 (1.6)	5 (2.8)
Total cholesterol (mmol/l)			
<5.17	36 (66.7)	80 (66.7)	116 (66.7)
5.17-6.19	14 (25.9)	30 (25.0)	44 (25.3)
>6.19	4 (7.4)	10 (8.3)	14 (8.0)
Triglyceride (mmol/l)			

	Male n (%)	Female n (%)	Total n (%)
<1.69	31 (58.5)	103 (89.6)	134 (79.8)
1.69-2.25	18 (34.0)	7 (6.1)	25 (14.9)
2.26-5.64	4 (7.5)	5 (4.3)	9 (5.4)
>5.64	-	-	-
LDLC (mmol/l)			
<2.59	11 (22.0)	43 (37.4)	54 (32.7)
2.59-3.35	20 (40.0)	46 (40.0)	66 (40.0)
3.36-4.13	12 (26.0)	17 (14.8)	30 (18.2)
4.14-4.90	2 (4.0)	8 (7.0)	10 (6.1)
>4.90	4 (8.0)	1 (0.9)	5 (3.0)
HDLC (mmol/l)			
>1.54	20 (37.7)	54 (45.8)	74 (43.3)
1.03-1.54	2 (3.8)	46 (39.0)	48 (28.1)
<1.03	31 (58.5)	18 (15.3)	49 (28.7)
Physical Activity Level (IPAQ)			
Sedentary	13 (21.7)	55 (39.0)	68 (33.8)
Moderate	26 (43.3)	63 (44.7)	89 (44.3)
High	21 (35.0)	23 (16.3)	44 (21.9)
WHtR			
<0.5	19 (32.8)	81 (61.8)	100 (52.9)
≥0.5	39 (67.2)	50 (38.2)	89 (47.1)

Based on previous studies, diabetes, hypertension, high total cholesterol, high triglycerides, and low HDL-cholesterol can be predicted by WHtR significantly better than by BMI or WC Li et al. [27]. Among Americans, non-Hispanic Whites and non-Hispanic Blacks, WHtR was associated with higher odds of type 2 diabetes compared to the odds of having type 2 diabetes based on WC. These results were in line with a study among adults in Taiwan that reported the adjusted ORs for any CVD risk factors in male and female are highest when assessed using WHtR as a filter, followed by WC, BMI, then WHR, respectively, and all are statistically significant (p<0.001) for both genders [28]. A study by Ashwell, Gunn and Gibson [29] also reported the results of discriminatory power analysis of BMI, WC, and WHtR data in differentiating adults with type-2 diabetes, dyslipidaemia, hypertension, metabolic syndrome and general CVD outcomes, clearly showing that WHtR had significantly greater discriminatory power compared with WC and BMI.

However, other meta-analysis, focused on hypertension, concluded that BMI, WHR, WC, or WHtR were not systematically better than others at the discrimination of hypertension [30]. On the

other hand, Liu et al. [31] reported that among 772 Chinese adult subjects, BMI, waist circumference and WHtR may equally predict multiple metabolic risk factors, such as blood pressure (systolic and diastolic blood pressure) and dyslipidaemia (triglyceride, HDL-C and plasma glucose). The relationship between WHtR, BMI, WC, and WHR with disease risk is still unclear; some of the studies found WHtR to be the best predictor compared to others, while other studies showed different results.

In our study, mean values of blood pressure, glucose level, and lipid profiles were higher among respondents with WHtR≥0.5, except for HDLC, which showed different results from expected. All of these factors were statistically significant. Results of this study showed that odds ratio of having high fasting glucose, triglyceride, systolic and diastolic blood pressure, and low HDLC were significantly higher among respondent with WHtR≥0.5 as compared to respondent with WHtR<0.5. Our study did not assess odds ratio of those risk factors with BMI, WHR, and WC, and therefore we could not compare the relationship between risk factors with studies measuring other indicators of obesity (WC, WHR, BMI).

Table 2. Mean, and standard deviation of waist to height ratio (WHtR), according to sociodemographic characteristics, anthropometric characteristics, blood pressure, blood glucose level, lipid profile, and physical activity level

	Mean	SD	p-value
Sex			
Male	0.540	0.080	.000
Female	0.497	0.064	
Age (year)			
<30	0.496	0.068	.001
≥30	0.533	0.073	
Occupation			
Non-professional	0.508	0.072	.516
Professional	0.515	0.072	
BMI (kg/m²)			
Underweight & Normal Weight (<25)	0.468	0.040	.000
Overweight & Obese (≥25)	0.570	0.065	
Fat Percentage			
Normal (<25% for male/ < 32% for female)	0.500	0.063	.207
High (≥25% for male/ ≥32% for female)	0.514	0.076	
Systolic Blood Pressure (mmHg)			
Normal (<135)	0.495	0.065	.000
Elevated (≥135)	0.561	0.076	
Diastolic Blood Pressure (mmHg)			
Normal (<85)	0.503	0.069	.000
Elevated (≥85)	0.572	0.074	
Systolic blood pressure ≥135 mmHg and/or diastolic blood pressure ≥85 mmHg			
Normal blood pressure	0.493	0.063	0.00
Elevated blood pressure	0.563	0.078	
Total Cholesterol (mmol/l)			
<5.17	0.500	0.063	.033
≥5.17	0.526	0.081	
Total glucose (mmol/l)			
<5.6	0.501	0.066	.001
≥5.6	0.555	0.080	
Triglyceride (mmol/l)			
<1.69	0.496	0.064	.000
≥1..69	0.569	0.078	
LDLC (mmol/l)			
<2.59	0.490	0.066	.010
≥2.59	0.520	0.071	
HDLC (mmol/l)			
≥1.03	0.534	0.076	.000
<1.03	0.488	0.059	
Physical Activity Level (IPAQ)			
Sedentary	0.499	0.067	.180
Moderate & Active	0.514	0.074	

Table 3. Correlation between glucose level, lipid profile, selected anthropometric indicators, blood pressure, physical activity level, with waist to height ratio (WHtR) and body mass index (BMI)

	Correlation (WHtR)	Correlation (BMI)
Percent body fat	0.538*	0.638*
Systolic blood pressure	0.509*	0.465*
Diastolic blood pressure	0.378*	0.402*
Triglyceride	0.396*	0.420*
HDLC	-0.384*	-0.430*
LDLC	0.254*	0.242*
Glucose level	0.186*	0.218*
Total cholesterol	0.174*	0.149*
Physical activity level	0.079	0.104

*p<0.05

Table 4. Relationship between glucose level, lipid profile, selected anthropometric indicators, blood pressure, physical activity level, and waist to height ratio (WHtR).

	Odds ratio	Low	High
Percent body fat	0.752	0.402	1.408
Systolic blood pressure	4.351*	2.026	9.344
Diastolic blood pressure	4.932*	1.571	15.484
Triglyceride	6.202*	2.517	15.281
HDLC	3.506*	1.862	6.600
LDLC	1.742	0.892	3.399
Glucose level	3.084*	1.186	7.831
Total cholesterol	1.843	0.973	3.488
Elevated blood pressure	4.162*	1.970	8.792
Physical activity level	0.839	0.452	1.556

*p<0.05

This study was cross sectional in nature and subjected to the limitations of cross sectional design. Limited sample size and sampling procedure suggested that the results of this study should not be generalized to others, but only respondents in this study. The uniqueness of our study is that we have shown that obesity prevalence as assessed by BMI, WHtR, WHR, and WC have portrayed differences as predictors. However, there is still uncertainty about which indicators are most sensitive and accurate among the population studies in relation to the disease risk, especially for chronic diseases.

5. CONCLUSION

About half of the respondents in this study were classified as high risk, based on WHtR as an indicator. The prevalence was higher among males compared to female respondents. The relationships between WHtR and lipid profile as well as fasting blood glucose were significant. Therefore, the results of the present study have supported the utility of the WHtR in relation to disease risk, specifically as they relate to lipid profiles and blood glucose.

COMPETING INTERESTS

Authors have declared that no competing interests exist.

REFERENCES

1. Zalesin KC, Franklin BA, Miller WM, Peterson ED, Mc Cullough PA. Impact of obesity on cardiovascular disease. Med Clin North Am. 2011;95(5):919-37.
2. Kurukulasuriya LR, Stas S, Lastra G, Manrique C, Sowers JR. Hypertension in obesity. Med Clin North Am. 2011;95(5): 903-17.
3. Franssen R, Monajemi H, Stroes ES, Kastelein JJ. Obesity and dyslipidemia. Med Clin North Am. 2011;95(5):893-902.
4. Schmandt RE, Iglesias DA, Co NN, Lu KH. Understanding obesity and endometrial cancer risk: Opportunities for prevention. Am J Obstet Gynecol. 2011;205(6):518-25.
5. Solomon CG, Manson JE. Obesity and mortality: A review of the epidemiologic data. Am J Clin Nutr. 1997;66:1044S–1050S.
6. Chouraki V, Wagner A, Ferrie`res J, Kee F, Bingham A, Haas B. Smoking habits, waist circumference and coronary artery disease risk relationship: The Prime study. Eur J Cardiovasc Prev Rehabil. 2008;15:625–630.
7. Qiao Q, Nyamdorj R. Is the association of type II diabetes with waist circumference or waist-to-hip ratio stronger than that with body mass index?. European Journal of Clinical Nutrition. 2010;64:30–34; DOI:10.1038/ejcn.2009.93.
8. Adams KF, Leitzmann MF, Albanes D, Kipnis V, Mouw T, Hollenbeck A, Schatzkin A. Body mass and colorectal cancer risk in the NIH-AARP cohort. Am J Epidemiol. 2007;1:166:36-45.
9. Seidell JC. Waist circumference and waist/hip ratio in relation to all-cause mortality, cancer and sleep apnea. Eur J Clin Nutr. 2010;64(1):35-41.
10. Coutinho T, Goel K, Corrêa de Sa´ D, Kragelund C, Kanaya AM, Zeller M, Park JS, Kober L, Torp-Pedersen C, Cottin Y, Lorgis L, Lee SH, Kim YJ, Thomas R, Roger VL, Somers VK, Lopez-Jimenez F. Central obesity and survival in subjects with coronary artery disease a systematic review of the literature and collaborative analysis with individual subject data. J Am Coll Cardiol. 2011;10(57):1877-86. DOI:10.1016/j.jacc.2010.11.058.
11. Huxley R, Mendis S, Zheleznyakov E, Reddy S, Chan J. Body mass index, waist circumference and waist: Hip ratio as predictors of cardiovascular risk-a review of the literature. European Journal of Clinical Nutrition. 2010;64:16–22. DOI:10.1038/ejcn.2009.68.
12. Lee CM, Huxley RR, Wildman RP, Woodward M. Indices of abdominal obesity are better discriminators of cardiovascular risk factors than BMI: A meta-analysis. J Clin Epidemiol. 2008;61(7):646-53.
13. Qiao Q, Nyamdorj R. The optimal cut off values and their performance of waist circumference and waist-to-hip ratio for diagnosing type II diabetes. European Journal of Clinical Nutrition. 2010;64:23-29. DOI:10.1038/ejcn.2009.92.
14. IPAQ. Guidelines for data processing and analysis of the international physical activity questionnaire (IPAQ)-short and long forms; 2005. Available:http://www.ipaq.ki.se/dloads/IPAQ%20LS%20Scoring%20Protocols_Nov05.pdf (Retrieved on 24 Dec 2011).
15. Gibson RS. Principles of nutritional assessment. New York: Oxford University Press; 1990.
16. World health organization. Preventing and managing the global epidemic: Report of a WHO consultation on obesity, Geneva, World Health Organization, Switzerland, Geneva. 1997;1998.
17. American College of Sports Medicine (ACSM). ACSM's guidelines for exercise testing & prescription (Ed 7). Philadelphia: Lippincott Williams & Wilkins; 2011.
18. WHO/IASO/IOTF. The Asia-pacific perspective: Redefining obesity and its treatment. Health Communications

Australia Pty Limited: Sydney; 2000.

19. World health organization. Definition, diagnosis and classification of diabetes mellitus and its complications. Part 1: Diagnosis and classification of diabetes mellitus. World health organization: Geneva; 1999.

20. Ashwell M, Hsieh SD. Six reasons why the waist-to-height ratio is a rapid and effective global indicator for health risks of obesity and how its use could simplify the international public health message on obesity. International Journal of Food Sciences and Nutrition. 2005;56(5):303-307.

21. American diabetes association. Diagnosis and classification of diabetes mellitus. Diabetes Care. 2004;27(1):s5-s10.

22. NCEP. Executive summary of the third report of the national cholesterol education program (NCEP) expert panel on detection, evaluation, and treatment of high blood cholesterol In adults (Adult treatment panel III). JAMA. 2001; 16:285(19):2486-97.

23. Ministry of Health Malaysia. Clinical practice guideline on management of hypertension–4th Edition. Kuala Lumpur: Ministry of Health Malaysia; 2013.

24. Flora MS, Mascie-Taylor CGN, Rahman M. Waist-to-height ratio and Socio-demographic characteristics of bangladeshi adults. Ibrahim Med. Coll. J. 2010:4(2):49-58.

25. Institute for Public Health. National Health and Morbidity Survey 2011. Putrajaya: Ministry of Health Malaysia; 2012.

26. Norfazilaha A, Julainaa MS, Azmawatia MN. Sex differences in correlates of obesity indices and blood pressure among Malay adults in Selangor, Malaysia. South African Family Practice. 2015;1(1):1–5.

27. Li W, Chen I, Chang Y, Loke S, Wang S, Hsiao K. Waist-to-height ratio, waist circumference, and body mass index as indices of cardiometabolic risk among Taiwanese adults. Eur J Nutr.2011;36:642. DOI:10.1007/s00394-011-0286-0.

28. Hsu H, Liu C, Pi-Sunyer FX, Lin C, Li C, Lin C, Li T, Lin W. The associations of different measurements of obesity with cardiovascular risk factors in Chinese. Eur J Clin Invest. 2011;41(4):393–404.

29. Ashwell M, Gunn P, Gibson S. Waist-to-height ratio is a better screening tool than waist circumference and BMI for adult cardio metabolic risk factors: Systematic review and meta-analysis. Obesity Reviews. 2012;13(3):275-286.

30. Obesity in Asia Collaboration. Is central obesity a better discriminator of the risk of hypertension than body mass index in ethnically diverse populations?. J Hypertens. 2008;26(2):169-77.

31. Liu Y, Tong G, Tong W, Lu L,Qin X. Can body mass index, waist circumference, waist-hip ratio and waist-height ratio predict the presence of multiple metabolic risk factors in Chinese subjects?. BMC Public Health. 2011;11:35.

16

Approach to Anaemia Diagnosis in Developing Countries: Focus on Aetiology and Laboratory Work-Up

S. Adewoyin Ademola[1*]

[1]*Department of Haematology and Blood Transfusion, University of Benin Teaching Hospital, PMB 1111, Benin City, Edo State, Nigeria.*

Author's contribution

The sole author designed, analyzed and interpreted and prepared the manuscript.

<u>Editor(s):</u>
(1) Dharmesh Chandra Sharma, Incharge Blood Component & Aphaeresis Unit, G. R. Medical College, Gwalior, India.
<u>Reviewers:</u>
(1) Luis Rodrigo, University of Oviedo, Spain.
(2) Anonymous, University of Baluchistan, Pakistan.
(3) Anonymous, Universidade do Estado do Rio de Janeiro, Brazil.
(4) J. A. Olaniyi, Department of Haematology, University of Ibadan, Nigeria.
(5) Irene Ule Ngole Sumbele, Department of Zoology and Animal Physiology, University of Buea, Cameroon.

ABSTRACT

Introduction: Anaemia is a significant public health problem in developing countries. Anaemia is never normal. The etiology of the anaemia should always be sought. Diagnosis of its cause and early treatment is crucial to improving the quality of life among affected persons. There is a need to provide practicing physicians with a good theoretical framework and a practical algorithm for arriving accurately at anaemia diagnosis.

Objective: This article seeks to collect, collate and concisely review anaemias with emphasis on the prevalent aetiologies and laboratory diagnosis in developing countries

Results: The etiology of anaemia in developing countries is myriad and requires accurate diagnosis. Nutritional (substrate) deficiencies and chronic diseases account for a significant proportion of acquired anaemias. The predominating inherited causes include haemoglobinopathies, red cell enzymopathies and membranopathies. A systematic approach will help the physician paddle through the large list of differentials, to cone down on precise diagnosis. Relevant clinical history, physical examination and baseline investigations are imperative. Further

---

Corresponding author: E-mail: drademola@yahoo.com

evaluations should be conducted in unresolved cases using suggested practical algorithms such as the morphologic and/or kinetic approach.

Conclusion: Baseline investigations including full blood count, reticulocyte count and peripheral blood film should be requested on patients presenting with anaemia. Relevant authorities should ensure availability of these basic tests in all health facilities. Consultations with hematology unit should be engaged when necessary.

Keywords: Anaemia; diagnosis; laboratory work-up; anaemia work-up; developing countries.

1. INTRODUCTION

The term, 'anaemia' is derived from two ancient Greek words, 'an' meaning 'without' and 'haima' meaning 'blood'. Literally, anaemia means bloodlessness or low blood level. Technically, anaemia describes a condition in which an individual's hemoglobin level (or hematocrit) falls two standard deviations below the average mean of normal for individuals of same age, sex and altitude [1,2]. The functional consequence of anaemia is decreased oxygen carrying capacity of the blood and general tissue hypoxia. Anaemia itself, is not a diagnosis, but rather a feature of an underlying disease.

The causes of anemia may be categorized in terms of patient's red cell appearance or size (cytometric or morphologic classification), the underlying patho-physiologic mechanism (aetiologic or erythrokinetic or biologic classification), marrow responsiveness or based on its biochemical or molecular basis [3]. Based on red cell morphology, anaemia may be described as microcytic-hypochromic, normocytic-normochromic or normochromic-macrocytic. From the kinetic stand-point, anaemias are grouped as anaemia of blood loss (haemorhage), haemolytic anaemia or anaemia of bone marrow failure. Based on marrow response to anaemia, anaemia may be grouped as hypo-regenerative (reticulocyte count < 50,000/ul), normo-regenerative (reticulocyte count between 50,000 and 100,000/ul), hyper-regenerative (> 100,000/ul) [4]. Normo-regenerative anaemia may often be difficult to diagnose and are often due to multiple aetiologies [4].

Undoubtedly, anaemia is the most common haematology laboratory feature among patients [4,5]. More than 90% of patients with primary haemopathies present with anaemia [5]. Anaemia is a feature of many topical diseases including Human immunodeficiency virus/Acquired Immunodeficiency syndrome (HIV/AIDS), malaria, and tuberculosis, parasitic infections such as schistosomiasis and hookworm infestations.

Making early and accurate diagnosis of tropical diseases, as well as prompt treatment decisions is related to the physician's ability to properly investigate anaemia. It is imperative for physicians, especially those in developing countries where the burden of anaemia is highest [4], to be equipped with requisite knowledge on how to investigate anaemia. Therefore, the objective of this article is to provide a general overview of anaemia, its causes and laboratory evaluation especially as it relates to developing countries. Relevant standard texts as well as journal articles on major databases including google scholar and pubmed were accessed, collated and summarized as appropriate sections.

2. ANAEMIA DEFINITIONS, DETERMINATION AND EPIDEMIOLOGY

The diagnosis of anaemia is established by low haemoglobin levels, haematocrit or reduced number of circulating red cells. In clinical practice, often times, anaemia is defined as blood haemoglobin concentration or haematocrit below established cut-offs. The lower cut-offs for definition of anaemia differs from individual to individual based on age, sex, geographical location, pregnancy status, smoking, altitude and ethnicity [6]. As such, there is need for clear definitions and reference intervals. According to the World Health Organisation (WHO), for non-smoking, non-African extraction individuals living at an altitude below 1000 meters, anaemia categories are presented in Table 1 [6-10].

According to Centre for Disease control and Prevention (CDC), anaemia in pregnancy is defined by Hb less than 11 g/dl in the first and third trimesters, and 10.5 g/dl in the second trimester [11]. Some authorities consider very severe anaemia to be Hb value less than 4 g/dl

Table 1. Who anaemia categories (haemoglobin cut-offs in g/dl)

Age groups:
Adult males above 15 years: Less than 13 g/dl
Non-Pregnant females above 15 years: Less than 12 g/dl
Teens aged 12 to 14.99 years: Less than 12 g/dl
Children aged 5 to 11.99 years: Less than 11.5 g/dl
Children aged 6 months to 4.99 years: Less than 11 g/dl
Pregnant women: Less than 11 g/dl
Severity of anaemia
Mild (10 to 10.9 g/dl)
Moderate (7 to 9.9 g/dl)
Severe (less than 7 g/dl)

while hyperanemia is haematocrit value less than 10% [12,13]. In individuals of African extraction, a cut-off of about 1 g/dl lower is recommended [6]. Even when haemoglobin value is not below the normal reference point, anaemia may be considered when haemoglobin level has significantly decreased below the individual's steady state value. Low borderline haemoglobin values may be seen in evolving disease conditions where there may still be adequate compensation or marrow reserves. Pseudoanaemia, otherwise referred to as relative or spurious anaemia is caused by expanded plasma volume due to haemodilution as in dilutional anaemia of pregnancy or a falsely reduced red cell mass due to redistribution as in splenomegaly.

The primary method for anaemia determination is haemoglobin testing. There are various methods for haemoglobin testing. The most accurate method is the colorimetric haemoglobinometry using cyanmethaemoglobin method [14]. Other less reliable methods include use of visual scales or haemoglobinometers. In developing countries, manual estimation of haematocrit (or packed cell volume) is commonly done using the micro-haematocrit (erythrocyte centrifugation) method. It is shown to be reliable for routine clinical purposes. A positive linear correlation exists between haematocrit and haemoglobin concentration. This has been validated with a correlation of 'Haematocrit = 2.62 x (haemoglobin level) + 3.67', coefficient of 0.98 and probability value less than 0.001 [15]. As a rule of thumb, packed red cell volume (PCV) is equivalent to 3 times the haemoglobin concentration levels.

An estimated two billion (more than one-third) of the world population are affected by anaemia [8, 16]. Its burden is higher in developing countries. Women of child bearing age and children bear the highest burden of anaemia [8,16,17]. WHO estimates that over 30% of all women and about 52.8 to 61.3% of pregnant women in developing nations are anaemic [8,16]. Similarly, among hospital patients, a high burden of anaemia has been reported [18-20]. In a recent retrospective study in Nigeria, the prevalence of anaemia among patients and clients receiving care in a tertiary hospital was observed to be 27.3% [21].

3. AETIOGENESIS OF ANAEMIA

All forms of anaemia may be categorized as haemolytic, hypoproliferative (aregenerative) or haemorrhagic. Haemolytic anaemia results from accelerated central or peripheral destruction of red cells. Hypoproliferative anaemia, otherwise called anaemia of bone marrow failure, results from decreased central production of red cells and/or its defective release from the bone marrow. Anaemia of blood loss or haemorrhage results from a breach in the integrity of blood vessels in the body, resulting in acute or chronic shortage of red cells/red cell mass. Hypoproliferative causes are either strictly production defects or maturation defects (otherwise called ineffective erythropoiesis). In terms of marrow reticulocyte response to anaemia, a list of its possible differentials is exemplified in Fig. 1.

Haemolysis describes a pathological state in which red cell survival is shortened below its normal interval [22,23]. Red cell life span is normally about 100 to 120 days in vivo. Haemolysis may be acute or chronic (depending on the rapidity of onset), inherited or acquired, immune or non-immune, intrinsic or extrinsic. Intrinsic causes are due to intracorpuscular defects in the red cells and they include red cell membranopathies and cytoplasmic defects. Examples of red cell membranopathies are hereditary spherocytosis, elliptocytosis, southeast Asian ovalocytosis, pyropoikilocytosis and others. Red cell cytoplasmic defects may further be grouped as haemoglobinopathies and enzymopathies. Two major broad forms of haemoglobinopathies include sickle cell disease and thalassemia. Enzymopathies include Glucose 6 Phosphate dehydrogenase (G6PD) deficiency, pyruvake kinase (PK) deficiency and others [24]. G6PD deficiency affects about 4 to 26% of Nigerians and 20 - 26% of the Nigerian male population [25-26]. In other developing African nations including Ghana, Kenya, Burkina Faso, Tanzania and Mali, frequency of G6PD deficiency ranges between 5 – 23.8% [27]. In India, prevalence of G6PD deficiency ranges from complete absence to as high as 27%, with average of about 10% [28]. On the other hand, extracorpuscular defects include immune and non-immune causes. Immune mediated haemolysis may be allo-immune, auto-immune or drug-induced in origin. In about 30 to 50% of cases, the cause of immune haemolysis is primary idiopathic, while others occur secondary to underlying diseases [22,29,30]. These secondary causes of immune haemolysis include neoplasms such as haematological malignancies and solid tumors, infections especially viral, connective tissue diseases or drugs [29]. Non-immune haemolysis may be due to exposure to toxins, infections, microangiopathy, as well as paroxysmal nocturnal haemoglobinuria (PNH). Toxaemias such as uraemia, snake and spider venoms are associated with reduced red cell lifespan [31]. Infections by microbes such as *Plasmodium falciparum, Babesia microti, Clostridium perfringens, Barthonella* species are known to cause direct lysis of red cells [22,23,32]. Malaria is a significant cause of anaemia in tropical Africa and other endemic areas, especially among under 5 children and pregnant women [33-38]. Micro-angiopathy may be caused by mucinous adenocarcinomas, haemolytic uraemic syndrome/thrombotic thrombocytopenic purpura (HUS/TTP), malignant hypertension, connective tissue diseases, burns, vasculitis, disseminated intravascular coagulopathy (DIC) [9,22]. It should be noted that HUS/TTP and DIC are thrombotic microangiopathies (TMA). Anaemia in TMA results from red cell lysis caused by the abnormal fibrin strand meshwork deposited within the microvasculature. DIC is a thrombo-haemorrhagic complication which occur secondary to several underlying disease processes. DIC is characterized by systemic (widespread) activation of coagulation system, resulting in obstruction of blood supply to vital

organs and overconsumption of coagulation proteins and platelets [39]. Known causes of DIC includes severe sepsis, acute haemolytic transfusion reaction, any form of shock, severe head injury or trauma, massive blood transfusion, vascular malformations, severe pancreatitis, obstetric complications such as intrauterine fetal demise, placental abruption, amniotic fluid embolism and others [39,40]. PNH is an acquired, progressive membrane defect that results from complement mediated lysis of red cells due to a defect in the PIG-A gene which anchors cyto-protective, complement regulating membrane surface proteins such as CD55 (decay accelerating factor, DAF), C8 binding protein (HRP) and most importantly, CD59 (membrane inhibitor of reactive lysis, MIRL) [41,42]. Most extracorpuscular defects are acquired, while most intracorpuscular defects are inherited except PNH.

Anaemia of bone marrow failure is a very significant cause of anaemia worldwide especially in developing countries largely due to nutritional deficiency anaemia. Marrow underproduction of red cells may occur at the stem cell, progenitor cell, or precursor cell pools. Known causes of marrow failure includes nutritional deficiencies, aplastic anaemia, sideroblastic anaemia, anaemia of chronic inflammation, myelophthisic anaemia, anaemia of renal failure, endocrine causes and congenital dyserythropoietic anaemias [9]. The highest burden of hypo-proliferative anaemia worldwide is caused by nutritional (substrate) deficiency (predominantly iron deficiency), closely followed by anaemia of chronic diseases [4,43]. Despite being the most abundant element/metal in the earth's crust, WHO estimates that approximately half (50%) of all cases of anaemia worldwide can be attributed to iron deficiency [43,44]. Micronutrients are necessary erythropoietic precursors required for normal haemopoiesis. They include vitamins B1, B2, B3, B6 (pyridoxine), B9 (folate), B12 (cobalamin) and trace metals such as iron, cobalt and copper [45]. Aplastic anaemia may be an inherited syndrome as in Fanconi'sanaemia, dyskeratosis congenital (DKC) or Schwachman diamond syndrome. In acquired aplastic anaemia, 60 to 70% (two-thirds) of cases are idiopathic, others are secondary to viral infections, irradiation, provocative drugs, pregnancy and graft versus host disease (GvHD) [46]. Anaemia of chronic inflammation, also known as anaemia of chronic disease, occurs in chronic inflammatory states such as autoimmune diseases, malignancies and chronic infections such as tuberculosis, HIV/AIDS and others [47]. Malignancies involving midline and paired organs such as breasts, lungs, prostate, and cervix have predilections for bone marrow involvement [48,49]. Bone marrow suppression resulting from marrow infiltration by ectopic tumor cells is termed myelophthisic anaemia. Hormones such as thyroxine and androgen are also important drivers of erythropoiesis. As such, endocrinopathies including addison's disease, hypothyroidism and hypogonadotrophic states are associated with hypoproliferative anaemia.

Please note that some forms of anaemia have multiple aetiologies. For instance, anaemia of chronic renal failure is associated with bone marrow underproduction owing to reduced erythropoietin drive alongside nutritional deficiencies (vitamin K deficiency), decreased red cell survival as well as haemorhage which may be precipitated by uraemic coagulopathy, gastritis and platelet dysfunction. Additionally, haemodialysis contributes to iron and folate deficiency, blood loss and ex-vivo red cell destruction [50].

4. PATHOPHYSIOLOGY AND CLINICAL ASPECTS OF ANAEMIA

Generally, symptomatology of anaemia among patients depends on its speed of onset, its clinical severity, patient's cardio-vascular reserve and presence of co-morbidities [9]. Clinical features of anaemia may be specific or non-specific. Non-specific features include hypoxia related effects of anaemia on organ systems most especially the brain, heart and muscles. Hypoxic effects of anaemia include physical fatigue, general malaise, dimness of vision, fainting spells, dizziness, tinnitus, palpitations, angina of efforts (if pre-existing heart disease), amenorhoea (in women), exercise intolerance, dyspnoea and paraesthesia [31]. Also, there will be pallor of mucous membrane surfaces of the eyes/conjunctiva, oral cavity, palms, sole of the feet, or the entire skin in newborns. However, clinical pallor may not be evident until haemoglobin levels less than 9 g/dl [51,52]. Specific features are related to the underling aetiology such as koilonychia in iron deficiency anaemia and atrophic painful glossitis in megaloblastic anaemia. Normally, a clinician will suspect anaemia based on one or more of the above listed symptoms and sign.

In anaemic conditions, host compensatory mechanisms are activated. These physiological adaptations include a hyperdynamic circulation, erythroid hyperactivity, increased 2, 3 DPG production, redistribution of blood flow from the peripheral (skin) to vital organs such as brain, heart and muscles [9,53]. Erythroid activity may be increased as much as 5 – 7 times normal. Decreased viscosity of anaemia blood and high levels of 2, 3 DPG helps to improve tissue perfusion by oxygen [53]. However, if hypoxia of vital organs persists for too long, compensatory mechanisms are lost. Cardiac decompensation culminates in anaemic heart failure. Features of anaemic heart failure include tachycardia, tachypnoea, dyspnoea, tender hepato-splenomegaly and bilateral pedal oedema [9]. If prompt appropriate intervention is not rendered, death ensues.

5. ANAEMIA WORK-UP

Laboratory evaluation of anaemia is crucial to diagnostic formulations in patient care. In clinical practice, accurate diagnosis relies on a tripod of clinical history, physical examination and laboratory investigations. Clinical history should include socio-demographic data noting age, sex, occupation, geographical location and ethnicity as it may have a bearing on the cause of anaemia. For instance, iron deficiency anaemia is more likely to be related to growth and development in children while chronic blood loss is a more likely cause in elderly persons. History suggestive of haemorhage or haemolysis, social history, family history, drug intake and nutritional history and other relevant details should also be elicited. A general physical examination and systemic examination especially cardiovascular and neurological systems are important. Physical signs such as jaundice and chronic leg ulcers may suggest a congenital haemolytic anaemia.

Anaemia may be multi-factorial in origin (anaemia of mixed origin). Sometimes, its cause may be obvious from clinical history alone, as in straight-forward acute blood loss. However, many cases of anaemia require more detailed history, physical examination and laboratory investigations to elucidate its cause(s) [5]. Laboratory investigations will often be required to establish or exclude possible differentials. Such investigation profiles engaged in the diagnosis and treatment of anaemia are termed anaemic work-up. Anaemia work-up investigations are intended to define anaemia, to establish its causes and to monitor response to treatment.

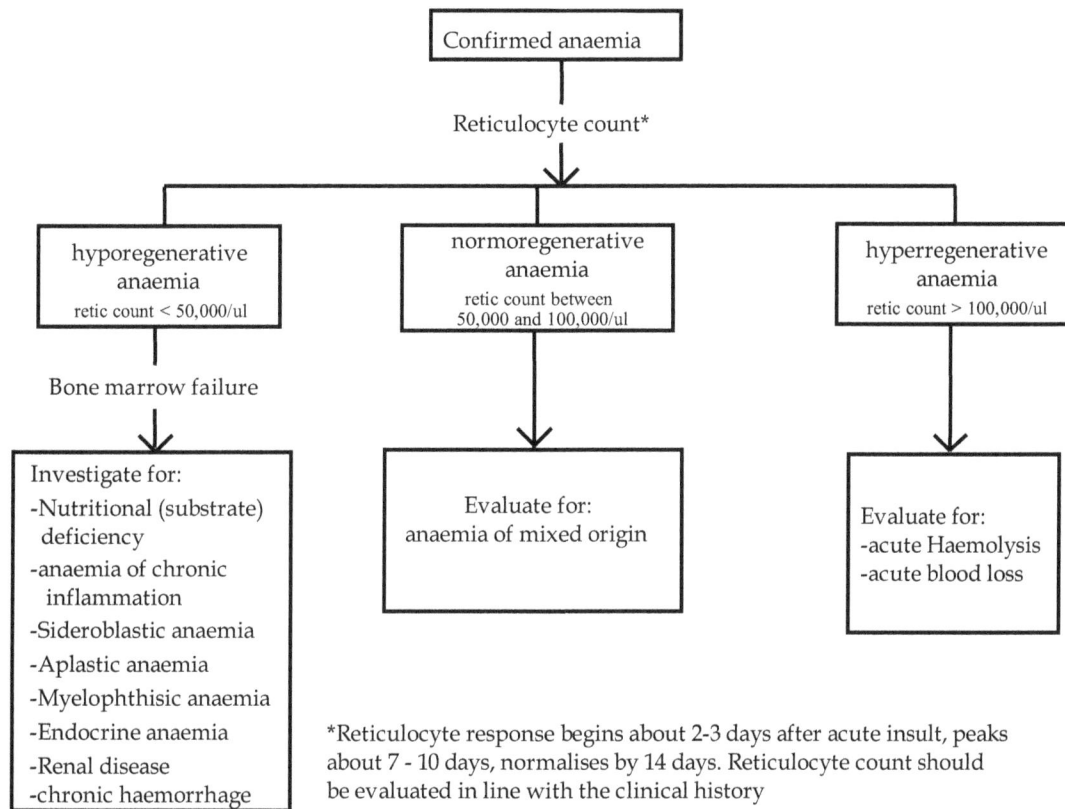

Fig. 1. Aetiologic classification of anaemia

Laboratory investigation of anaemia should never be in isolation, rather it should be directed by a patient's clinical history and physical examination findings. For instance, it would be clinically absurd to request bone marrow aspiration (BMA) plus biopsy or immunophenotyping/flow cytometry or even haematinic assays at first clinical interview with a paediatric patient presenting to you with a history of delayed growth, chronic anaemia/pallor, jaundice and recurrent bone pains. Such a patient would rather benefit from a full blood count (FBC), reticulocyte count, peripheral blood film (PBF), haemoglobin electrophoresis, high performance liquid chromatography (HPLC), biochemical markers of haemolysis, as the history points toward sickle cell disease as a top differential.

As a baseline, initial laboratory work-up when investigating anaemia should include full blood count (including red cell indices), reticulocyte count and peripheral blood film [54-56]. Arguably, reticulocyte count is the single most important laboratory investigation in any case of anaemia. Reticulocytes are the youngest anucleate red cells in the peripheral circulation and they take

about 1- 2 days for maturation in the periphery [54]. Normally, in anaemic conditions, reticulocyte production is increased in order to compensate for the decreased red cell mass. Normal reticulocyte count in adults is 0.5-1.5% and 2-5% in newborns [23,45]. Increased reticulocyte count is a sign of adequate marrow regeneration in response to anaemia following haemolysis or haemorrhage or haematinic therapy. Poor reticulocyte response suggests a hypoproliferate anaemia or bone marrow failure [57]. Reticulocyte count may be reported as percentage or absolute counts or corrected for the degree of anaemia. Evaluation of anaemia using reticulocyte count is more reliable through the use of indices such as the reticulocyte production index (RPI). In severe anaemia, the rate of red cell release from the marrow exceeds the normal rate and this gives a false impression of increased production. To correct for this phenomenon (where release exceeds production), RPI is more sensitive and is used for shift correction. Generally, normal RPI is 1. RPI > 3 suggests anaemia with adequate regeneration. RPI < 2 suggests anaemia with inadequate regeneration [58]. A full blood count (FBC) is important because anaemia is not always isolated. Bi- or pancytopenia may suggest underlying diseases causing central suppression of haemopoiesis such as malignancies, nutritional deficiencies or HIV/AIDS. It is therefore important to request a FBC rather than just a PCV (haematocrit). Red cell indices such as mean corpuscular volume(MCV), mean corpuscular haemoglobin (MCH) and mean corpuscular haemoglobin concentration(MCHC) are a part of full blood count.They are useful in categorizing anaemia as either normocytic, microcytic or macrocytic (Fig. 2). Major differentials of microcytic hypochromic anaemia are iron deficiency anaemia, thalassemias, sideroblastic anaemia and occasionally, anaemia of chronic diseases [9,59].

Normocytic anaemia may be seen in combined (mixed) nutritional deficiency states, acute blood loss, anaemia of chronic diseases and anaemias due to endocrine dysfunction [60]. Macrocytic anaemias may be megaloblastic or non-megaloblastic [61,62]. Megaloblastic causes include folate and B12 deficiency, as well as acute nitrous oxide poisoning. Whereas, non-megaloblastic macrocytosis is observed in alcoholism, neonates, myeloma, hypothyroidism, liver disease, pregnancy, aplastic anaemia and myelodysplastic syndrome [61,62]. Clinical indications for a peripheral blood film (PBF) request are myriad and they include cases listed in Table 2 [63,64].

PBF should be reported by a haemato-morphologist. This requires that adequate clinical details should be provided by the requesting clinician, in order to facilitate holistic review of patient's blood smear by the haemotologist.

Further laboratory evaluations would include specific investigations to pin down the exact cause of the anaemia. Further anaemia work-ups include other haematological, biochemical, microbiology or histo-pathological tests. They include C-reactive protein/Erythrocyte Sedimentation Rate (CRP/ESR), renal function test (E/U/Cr), liver function test (LFT), anti-globulin test, haemoglobin electrophoresis, G6PD assay, stool for occult blood, flow cytometry for CD55/59, bone marrow cytology and histology, lymph node histology, haematinic assays, prussian blue reaction, cytogenetic studies, erythropoietin assay, serum hepcidin levels, hormone assays (serum androgen and thyroxine levels), GIT studies and so on [5,9,55,65,66]. Erythrocyte sedimentation rate (ESR) is raised in chronic inflammation. ESR is

rather an unspecific marker. However, a very high ESR (above 100 mm in 1 hour) may be seen in multiple myeloma and other plasma cell dyscrasia, as well as polymyalgia rheumatica and tuberculosis. Normal ESR level (Westergren method) is less than 15 mm in one hour in adult males and less than 20 mm in one hour in adult females. ESR may be slightly reduced in sickle cell disease and slightly increased in the elderly. On the other hand, C-reactive protein (CRP) gives a more sensitive and accurate reflection of acute inflammation. Normal adult CRP levels is about 1 to 5 mg/l. Deranged renal function and liver function tests may point to anaemia of chronic renal failure and liver disease respectively. Direct and indirect antiglobulin tests, also called Coomb's test were designed by Coombs and colleagues in 1945 for detection of non-agglutinating antibodies in the serum. Coombs test are useful in investigating immune related causes such as auto-immune anaemias and haemolytic transfusion reactions [67]. Haemoglobin electrophoresis and HPLC are highly informative in diagnosis or exclusion of abnormal haemoglobin variants such as sickle cell disease and thalassemia [56,68,69]. G6PD assay should be requested in suspected cases of haemolytic anaemia especially in males. Patients with history of chronic cough, chronic diarrhoea and significant weight loss, as well as individuals with history of sexually risky behaviors should be referred for retroviral screening (RVS) following proper counseling and consent. Stool test for occult blood is unspecific and may be associated with false-positives depending on the individual's diet or use of iron containing tablets. However, true-positive result suggests some sort of GI bleeding, maybe peptic ulcer disease or gastro-intestinal malignancy. Gastro-intestinal endoscopies and CT/MRI may be required for further evaluation. Lymph node biopsy histology is indicated in suspected lymphomas or metastatic lymphadenopathy. Bone marrow aspiration and biopsy is an invasive procedure, as such patients should be carefully selected, educated and consenting. Not all cases of anaemia will require bone marrow examinations. BMA and biopsy is indicated in cases of unexplained anaemia or leukocytosis despite peripheral blood analysis, unexplained lymphadenopathy or splenomegaly, suspected acute leukaemias, megaloblastic anaemia, advanced lymphomas or non-haematologic malignancies with marrow involvement and so on [55,70]. Marrow blood is also useful for microbiological cultures, cytogenetic studies and Perl's staining (Prussian blue reaction) for marrow iron stores. Haematinic assays include serum iron levels, total iron binding capacity (TIBC), percentage transferrin saturation (TSAT), serum ferritin levels, serum transferrin receptor levels, serum folate and red cell folate levels as well as serum cobalamin levels. These assays, with their respective limits and pitfalls, are engaged in assessing iron, folate or cobalamin deficiency anaemias. In suspected haemolytic anaemia, relevant biochemical tests for haemolysis includes serum bilirubin levels, serum enzymes including aspartate transaminase and lactate dehydrogenase, haptoglobin and haemopexin levels [60]. Haptoglobin is more sensitive and specific than indirect bilirubin assay. A combination of raised lactate dehydrogenase (LDH) levels alongside reduced serum haptoglobin is 90% specific for diagnosing haemolysis. Normal serum LDH coupled with serum haptoglobin level above 25 mg/dl is 92% sensitive to exclude haemolysis [71]. Haptoglobin level (in the absence of liver cirrhosis) below 28mg/d is 92% sensitive and 98% specific for predicting haemolysis [72]. A practical schema for evaluation of haemolytic anaemia is provided in Fig. 3. Examination of the peripheral blood is usually sufficient in diagnosis of haemolytic anaemia. However, most cases of reticulocytopenic anaemia or pancytopenic anaemia resulting from marrow failure will require bone marrow examination for adequate diagnosis.

In steady state, normal non-anaemic serum erythropoietin (EPO) level is about 5 to 20 milliunits/ml [73]. Low EPO levels suggest renal disease. In response to anaemia in absence of renal damage, endogenous EPO levels increase exponentially in order to compensate and promote production of red cells. However, significant anaemia especially in HIV/AIDS with serum endogenous EPO levels below 500 mu/ml may be corrected with exogenous (recombinant) EPO treatment [74].

Detection of rheumatoid factor and anti-nuclear antibodies are relevant in investigation of auto-immune diseases/connective tissue diseases. Radiological studies such as abdominal X-rays, abdominal ultrasonography and CT scan may be used to delineate occult intra-abdominal malignancies. Work-ups such as blood culture and other microbiological cultures, blood film for malaria parasite, stool for ova and parasite, retroviral screening, urine m/c/s, lumber puncture (CSF) analysis are relevant to evaluating infection/infestation associated anaemia.

Advanced techniques including cytogenetics and nucleic acid amplication protocols such as PCR are required for evaluation of primary haemopathies especially haematological malignancy.

This list of anaemia work-up investigations is by no means exhaustive. However, anaemic work-ups should be targeted towards confirming or refuting its likely aetiology in a systemic unprejudiced manner, considering the high cost of laboratory tests. A physicians ability to select the most appropriate and relevant investigations in anaemia work-up depends on the depth of his knowledge database and clinical experience. A good physician is one who knows his limits. Consultations should be sought or referrals made to appropriate specialist teams where and when necessary.

6. GENERAL APPROACH TO ANAEMIA TREATMENT

General approach to treating anaemia include methods for promotion of red cell production in hypoproliferative anaemia such nutritional supplements in nutritional anaemia, limitation of red cell destruction in haemolytic anaemia such as immunosuppressive therapy in auto-immune haemolytic anaemia and arrest of bleeding in anaemia of blood loss. Severe symptomatic anaemia requires replacement with red cell concentrate (packed red cells). Specialist blood component should be prescribed as the situation warrants. Haematology consultations should be sought when in doubt.

Blood transfusion is not totally innocuous and should not be undertaken lightly. There must be a clear indication for every transfusion event. Transfusion should be withheld except the anaemia is severe (haemoglobin less than 7 g/dl), symptomatic at any level, evidence for continuing blood loss or in pre-operative/procedure/surgical preparations. In disease conditions associated with lower affinity haemoglobins such as sickle cell disease, transfusions should be withheld except in occasions of very severe anaemia (haemoglobin level less than 4 g/dl) or acute worsening anaemia. While symptomatic relief with blood transfusion is offered, the cause of the anaemia should be pursued. Erythropoiesis stimulating agents such as erythropoietin and haematinics should be administered where indicated. Tactful skills (bloodless surgeries) should be engaged at surgeries. Definitive treatment should be directed at the underlying disease.

Table 2. Indications for peripheral blood film

Unexplained peripheral blood cytopenias	Anaemia
	Leucopenia
	Thrombocytopenia

Unexplained high leucocyte counts
Jaundice or haemolysis
Features suggestive of an inherited haemolytic anaemia
Suspected leukaemias or lymphomas
Liver or renal failures
Severe bacterial sepsis and parasitic infections
Advanced cancers with possible bone marrow involvement
Cases of nutritional anaemias
Others

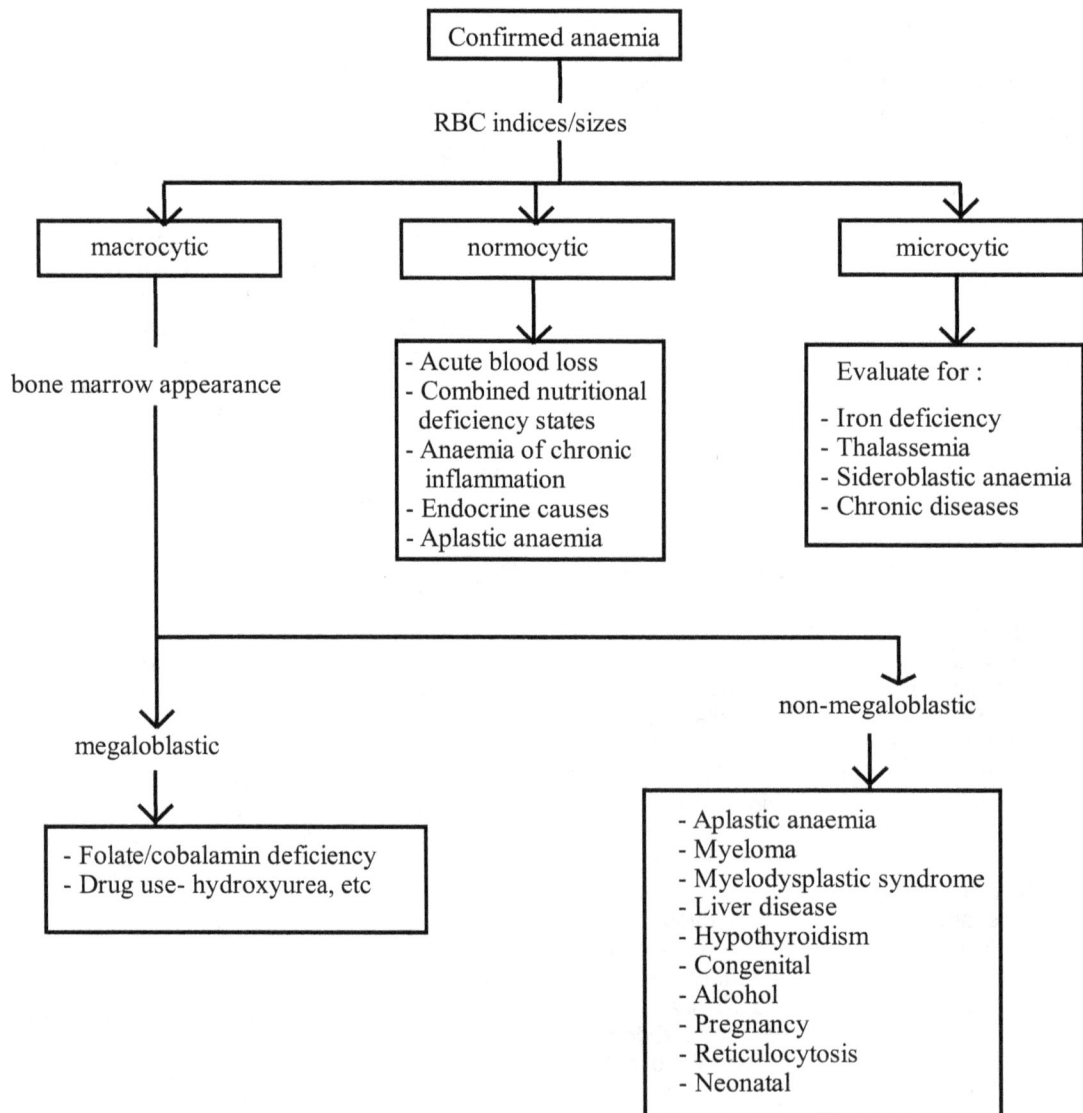

Fig. 2. Diagnostic algorithm for anaemia evalution

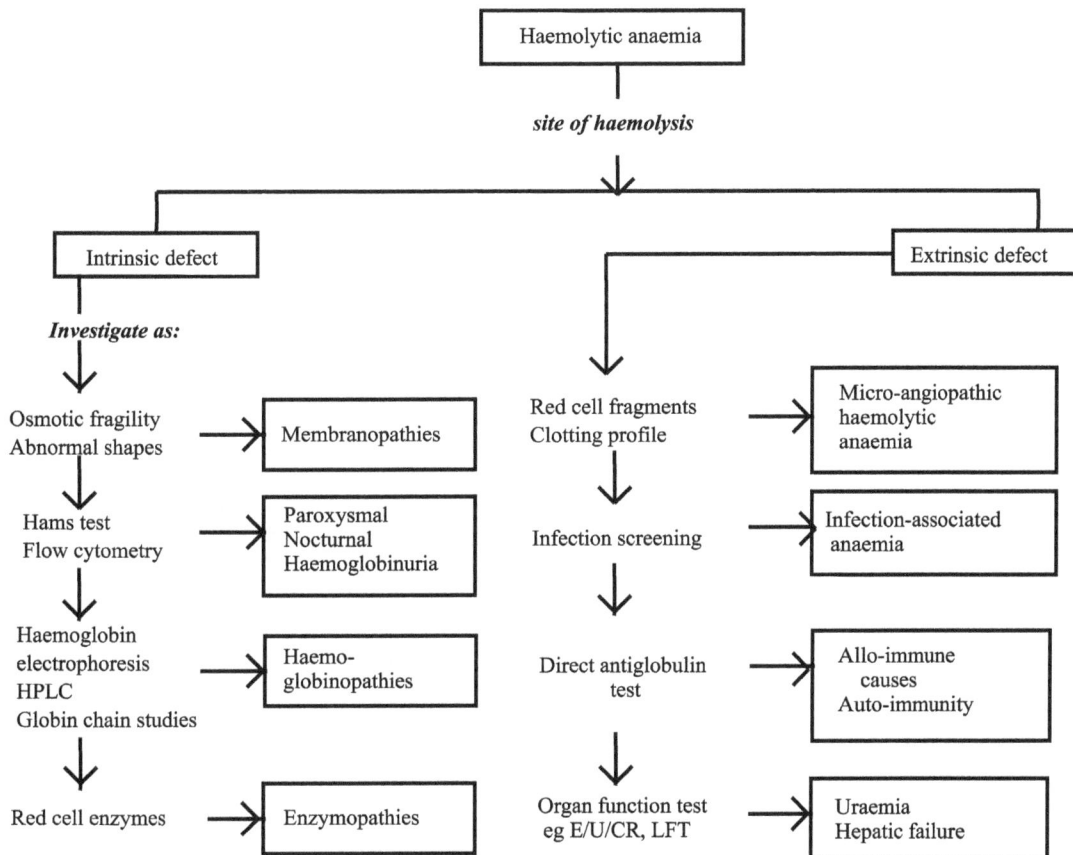

Fig. 3. Evaluation of haemolytic anaemia

7. CONCLUSION

Laboratory investigations are not substitutes for good clinical skills in patient interview and physical examination. Physicians should treat patients, not laboratory tests. However, in appropriate situations, relevant laboratory investigations that would facilitate patient care should be requested.

The author also recommends that FBC, reticulocyte count and PBF should be requested on any patients presenting with anaemia as initial baseline investigations. Relevant authorities and stakeholders should ensure that these tests are routinely available in all health facilities. This therefore calls for improvements in diagnostic services especially in developing nations. Automation of medical laboratories is highly desirable as it reduces processing time and manpower needs and improves diagnostic accuracy. Though more expensive to install and operate, automation is a more suitable alternative for laboratories with high sample volume.

Blood transfusion is never a quick-fix unless the cause of anaemia is found and treated. As such, the cause of anaemia should always be sought by the attending physicians at all levels of health-care. Prompt actions should be taken as anaemia may portray life threatening causes such as malignancies. Difficult cases should be referred to a haematologist and other appropriate specialists.

CONSENT

It is not applicable.

ETHICAL APPROVAL

It is not applicable.

COMPETING INTERESTS

Author has declared that no competing interests exist.

REFERENCES

1. Wiwanitkit V. Introduction to tropical anemia. In: Tropical Anaemia. Nova Science Publishers. New York. 2007;1:1–17.

2. Sullivan KM, Mei Z, Grummer-Straw L, Parvanta I. Haemoglobin adjustments to define anaemia. Tropical Medicine and International Health. 2008;13(10):1267-1271.

3. Risch L, Herklotz R, Huber AR. Differential diagnosis of anemia. TherUmsch. 2004; 61:103-115.

4. Jean-François L, Photis B. Pathophysiology and differential diagnosis of anaemia. In: Beaumont C, Beris P, Beuzard Y, Brugnara C (eds). ESH Handbook on Disorders of erythropoiesis, erythrocytes and iron metabolism. 2009;4:108-141.

5. Beck ON. Anaemia: General considerations. Diagnostic Hematology. Springer-Verlag London Ltd. London. 2009;7:199-218.

6. Sullivan KM, Mei Z, Grummer-Straw L, Parvanta I. Haemoglobin adjustments to define anaemia. Tropical Medicine and International Health. 2008;13(10):1267-1271.

7. World Health Organisation. Haemoglobin concentrations for the diagnosis of anaemia and assessment of severity. 2011, WHO/NMH/NHD/MNM/11.1

8. World Health Organization. Worldwide prevalence of anaemia 1993 – 2005. WHO, Geneva; 2008. ISBN 978-92-4-159665-7.

9. Glader B. Anaemia: general considerations. In: Greer JP, Foerster J, Lukens JN (eds). Wintrobe's Clinical Haematology. Lippincott Williams & Wilkins Publishers; 11th ed. 2004;27:770-793.

10. Nutritional anaemias. Report of a WHO scientific group. Geneva, World Health Organization, 1968. (WHO Technical Report Series, No. 405). Available:http://whqlibdoc.who.int/trs/WHO_TRS_405.pdf

11. Centers for Disease Control and Prevention. Recommendations to prevent and control Iron deficiency in the United States. Morbidity and Mortality Weekly report. 1998;47(No. RR – 3).

12. Indian Council of Medical Research. Evaluation of the National Nutritional Anaemia Prophylaxis Programme. Task Force Study. New Delhi: ICMR; 1989

13. Sharma JB, Shankar M. Anemia in Pregnancy. Journal internal medical sciences academy. 2010;23(4):253-260.

14. Briggs C, Bain BJ. Basic Haematological techniques. Bain BJ, Bates I, Laffan MA, Lewis SM (eds). Dacie and Lewis Practical Haematology. 11 ed. Elsevier Churchill Livingstone. 2012;3:23-56.

15. Bhokaisawan N, Chinayon S. The correlation between haematocrit and haemoglobin. Chula Med J. 1982;26:15-21.

16. World Health Organisation. The prevalence of Anaemia in Women: A tabulation of Available information. Geneva: WHO; 1992. (WHO/MCH/MSM/92.2)

17. El Kishawi RR, Soo KL, Abed YA,Muda WA. Anemia among children aged 2-5 years in the Gaza Strip- Palestinian: A cross sectional study. BMC Public Health 2015;1(15):319. DOI:10.1186/s12889-015-1652-2.

18. George IO, Otaigbe BE. Anaemia in Critically Ill Children - A Case Study from Nigeria. International Journal of tropical disease & health. 2012;2(1):55-61.

19. Rong M, Tay J, Ong YY. Prevalence and Risk Factors of Anaemia in Older Hospitalised Patients. Proceedings of Singapore Healthcare. 2011;20(2):71-79.

20. Brown BJ, Oladokun RE. Health status of children in institutionalized homes in South West Nigeria. The Nigerian postgraduate medical Journal. 2013;20 (3):168-173.

21. Adewoyin AS, Bazuaye GN, Enabudoso E. Burden of anaemia among In- and Out-patients seen at the University of Benin Teaching Hospital, Benin City. Annals of Tropical Pathology. 2014;5(2):99-105.

22. Dhaliwal G, Cornett PA, Tierney LM. Haemolytic anaemia. Am Fam Physician. 2004;69(11):2599-2606.

23. O'neal PA, Schechter GP, Rodgers GP, Miller JL. Haemolytic anaemia. In: Rodgers GP, Young NS. The Bethesda Handbook of Clinical Haematology. 3 ed, 3:22-36.

24. Joan-Luis Vives Corrons. Red blood cell enzyme defects. In: Beaumont C, Beris P, Beuzard Y, Brugnara C (eds). ESH Handbook on Disorders of Erythropoiesis, Erythrocytes and Iron Metabolism. 2009;17:436-453.

25. Ademowo OG, Falusi AG. Molecular epidemiology and activity of erythrocyte

G6PD variants in a homogenous Nigerian population. East Afr. Med. J. 2002;79:42-44.

26. Egesie OJ, Joseph DE, Isiguzoro I, Egesie UG. G6PD activity and deficiency in a population of Nigerian Males Resident in Jos. Nigerian Journal of physiological Sciences. 2008;23(1-2):9-11.

27. Carter N, Pamba A, Duparc S, Waitumbi JN. Frequency of glucose 6 phosphate dehydrogenase deficiency in malaria patients from six African countries enrolled in two randomized anti-malarial clinical trials. Malar J. 2011;10:241. DOI:10.1186/1475-2875-10-241.

28. Rai V, Kumar P. Epidemiological study of Glucose 6 Phosphate Dehydrogenase Deficiency in scheduled caste population of India. Journal of Anthropology; 2012. Available:http://dx.doi.org/10.1155/2012/984180.

29. Gordon – Smith EC, Elebute MO. Acquired haemolytic anaemias. In: Hoffbrand AV, Catovsky D, et al. (eds), Postgraduate Haematology, 6 ed. West Sussex. Wiley-Blackwell. 2011;10:158-175.

30. Zeerleder S. Autoimmune haemolytic anaemia – a practical guide to cope with a diagnostic and therapeutic challenge. The Journal of medicine. 2011;69(4):177-184.

31. Murphy MF, Wainscoat J, Pasi KJ. Haematological disease. Kumar P, Clark M (eds). Kumar and Clark's clinical medicine. Saunders Elsevier Publishers, Spain. 7 ed. 2009;8:387-447.

32. Berkowitz FE. Hemolysis and infection: Categories and mechanisms of their relationship. Rev Infect Dis. 1991;13:1151-1162.

33. Fowowe AA. Malaria: A Major Cause of Anemia Among Under 5 Children on Hospital Bed in State Specialist Hospital, Ondo, Ondo State, Nigeria. Available:www.agpmpn.org/.../9716134Malaria.pdf (Last accessed on 01-06-2014).

34. Guyatt HL, Snow RW. The epidemiology and burden of Plasmodium falciparum-related anemia among pregnant women in sub-Saharan Africa. Am J Trop Med Hyg. 2001;64(1-2 Suppl):36-44.

35. Verhoeff FH, Brabin BJ, Chimsuku L, et al. Malaria in pregnancy and its consequences for the infant in rural Malawi. Ann Trop Med Parasitol. 1999; 93(1):S25-33.

36. Madukaku CU, Nosike DI, Chukwuocha AN. Malaria and its burden among pregnant women in parts of the Niger-Delta area of Nigeria. Asian Pacific Journal of Reproduction. 2012;1(2):147-151

37. Osazuwa F, Ayo OM, Imade P. Contribution of malnutrition and malaria to anaemia in children in rural communities of Edo state, Nigeria. N Am J Med Sci. 2010;2(1):532-536.

38. Bashawri LAM, Mandil AA, Bahnassy AA, Ahmed MA. Malaria: Haematological aspects. Annals of Saudi Medicine. 2002;22(5-6):372-377

39. Collins PW, Thachil J, Cheng - Hock T. Acquired coagulation disorders. In: Hoffbrand AV, Catovsky D, et al. (eds), Postgraduate Haematology, 6 ed. West Sussex. Wiley-Blackwell. 2011;43:839-859.

40. Dalainas I. Pathogenesis, diagnosis and management of disseminated intravascular coagulation: A literature review. European Review for Medical and Pharmacological Sciences. 2008;12:19-31.

41. Hillmen P. Paroxysmal nocturnal haemoglobinuria. In: Hoffbrand AV, Catovsky D, et al. (eds), Postgraduate Haematology, 6 ed. West Sussex. Wiley-Blackwell. 2011;11:176-185.

42. Rosse WF. Paroxysmal nocturnal haemoglobinuria; 2004. Available:http://www.orpha.net/data/patho/GB/uk-PNH.pdf. (Last assessed on 9th September, 2014).

43. Dahlerup JF, Eivindson M,Jacobsen BA, Jensen NM,Jorgensen SP, Laursen SP, et al. Diagnosis and treatment of unexplained anemia with irondeficiency without overt bleeding. Dan Med J. 2015;61(4).pii: C5072.

44. WHO/UNICEF/UNU. Iron deficiency anaemia: Assessment, prevention and control. Geneva: World Health Organization; 2001.

45. Erythropoiesis and general aspects of anaemia. In: AV Hoffbrand, PAH Moss, JE Pettit. Essential Haematology. 5th edition. 2006;2:12-27

46. Marsh JCW, Ball SE, Cavenagh J, et al. Guidelines for the diagnosis and management of aplastic anaemia. Br J Haematol. 2009;147:43-70.

47. Weiss G, Goodnough LT. Anemia of Chronic Disease. N Engl J Med. 2005; 352:1011-1023.

48. Besa EC. Myelophthisic anemia. Emedicine; 2013

49. Makoni SN, Laber DA. Clinical spectrum of myelophthisis in Cancer patients. American Journal of Hematology. 2004; 76:92-93.

50. Nurko S. Anemia in chronic kidney disease: Causes, diagnosis, treatment. Clevaland Clinic J Med. 2006;3:289-97.

51. Sheth TN, Choudhry NK, Bowes M, Detsky AS. The relation of conjunctival pallor to the presence of anemia. J Gen Intern Med. 1997;12:102-106.

52. Nardone DA, Roth M, Mazur DJ, McAfee JH. Usefulness of physical examination in detecting the presence or absence of anemia. Arch. Intern. Med. 1990;150:201-204.

53. Metivier F, Marchais SJ, Guerin AP, Pannier B, London GM. Pathophysiology of anaemia: focus on the heart and blood vessels. Nephrol Dial Transplant. 2000; 15(3):14-18.

54. Barth D, Hirschmann JV. Anaemia. In: Tkachuk, Douglas C, Hirschmann JV, (eds). Wintrobe's Atlas of Clinical Hematology, Lippincott Williams & Wilkins. 2007;1.

55. Perkins S. Diagnosis of anemia. In: Carl R. Kjeldsberg(ed) Practical Diagnosis of Hematologic Disorders. 4ed ASCP Press, Singapore. 2006;1:1-16.

56. Thomas AE. Investigation of anaemia. Current Paediatrics. 2005;15:44-49.

57. Lee GR, Foerster J, Lukens J, Paraskevas F, Greer JP, Rodgers GM. Wintrobe's Clinical Hematology. 10th ed. Baltimore: Williams and Wilkins; 1999.

58. Reticulocytes and their significance; 2010. Available:www.sysmex.ru/files/articles/Xtra_online_reticulocytes.pdf.
(Accessed on december 15th, 2013).

59. Hypochromic anaemia and iron overload. In: AV Hoffbrand, PAH Moss, JE Pettit. Essential Haematology. 5th edition. 2006; 3:28-43.

60. Wall M, Street A. Investigation of normocytic normochromic anaemia in adults. Medicine Today 2006;7(3):43-47.

61. Kaferle J, Strzoda CE. Evaluation of macrocytosis. Am Fam Physician. 2009; 79(3):203-208.

62. Hoffbrand AV. Megaloblastic anaemias. In: Hoffbrand AV, Catovsky D, et al (eds), Postgraduate Haematology, 6 ed. West Sussex. Wiley-Blackwell. 2011;5:61–82.

63. Barbara J Bain; Diagnosis from the blood Smear. N Engl J Med2005, 353:498 – 507.

64. Adewoyin AS, Nwogoh B. Peripheral Blood film: A review. Annals of Ibadan postgraduate Medicine. 2014;12(2):71-79.

65. Roy CN. Anemia of inflammation. Hematology. 2010;276-280.

66. Ogedegbe HO, Csury L, Simmons BH. Anaemia: A clinical laboratory perspective. Laboratory medicine. 2004;35(3):177-185.

67. Bain BJ, Win N. Acquired haemolyticanaemias: In: Bain BJ, Bates I, Laffan MA, Lewis SM (eds). Dacie and Lewis Practical haematology. Churchill Livingstone 11 ed. 2012;13:273-300.

68. Wajcman H, Moradkhani K. Abnormal haemoglobins: Detection and characterization. Indian J Med Res. 2011; 134:538-546.

69. Bain BJ. Laboratory techniques for the identification of abnormalities of globin chain synthesis. In: Bain BJ(ed). Haemoglobinopathy diagnosis. Blackwell Publishing Oxford. 2006;2ed. 2:26-62.

70. Bain BJ. Bone marrow aspiration. J Clin Pathol. 2001;54:657-663.

71. Kale V, Aftab A. Diagnostic evaluation of anaemia. In: Silverberg DS(ed). Anaemia. InTech Publishers, Rijeka Croatia. 2012;6:75-92.

72. Kormoczi GF, Saemann MD, Buchta C, et al. Influence of clinical factors on the haemolysis marker haptoglobin. Eur J Clin Invest. 2006;36:202-209.

73. Musicant J. Clinical indications for measuring endogenous erythropoietin levels. Critical Review. 1990;1-8.

74. Ng T, Marx G, Littlewood T, Macdougall I. Recombinant erythropoietin in clinical practice. Postgrad Med J. 2003;79:367-376.

17

Appropriateness of Use of Blood Products in Tertiary Hospitals

Jerold C. Alcantara[1*], Ann P. Opiña[1] and Rhashani Arjay M. Alcantara[2]

[1]Saint Louis University, School of Natural Sciences, Baguio City, Philippines.
[2]Lorma Medical Center, Clinical Laboratory Department, San Fernando City, Philippines.

Authors' contributions

All authors have equally contributed in the conceptualization and study design; acquisition, analysis and interpretation of data; and in drafting and critical revision of the manuscript. All authors read and approved the final manuscript.

Editor(s):
(1) Salah Aref, Department of Hematology, Mansoura University, Egypt.
(2) Dharmesh Chandra Sharma, Incharge Blood Component & Aphaeresis Unit, G. R. Medical College, Gwalior, India.
Reviewers:
(1) Anonymous, USA.
(2) Celso Eduardo Olivier, Department of allergy and immunology, Instituto Alergoimuno de Americana, Brazil.
(3) Phuong-Thu Pham, David Geffen School of Medicine at UCLA, Nephrology Division, Kidney Transplant Program Los Angeles, CA 90095, USA.
(4) Anonymous, Denmark.

ABSTRACT

Aims: This study aimed at evaluating the appropriateness of use of blood products in Northern Philippines and sought to find out if significant differences exist on the appropriateness of use of the blood products among the different departments and the tertiary hospitals.

Methodology: The appropriateness of use was determined by the criteria of the joint initiative of the National Health and Medical Research Council (NHMRC) and the Australasian Society of Blood Transfusion (ASBT). The frequency of utilization and the percentage of appropriateness were determined to compare the use of blood products among the different departments and the tertiary hospitals. Contingence tables were formed to test the associations between the categorical variables. The statistical significance was determined by Chi square test when p value <0.05.

Results: A total of 1,075 transfusion events were evaluated with a mean number of 2.43 transfusions per patient. Forty-one percent (41%) received two transfusions, 22% received one, and 37% received three or more transfusions. Five hundred eighty-three (583) transfusions were in the Medicine, 215 in Surgery, 218 in Obstetrics and 59 in Pediatrics. The overall prevalence of

Corresponding author: E-mail: jerold.alcantara@yahoo.com

appropriate use among the different departments was 65%, and 59% among the tertiary hospitals. Appropriateness of use was statistically different among departments. A significant association also exist between the percentages of appropriate use of the blood products among the tertiary hospitals.

Conclusion: The study revealed that there was substantial variation in the appropriate transfusion practices across study hospitals and appropriateness of use was influenced by the departments regardless of the blood products.

Keywords: Appropriateness of use; blood transfusion; blood products; tertiary hospital.

1. INTRODUCTION

In modern health care today, blood transfusion plays a vital role. Blood transfusion can alleviate health and save life if used appropriately. According to WHO [1], appropriate use of blood products is defined as "the transfusion of safe blood products only to treat a condition leading to significant morbidity or mortality that cannot be prevented or managed effectively by other means".

There are two crucial factors that determines the safety and effectiveness of transfusions. First is the accessibility(with reasonable cost) and adequacy of supply of safe blood and blood products to meet the national needs; and second, the appropriate clinical use of blood and blood products. However, the clinical use of blood between different hospitals, different clinical specialties and different clinicians with in the same team, evidently showed that there is substantial disparities on the pattern of clinical blood use from every region of the world [2].

High proportion of unnecessary blood transfusions have constantly revealed from various studies despite of publishedguidelines. The wide variation in the transfusion practice was due to the absence of consensus on the most appropriate criteria for blood transfusion therapy; the differences on blood component therapy guidelines; and the mixed effectiveness on the strategies in changing transfusion practice. Overall, there is difficulty in changing and maintaining the change in practice which is more difficult especially if no sustainability of the strategies [3].

In the Philippines, there is paucity of published papers, studies and data with regard to appropriateness of use of each blood products. Hence, such studies like this should be conducted to evaluate or assess rational and optimal utilization of blood products. Moreover, it would provide data for future studies or

references and may serve as one of the bases in developing a blood management oversight program so as to promote safe and judicious use of blood. Such an oversight program serves to reduce variation in transfusion practice and inappropriate use, and implement more efficient methods to manage patients at risk for transfusion.

A significant function of transfusion committee is to review the appropriateness of use of blood products. Five percent (5%) of all transfusion should be audited on a quarterly basis as a requirement. They are three forms of review that can be used: prospective, concurrent or retrospective review [4]. There is a need for continuous evaluation in blood transfusions and audit of the use of blood products as therapy, mainly in hospitals where no transfusion committee exists. Hence, this study aimed at evaluating the appropriateness of use of blood products among the different tertiary hospitals and sought to find out if significant differences exist on the appropriateness of use of the blood products among the different departments and the tertiary hospitals.

2. MATERIALS AND METHODS

The study employed a retrospective design guided with preset criteria and carried out among the tertiary hospitals in Northern Philippines. All consecutive requests for blood transfusions in a three month period from January to March 2010 were analyzed.

The study included records of all patients aged 12 years old or older from the Medicine, Surgery, Obstetrics, and Pediatrics departments of the different tertiary hospitals who underwent blood transfusion. Selection of hospital departments as the subjects of the study was done through survey with the most blood transfusion cases.

Patient's medical history was reviewed for each request of blood product. Factors including age, current diagnosis, department, type and amount of blood products, and the reasons or stated indication for the transfusion of a blood product were analyzed using their patient's records. When information was not available or if the reason for the transfusion was unclear, the researchers considered the transfusion as inappropriate. The researchers sought a hematologist for assistance as needed.

Appropriate use of blood products and their therapeutic effect was assessed by using pre-set criteria (Appendix). Violation of the established pre-set criteria was considered as "inappropriate" use of blood product for a particular subject.

The appropriateness of use was determined by the criteria of the joint initiative of the National Health and Medical Research Council (NHMRC) and the Australasian Society of Blood Transfusion (ASBT) [5]. The frequency of utilization and the percentage of appropriateness were determined to compare the use of blood products among the different departments and the tertiary hospitals. Contingence tables were formed to test the associations between the categorical variables. The statistical significance was determined by Chi square test when p value <0.05.

3. RESULTS

A total of 1,075 transfusion events were evaluated among the tertiary hospitals, with a mean number of 2.43 transfusions per patient. Forty one percent (41%) received two transfusions, 22% received one, and 37% received three or more transfusions. Of the total transfusion events, 583 were from the Medicine, 215 from Surgery, 218 from Obstetrics and 59 from Pediatrics.

Among the selected blood products, packed red blood cells (841) was the most frequently utilized, followed by whole blood (127), platelet concentrates (91) and fresh frozen plasma (16). Although cryoprecipitate was included in study, there was no demand of use that was recorded among the different departments to all the tertiary hospitals. Frequency of utilization of the blood products is shown in Table 1.

The overall prevalence of appropriate use among the different departments was 65%. Along with the department, the Paediatrics had the highest percentage of appropriateness with 86%. It should be pointed out that there was minimal utilization of the different blood products in this department given the reason that the criteria for the evaluation for transfusion in such patients are different from those used in adult patients. The department of Medicine had 75% of appropriateness, Obstetrics with 52% and least to Surgery with 48%. These departments are associated with high inappropriate transfusions especially to Surgery and Obstetrics departments. Percentage of appropriateness of the blood products is shown in Table 2.

Table 1. Frequency of utilization of the blood products among the different departments

Department	Whole blood	Packed red cells	Platelet concentrate	Fresh frozen plasma	Overall
Medicine	58	468	41	16	583
Surgery	56	149	10	_*	215
Obstetrics	12	191	15	_*	218
Pediatrics	1	33	25	_*	59
Overall	127	841	91	16	1075

_ no demand

Table 2. Appropriateness of use of the blood products among the different departments

Department	Appropriate	Whole blood	Packed red cells	Platelet concentrate	Fresh frozen plasma
Medicine	75%	54%	67%	79%	100%
Surgery	48%	0%	45%	100%	_*
Obstetrics	52%	0%	77%	79%	_
Pediatrics	86%	100%	83%	76%	_
Overall	65%	39%	68%	84%	100%

_ no demand

Among the tertiary hospitals, Hospital B had the most prevalence of appropriate use with 75%, Hospital C with 53% and 48% to Hospital A. Neither of the tertiary hospitals projected a good percentage of appropriate use (shown in Table 3). This indicates a high proportion of unnecessary or inappropriate transfusions practices across study hospitals.

Analysis of the data showed that appropriateness of use was statistically different among departments. Moreover, there is significant association exist between the percentage of appropriate use of blood products among the tertiary hospitals as P values were .04 and .005 respectively.

4. DISCUSSION

4.1 Whole Blood

In an Indian tertiary care hospital audit, there was an increased prevalence of inadequate use of whole blood [6]. In the evaluation done using pre-set criteria, the study found that the overall percentage of appropriate use is 40.7; it was unnecessary in 19.2% of cases (hemoglobin >11 g/dl). In 16.5% of cases, blood was transfused despite the absence of any of these indications, on the advice of the anaesthetist or surgeon responsible for the patient (clinician choice).

In our study, there are 127 transfusion cases of whole blood. Overall, 39% of these were classified as "appropriate". The primary trigger for transfusion was low haemoglobin. Without taking the post transfusion hemoglobin as another criterion for appropriateness, there is an increase in the percentage of appropriate use (43%). In 23% of these cases, blood was used appropriately but the response therapeutically was non-efficacious. Other triggers for transfusion were active bleeding and some were no indication at all but rather a clinician choice. The study of Niraj et al. [6], substantiated that this group of transfusions had a very high rate of inappropriate use (52%).

Using both pre-set criteria, blood was used inappropriately in 61% of cases. In 52% of these cases, the transfusion triggers were inappropriate however, the post hemoglobin results among these cases showed therapeutically efficacious. On the other hand, 15% of cases were transfused appropriately but was therapeutically non-efficacious. Moreover, 33% of cases were inappropriately used and were non-efficacious at the same time.

The departments of Medicine and Surgery have the most number of consumption with 58 and 56 units utilized, respectively. However, results showed that Surgery and Obstetrics departments had high percentage of inappropriate use of whole blood. In fact, all transfusions in both departments were inappropriate. The department of Medicine had 54% while in Pediatrics all uses were considered as appropriate (100%) though there was only 1 unit of whole blood utilized in this department. The study of Marti-Carvajal et al. [7], on the appropriate use of blood products in paediatrics patients, found out that whole blood had the most prevalence of appropriate use (83%). The result is comparable to the findings of this study as they both projected a good and high percentage of appropriateness. This reflects a rational and judicious use of whole blood to paediatric patients.

Among the tertiary hospitals, the study showed an overall low percentage of appropriate use (23%). In one of the tertiary hospital (Hospital A), all transfusion cases were classified as inappropriate despite of the very minimal number of utilization (6 units). It is noticeable also that the other two hospitals had increased number of utilization however; the prevalence of appropriate use was low with 38% to Hospital B and 30% to Hospital C.

Table 3. Appropriateness of use of the blood products among the tertiary hospitals

Department	Appropriate	Whole blood	Packed red cells	Platelet concentrate	Fresh frozen plasma
Hospital A	48%	0%	66%	78%	_
Hospital B	75%	38%	61%	100%	100%
Hospital C	53%	30%	76%	_	_
Overall	59%	23%	68%	89%	100%

_ *no demand*

The objective of blood transfusion, as specified by the American Society of Anesthesiologists (ASA) [8] guidelines, is to improve inadequate oxygen delivery secondary to anemia. The primary trigger for transfusions of whole blood is low hemoglobin. The other two common but inappropriate triggers are hypovolemic and the clinician choice. The use of whole blood as a volume substitute, though inappropriate, is still being practiced. The reason for this may be the availability of blood, and the belief that complications of transfusion occur infrequently and are usually benign [6].

Unfortunately, there are hospitals in the study which have no oversight programme for monitoring quality of transfusion practices, which may be one of the reasons for having such a low percentage of appropriate use yet, with high number of utilization. There might be a so called transfusion committee but does not work efficiently or effectively. There might be a need to evaluate the program in order to assess its effectiveness. Grindon et al. [9] pointed out that the presence of a transfusion committee assures consultation in haemotherapy: It evaluates effectiveness of transfusion practices with blood products. Blood safety survey of WHO [10] found that only 25% hospitals performing transfusions in developing countries and 33% hospitals in transitional countries have a transfusion committee to monitor transfusion practices and to review blood utilization; as compared to 88% hospitals in developed countries.

4.2 Packed Red Cells

Several studies showed that the bloods with greatest prevalence of inappropriate use were packed red cells and fresh frozen plasma [7,11,12]. In an evaluation of red blood cell transfusion practices with the use of pre-set criteria, Ghali, Palepu & Paterson [13], found that in 55.3% of cases packed red cells was transfused unnecessarily.

Similar result was obtained in our study. Packed red cells and whole blood had the most prevalence of inappropriate use. Of 721 transfusions with packed red cells, 68% of these were considered as appropriate. Triggers for transfusion were symptomatic anaemia and low haemoglobin (including preoperative haemoglobin). Without considering the therapeutic effect criteria, appropriate transfusion trigger showed a higher percentage of 78%. The study of Schot & Steenssens [12] also found out

that 4% of packed red cells were inappropriate in terms of effectiveness of transfusion. Similarly, from 78% appropriate use, only 15% of these cases were non-efficacious using the pre-set therapeutic effect criteria.

The study also found several cases of transfusions with a single unit of packed red cells, and of these, 66% belonged to the group of inappropriate use. Metz et al. [14], also found a high proportion of inappropriate use of single-unit transfusion. Transfusion of a single unit of packed red blood cells (PRBC) should not be considered inappropriate by itself; however, its use without an appropriate clinical judgement is not acceptable.

Following the guidelines, only the department of Paediatrics present a good percentage of appropriateness (83%). The departments of Medicine and Obstetrics showed a high percentage of appropriateness with 67% and 77% respectively however, low percentage to Surgery department (45%). The study of Marti-Carvajal et al. [7] also found that a high proportion of inappropriate use to Surgery department (62%). Preference of alleviation of symptoms over prevention of latter complications has been postulated as one of the causes of this phenomenon. In many instances a low haematocrit count is used to determine a request for a transfusion of PRBC; the correct approach is to combine the laboratory criteria with the symptoms of the patient. The New South Wales study also found that more of red blood cells were used inappropriately for surgical than for other admissions [15].

Among the tertiary hospitals, the study showed an overall of 68% of appropriate use. Noticeably, percentage of appropriateness among these hospitals was quite close and comparable to each other. Hospital A has 66% of appropriateness of use; Hospital B has 61% while Hospital C has 76%. Neither of the hospitals obtained a good percentage of appropriateness. Thus, reflecting a high proportion of inappropriate transfusions of such blood products across study hospitals.

Similar to the findings with whole blood, the same reason can be given as explanation for the high percentage of inappropriate use of this blood product. Consistent with the findings in whole blood, Surgery is likely associated with higher risk of inappropriate used. It is likely that Surgery was responsible of this phenomenon.

Marti-Carvajal et al. [7] affirmed in their study that Surgery was associated with higher risk of inappropriate transfusion than the Medicine department.

From a general point of view, a decision to transfuse should always be based on an analysis of risk and benefit, and should consider two factors: (1) evaluation of the physiological needs of the patient; and (2) transfusing only blood products that satisfy those physiological needs [16]. As in Metz et al. [14], the study found that many inappropriate transfusions of packed red cells were carried out on asymptomatic patients in the perioperative period, although there is no evidence that mild or moderate anaemia contributes to perioperative morbidity and mortality [17,18].

4.3 Platelets

According to pre-set criteria, this study showed overall high percentage of appropriate use of platelets (84%). This reflects good knowledge on the rational use of this blood product, as unnecessary platelet transfusion poses health risks and there are precise indications for its use. The main indication for platelets transfusion is to prevent bleeding in patients with marrow failure. There is a hypothesis that, regardless of the weight of the recipient, transfusion of over 2 platelet units would be excessive [19]. When deciding to transfuse platelets, physician must consider other factors that increase the risk of bleeding in patients with thrombocytopenia and might suggest reduction in the use of platelets [20]. Ancliff and Machin [21] reviewed data about the threshold for prophylactic platelet transfusion and pointed out that a threshold of $10 \times 10^9/l$ is safe in stable patients. However, according to Contreras [22] there is a need to define precise indications for use of platelet transfusion and this could be achieve by conducting randomized trials and effective and efficient audit.

There are 91 transfusion cases of platelet concentrates included in the study. Common transfusion triggers were the following: Active bleeding with thrombocytopenia; prophylactic administration with severe thrombocytopenia; and thrombocytopenia in patients undergoing surgery on critical area or in patients undergoing invasive procedure. Overall, 84% of transfusions were deemed appropriate. However, with no consideration to therapeutic effect criteria for appropriateness, there was even higher percentage of appropriate use (91%). In 14% of

these cases, blood was used appropriately but the therapeutic response was non-efficacious. This implies a poor response to platelet transfusion therapy. Percentage of appropraiteness among the different departments is as follows: 79% in Medicine and Obstetrics, 100% in Surgery, 76% in Pediatrics.

Using both pre-set criteria, this blood product was used inappropriately in 16%. In 18% of these cases, the transfusion trigger was inappropriate however, the therapeutic effect was efficacious. On the other hand, 59% of cases was transfused appropriately but the response was non-efficacious. Moreover, 23% of cases was transfused inappropriately and were non-efficaciuos at the same time.

Among the tertiary hospitals, the study showed an overall good percentage of appropriate use (89%). In Hospital A, 78% of transfusion cases were classified as appropriate. In Hospital B, all transfusions were deemed appropriate (100%). However, in Hospital C, there was no demand of transfusion of this product. The high percentage of appropriateness reflects a good transfusion practice of such blood product.

4.4 Fresh Frozen Plasma

Despite clear guidelines, requests for fresh frozen plasma (FFP) are the most frequent inappropriate orders received by the blood bank. Many authors found in their studies a greater prevalence of inadequate use of FFP [11,12,14]. This reflects little knowledge about the rational use of this blood product, as FFP has risks and there are precise indications for its use [18]. The most frequent reason for these inappropriate orders, accounting for at least a third of them, is for correction of a prolonged International Normalized Ratio (INR) in the absence of bleeding [23-26]. This prophylactic correction of minor laboratory coagulation abnormalities continues in the absence of evidence of its benefit [27]. Segal and Dzik [28] had suggested that inappropriate FFP orders occur because of 3 assumptions: (1) Elevation of the prothrombin time (PT)/INR will predict bleeding in the setting of a procedure. (2) Preprocedure administration of FFP will correct the prolonged clotting time results. (3) Prophylactic transfusion results in fewer bleeding events.

Conversely in this study, following both the pre-set criteria, all uses of this blood product were classified as appropriate (100%). The main reason for transfusion was prolonged PT/INR. However, there was very minimal number of use (16 units) to this blood product as observed among the different tertiary hospitals. The possible explanation to this could be due to unavailability of this blood product at that time of the study or could be due to little knowledge on its rational use. In addition, it was found out that during the conduct of the study, the nearest blood center was not preparing such component because of equipment problem concerning their blood bank freezer.

The study of Brein, Butler & Inwood [29] in a Canadian General Teaching Hospital, found out that 95% of the units of fresh frozen plasma was transfused appropriately in 90% of the transfusion episodes and that the transfusions were appropriate in 85% or more of the episodes on the various services.

In this study, the percentage of appropriateness among the different departments was as follows: Medicine 95%, Surgery 85%, Obstetrics 89%, and Paediatrics 100%. The study by Ali and colleagues [26], 70% of the transfusion episodes with fresh frozen plasma was considered appropriate. Other studies found that 62% to 70% of transfusions of fresh frozen plasma was deemed appropriate [25,30-32]. The high percentage of appropriate transfusions in this study can be attributed to several factors. First, the minimal availability of this blood product hence, it was only requested as deemed necessary and appropriate. Second, it reflects that clinicians have good orientation on the rational and optimal use, as FFP transfusions poses risks to patients.

Among the different departments included in this study, only Medicine had the demand of use for this blood product and all uses were classified as appropriate and efficacious. Before examining the effect of FFP on mildly elevated INRs, one must consider the effect of medical treatment without FFP on mildly prolonged coagulation test results. The findings in the study of Holland and Brooks [33] suggest that the natural course of high-normal to mildly elevated INRs (1.3-1.6) is to decrease with supportive care and treatment of the underlying condition alone. The exact reasons for this natural correction are unclear but could relate to correction of the following: (1) dehydration causing hypoperfusion of the liver, (2) anemia causing systemic hypoxia, and/or (3) metabolic disturbances causing pH changes.

Although cryoprecipitate was included in the study, there was no recorded demand of use of this blood product to any of the tertiary hospitals. The possible reasons for this were the same as those described for FFP: problems on the access of blood product at that time of study due to unavailability of this blood product at the nearest blood center and insufficient or limited knowledge on its rational use. This blood product is indicated for use only in specific illnesses.

In summary, results of the study showed that overall, only the Paediatrics department had obtained a good percentage of appropriateness among the different department. Surgery and Obstetrics departments were associated with higher risk of inappropriate transfusion than Medicine and Paediatric departments. Similar results were found in the study of Marti-Carvajal et al. [7] showing that Surgery, Emergency and Obstetrics departments were associated with higher risk of inappropriate transfusion than the Medicine department. In contrast, Mozes et al. [11] reported no relationship between inappropriate transfusion in the Surgery, Medicine and Paediatrics departments.

4.5 Significant Associations on the Appropriateness of Use among the Different Departments and among the Tertiary Hospitals

Clinicians at different departments and specialties may vary on how they use blood products clinically. The European Community (EC) reports found substantial differences in the clinical use of blood components in Australia, New Zealand and overseas [5]. On the report given, EC identified three main problems: (1) significant variability in the use of blood in the same clinical situations, implying that there is both overuse and potential under-use of blood; (2) misuse of blood components (with the rate of transfusion errors being higher than that of transfusion-transmitted viral diseases); and (3) lack of documentation about the process, rationale and outcomes of blood component therapy.

Similarly, this study found that appropriateness of use was statistically different among the different departments and that a significant association exist between the percentages of appropriate use of blood products among the tertiary hospitals. Thereby, further claim that appropriateness of use is influenced by the hospital department regardless of the blood products. It strongly asserts, as well, that appropriate use of blood products varies among tertiary hospitals. The study of Rubin, Schofield, Dean, Shakeshaft, & Frommer [15], concluded that there was substantial variation in inappropriate practice across study hospitals. Substantiated further by several studies in Australia and New Zealand, they found that the amount of blood used and the percentage of admissions involving the use of blood components vary across different types of hospitals, even for the same procedure or diagnosis, and that the percentage of use that can be classed as inappropriate was unacceptably high. These results were consistent with studies from Europe and the United States [5].

Along with the departments, Paediatrics has the highest percentage of appropriateness. In fact it is only the department which revealed a good percentage of appropriateness. On the other hand, Surgery is significantly associated with higher risk of inappropriate transfusion. Statistical data imply that Obstetrics and Paediatrics have better transfusion practices as compared to Surgery. Tertiary hospitals have comparable transfusion practices as revealed by data in the study. In terms of appropriateness of use among blood products, a significant association was found in the use of whole blood and packed red cells implying variation of transfusion practices to such blood products among the different departments.

Differences in transfusion practices between different departments among the tertiary hospital could be explained by the following reasons: The difficulty in evaluating appropriate use of blood products in patients with bleeding in different surgical services; Differences among clinicians transfusion practice in different departments, at different fields of specialty; The differences in existing guidelines reflect the difficulty in defining clear evidence-based parameters as a uniform trigger. Lastly, the lack of orientation, updates and/or little knowledge according to the most current clinical transfusion practice guidelines on the rational use of blood products [5].

5. CONCLUSION

In the light of the foregoing findings of this study, a high prevalence of inappropriate use of blood products was found among the tertiary hospitals. Higher risk of inappropriateness was observed in the Medicine, Surgery and Obstetrics

departments while Pediatrics revealed a good percentage of appropriateness. There was substantial variation in the appropriate transfusion practices across tertiary hospitals and appropriateness was influenced by the departments.

6. STUDY LIMITATIONS

This was a retrospective review on the appropriateness of transfusion of blood products. Appropriateness was reviewed based only on the information available in the medical charts, thus, percentage of inappropriateness may be overestimated. However, we believe that this was the first audit that has been carried out, more strongly that several tertiary hospitals were involved. Results may serve as an initial basis for the improvement of transfusion practices. The study proposes that a quality monitoring system such as medical audit and continuing medical education be initiated into each hospital.

CONSENT

It is not applicable.

ETHICAL APPROVAL

It is not applicable.

COMPETING INTERESTS

Authors have declared that no competing interests exist.

REFERENCES

1. World Health Organization. The clinical use of blood in obstetrics, pediatrics. Surgery & Anaesthesia, Trauma & Burns; 2001.
2. World Health Organization. Blood Transfusion Safety: Safe and Appropriate Use; 2002.
3. McGrath KM, Hancock L, Foster KM. Compliance with clinical guidelines for blood transfusion practice: How can changes be maintained? Medical Journal of Australia. 2001;174:435.
4. Hillyer CD, Silbertein LE, Ness PM, Anderson KC. Blood banking and transfusion medicine: Basic principles and practice. Singapore: Elsevier Science; 2003.

5. National Health and Medical Regional Council (NHMRC)/ Australasian Society of Blood Transfusion (ASBT). Clinical practice guidelines on the use of blood components; 2002.

6. Niraj G, Puri GD, Arun D, Chakravarty V, Aveek J, Chari P. Assessment of intraoperative blood transfusion practice during elective non-cardiac surgery in an Indian tertiary care hospital. British Journal of Anaesthesia. 2003;91(4):586-589.

7. Martí-Carvajal AJ, Muñoz-Navarro SR, Peña-Marti GE, Comunian G. An audit of appropriate use of blood products in adult patients in a Venezuelan general university hospital. International Journal for Quality Health Care. 1999;11(5):391-395.

8. American Society of Anesthesiologists. Practice guidelines for blood component therapy: A report by the american society of anesthesiologists task force on blood component therapy. Anesthesiology. 1996;84(3):732-747.

9. Grindon AJ, Tomasulo PS, Bergin JJ, Klein HG, Miller JD, Mintz PD. The hospital transfusion committee. Guidelines for improving practice. JAMA. 1985;253:540-543.

10. World Health Organization. Global Database on Blood Safety (GBDS), 2007 Survey; 2007.

11. Mozes B, Epstein M, Ben-Bassat I, Modan B, Halkin H. Evaluation of the appropriateness of blood and blood product transfusion using preset criteria. Transfusion. 1989;29:473-476.

12. Schot J, Steensens L. Blood usage review in a Belgian University Hospital. Int. Journal Quality Health Care. 1994;6:41-45.

13. Ghali WA, Palepu A, Paterson WG. Evaluation of red blood cell transfusion practices with the use of preset criteria. Canada Medical Association Journal (CMAJ). 1994;150:1449-1454.

14. Metz J, McGrath KM, Copperchini ML, Haeusler M, Haysom HE, Gibson PR, Millar RJ, Babarczy A, Ferris L, Grigg AP. Appropriateness of transfusions of red cells, platelets and fresh frozen plasma. An audit in a tertiary care teaching hospital. Medical Journal of Australia. 1995; 162:572-77.

15. Rubin G, Schofield W, Dean M, Shakeshaft A. Frommer M. Red blood cell transfusion practices in New South Wales. Australian Center for Effective Health Care; 2009.

16. Gould SA, Forbes JM. Controversies in transfusion medicine: Indications for autologous and allogeneic transfusion should be the same: Pro. Transfusion. 1995;35:446-449.

17. Carson J, Duff A, Berlin J, Lawrence V, Poses R, Huber E, O'Hara D, Noveck H, Strom B. Perioperative blood transfusion and postoperative mortality. Journal of American Medical Association. 1998;279:199-205.

18. National Institute of Health (NIH) Consensus development conference. Fresh frozen plasma. Indications and risks. Journal of American Medical Association. 1986;253:551-553.

19. Slichter S, Corash L, Schiffer C, Schecter GP, McArthur JR. The education program of the American society of hematology. Orlando, Florida. 1996;119-131.

20. McCullough J, Steeper T, Connelly D, Jackson B, Huntington S, Scott E. Platelet utilization in a University Hospital. Journal of American Medical Association. 1988;259:2414-2418.

21. Ancliff P, Machin S. Trigger factors for prophylactic platelet transfusion. Blood Reviews. 1998;12:234-238.

22. Contreras M. Consensus conference on platelet transfusion. Final Statement. Blood Reviews. 1998;12:239-240.

23. Dzik W, Rao A. Why do physicians request fresh frozen plasma [letter]? Transfusion 2004;44:1393-1394.

24. Tuckfield A, Haeusler MN, Grigg AP, Metz J. Reduction of inappropriate use of blood products by prospective monitoring of transfusion request forms. Medical Journal of Australia. 1997;67:473-476.

25. Snyder AJ, Gottschall JL, Menitove JE. Why is fresh-frozen plasma transfused? Transfusion. 1986;26:107-112.

26. Ali A, Vander B, Blajchman M. Quality assurance in the use of blood products: Report of a pilot study. Presented at fourth scientific session. Canadian Red Cross Society Blood Transfusion Service; 1986.

27. Stanworth SJ, Brunskill SJ, Hyde CJ. Is fresh frozen plasma clinically effective? A systematic review of randomized controlled trials. British Journal of Haematology. 2004;126:139-152.

28. Segal JB, Dzik WH. Transfusion Medicine/Hemostasis clinical trials network. Paucity of studies to support that abnormal coagulation test results predict bleeding in the setting of invasive

procedures: An evidence-based review. Transfusion. 2005;45:1413-1425.

29. Brein W, Butler R, Inwood M. An audit of blood component therapy in a Canadian general teaching hospital. Canada Medical Association Journal (CMAJ). 1989;140:812-815.

30. Blumberg N, Laczin J, McMican A, Heal J, Arvan D. A critical survey of fresh frozen plasma use. Transfusion. 1986;26(6):511-513.

31. Shaikh BS, Wagar D, Lau PM, Campbell E. Transfusion pattern of fresh frozen plasma in a medical school hospital. Vox Sanguinis. 1985;48:366-369.

32. Jones J. Abuse of fresh frozen plasma. British Medical Journal. 1987;295:287.

33. Holland L, Brooks J. Toward rational fresh frozen plasma transfusion. The effect of plasma transfusion on coagulation test results. American Society for Clinical Pathology. 2006;126:133-139.

34. Sacher RA, McPherson RA. Widmann's clinical interpretation of laboratory tests. 11th ed. Philadelphia: FA Davis Company; 2000.

APPENDIX

APPROPRIATENESS CRITERIA

Whole Blood

Appropriate if any one of the following applicable, likely to be inappropriate if none applicable:

- Hb is <80 g/L
- Hb<100 g/Lin patients with medical co-morbidities (such as coronary artery disease, renal dysfunction, left ventricular dysfunction, and chronic obstructive airway disease)
- Blood loss >20% of blood volume when more than 1000 ml

Red Blood Cells

Appropriate if any one of the following applicable, likely to be inappropriate if none applicable:

- Hb is <70g/L.
- Hb range of 70–100g/L during surgery associated with major blood loss
- Hb range of 70–100g/L during surgery with signs or symptoms of impaired oxygen transport
- Hb is <80g/L in a patient on a chronic transfusion regimen or during marrow suppressive therapy

Platelets

Appropriate if any one of the following applicable, likely to be inappropriate if none applicable:

- Prophylaxis for major surgery or invasive procedure and platelet count < 50×10^9/L
- Massive haemorrhage/transfusion and platelet count < 50×10^9/L
- Bone marrow failure and platelet count < 10×10^9/L
- Bone marrow failure and platelet count < 20×10^9/L with risk factors
- Bleeding or massive hemorrhage

Fresh Frozen Plasma

Appropriate if any one of the following applicable, likely to be inappropriate if none applicable:

- INR or APTT high* and liver disease before major surgery or invasive procedure
- INR or APTT high and liver failure
- INR or APTT high and acute disseminated intravascular coagulation
- INR or APTT high and excessive bleeding
- INR or APTT high before an invasive procedure
- INR or APTT high before, during or after major surgery
- INR high and warfarin effect present and massive blood loss or emergency surgery
- Correction of single factor deficiency when a specific factor was not available
- Treatment of thrombotic thrombocytopenic purpura.

Cryoprecipitate

- Appropriate if fibrinogen test result available and fibrinogen level < 1.0 g/L and where there is clinical bleeding or trauma or invasive procedure or disseminated intravascular coagulation.

*APTT - activated partial thromboplastin time. INR - International normalised ratio of prothrombin time.
* "High" - above the hospital's normal range*

Adapted from the literature of NHMRC/ASBT Clinical Practice Guidelines on the Appropriate Use of Blood and Blood Products [5].

THERAPEUTIC EFFECT CRITERIA

Whole Blood

- Increase of 3% hct level or 1g/dL on hb level per unit (increase may not be apparent for 48 to 72 hours.

Red Blood Cells

- Increase of 3% hct level per unit

Platelets

- Increase of 5000-8000 platelet count per concentrate

Fresh Frozen Plasma

- Increase of 20-30% in coagulation factor activity per dose of 10-15ml of plasma per kg body weight

Cryoprecipitate

- Increase of 50-100 units of factor VIII per unit (about 10 ml volume)
- Increase plasma fibrinogen concentration by approximately 50 mg/dL

Adapted from the book of Sacher, & McPherson Widmann's Clinical Interpretation of Laboratory Tests [34].

18

The Evaluation of Blood Requests for Transfusion and It's Utilization in Four Iranian Hospitals

Azita Chegini[1*], Alireza Ebrahimi[2] and Amirhossein Maghari[3]

[1]Blood Transfusion Research Center, High Institute for Research and Education in Transfusion Medicine, Tehran, Iran.
[2]Department of Hematology, Faculty of Medical Sciences, Tarbiat Modares University, Tehran, Iran.
[3]Department of Biostatistics, New Hearing Technologies Research Center, Baqiyatallah University of Medical Science, Tehran, Iran.

Authors' contributions

This work was carried out in collaboration between all authors. Author AC designed the study, wrote the protocol, and wrote the first draft of the manuscript. Authors AC, AE and AM managed the literature searches, analyses of the study performed the spectroscopy analysis and managed the experimental process and identified the species of plant. All authors read and approved the final manuscript.

Editor(s):
(1) Dharmesh Chandra Sharma, Incharge Blood Component and Aphaeresis Unit, G. R. Medical College, Gwalior, India.
Reviewers:
(1) Sandro Percario, Federal University of Pará, Brazil.
(2) Anonymous, Instituto Alergoimuno de Americana, Brazil.
(3) Adewoyin Ademola Samson, University of Benin Teaching Hospital, Nigeria.
(4) Katsuyasu Saigo, Himeji Dokkyo University, Japan.

ABSTRACT

Background: Transfusion is one of the most important elements of healthcare. In order to save human lives, 85 million blood units are used in the world annually. Access to blood products is a common problem throughout the world. Presently, demand is increasing significantly for blood usage. The main goal is to evaluate blood usage in four hospitals by comparing them with international standards and utilization of efficient methods to prevent unnecessary transfusions.
Materials and Methods: This is a retrospective hospital based survey carried out at Tehran Blood Transfusion Centre. Data regarding blood transfusion requests, units requested, units cross matched, unused units returned and other details were collected from the blood bank laboratory records in four Iranian hospitals. The crossmatched to transfusion ratio was evaluated.

Corresponding author: E-mail: azita_chegini@yahoo.com

Results: There were a total of 548,568 requests for units of blood in total. 196, 059 units were crossmatched and 82,320 units were transfused. The proportion of C/T (total) was 2.38 and the proportion of transfusions to the number of beds was 16. The C/T ratios for all hospitals were 2.38. Only 42% of blood cross matched units was utilized. One of four hospitals in our survey which specializes in cardiac the C/T ratio is 1.86 and the ratio of blood infusion to hospital bed is 19.7. Another hospital specializes in pediatric hematology oncology and C/T ratio is 1.04 (the ratio of blood infusion to hospital bed=19.6). A 1,000 bed general hospital with cardiac and oncology departments in which C/T ratio is 2.94.

Conclusion: We saw over ordering requests of blood units which is different in 4 hospitals. The number of beds and departments can have a direct effect on the C/T ratio. The quantity of blood used depends on the number of beds and fields of specialization present at the hospital.

Suitable usage of blood depends on great hospital and number of expertise. There is a need to expand our hemovigilance teaching program. Use of abscreening helps to achieve a more efficient blood utilization and should be engaged in our locality to prevent unnecessary demands.

Keywords: Blood component transfusions; blood grouping and cross matching; erythrocyte transfusions.

1. BACKGROUND

Transfusion is one of the most important elements of modern healthcare. In order to save human lives 85 million blood units are used in the world annually [1]. According to World Health Organization the amount of required blood in Southeast Asia is around 16 million units per year from which 9.4 million units are collected [2]. The improper use of medical technology plays a vital role in the escalation of treatment costs. Inappropriate blood usage is another major factor. Other factors contributing to the rising expenditures are infusions of blood products, collection, logistics, laboratory tests and prescriptions [3].

Access to blood products is a common problem all over the world. At the moment demand has increased significantly for blood usage. A high percentage of blood products are wasted due to excess demand for blood products in elective surgeries and a lot of time and a very high quantity of reagent is wasted. Extensive research in the United States of America and Australia has shown that with proper usage, collection of information from blood banks and routine training, expenditures can be significantly reduced. It is possible to avoid unnecessary cross matches through blood group tests and Ab-screening in low risk surgeries and following maximum surgical blood order schedule standards [4].

In 1975, Henry Boral suggested that utilization of cross matched units to transfusion units ratio would be effective in the application of blood products. American Association of Blood Banks recommends that cross matched units to transfusion units ratio should equal 2 or less for surgical patients and almost 1 for medical patients [5,6]. In some other sources the cross matched units to transfusion units ratio standard is mentioned as less than 1.5 for medical patients. The ideal ratio for cross matched units to transfusion units ratio is equal to 1 and if the C/T ratio is more than 2.5, it means there are unnecessary cross matches and demonstrates that less than 40% of cross matched units are injected. The standard according to World Health Organization is 6-16 blood units per hospital bed [7]. The purpose of this survey is to evaluate cross matched to transfusion ratio as a measure or efficient blood utilization in Tehran.

2. MATERIALS AND METHODS

This is a retrospective study carried out at Tehran blood transfusion Centre. Data was collected on blood product pattern of requests and utilization from different blood bank's hospitals in the region over a period of three years, between 2010 and 2012 were retrieved. Blood Bank's hospitals sent completed forms monthly. Information in the form included: units requested, units cross matched, units transfused, units returned unutilized and Blood groups of transfused. Four hospitals had selected included:

A- University hospital specialized in cardiac surgery with 460 active beds.
B- General hospital with 1000 active beds.
C- Private General Hospital with 150 beds.
D- Private pediatric hematologic hospital with 100 beds.

This data was used to evaluate the C:T ratio, which was described as the number of cross match units transfused/ number of cross matched units requested. Data is analyzed by using IBM SPSS (ver.21) software.

3. RESULTS

Four hospitals were studied; two private and two public. They had requests for 548,568 units of blood in total. Out of 548,568 units of blood, 196,059 units were cross matched and 82,320 units were transfused. The proportion of C/T (total) is 2.38 and the proportion of transfusion to the number of beds is 16. Only 42% of blood cross matched units was utilized.

Hospital A- University hospital has 460 beds and specializes in cardiovascular surgery. The total blood request for a 3 year period was 79,411. Number of cross matched, transfused and returns are present in Table 1. During the stated three years the number of transfusions per bed was reduced but the number of returns increased. A noticeable difference is apparent during these 3 years (p=0.008).

Hospital B is a general hospital with 1,000 beds. The total blood requests for a 3 year period were 456,265. Number of cross matched, transfused and returns are seen in Table 2. The proportion

of cross matched units to transfusion units ratio is 2.94. The proportion of transfusion to the number of beds is 15. But the number of transfusions during the three years of the study is not statistically significant, however, there is a noticeable difference in the number of returns for the 3 year period with hemovigilance education (p=0.002).

Hospital C is a general private hospital with only major departments. Total blood requests for a 3 year period were 6,755. Number of cross matched, transfused and returned units are seen in Table 3. The proportion of cross matched units to transfusion units ratio was 1.79. The proportion of transfusions to the number of beds is 8.7. But the number of transfusions did not vary enough to be of statistical importance. However, there is a noticeable difference in the number of returns for the 3 year period (p=0.002).

Hospital D has 100 beds and specializes only in pediatric hematologic and oncology. The proportion of C/T is 1.04. The proportion of transfusions to the number of beds is19.6. The proportion of transfusions to the number of beds increased in the third year and reached 21.03, but there is no noticeable difference in the number of returns (Table 4).

Table 1. Distribution of requested, cross matched, transfused, returned packed cell units in a university hospital specialized in cardiac surgery with 460 active beds during 2010-1012

	Requested units	Cross matched units	Transfused units	Returned units	Ratio C/T	Transfused to beds ratio
2010	26236	16555(63%)	9443(36%)	3815(23%)	1.75	21.46
2011	27584	17178(62%)	9409(37%)	4204(24.5%)	1.82	21.38
2012	25591	16643(65%)	8336(50%)	4920(29.6%)	2	18.95
Total	79411	50376(63.4%)	27188(54%)	12939(25.7%)	-	-

Table 2. Distribution of requested, cross matched, transfused, returned packed cell units in hospital B-general hospital with 150 beds during 2010-2012

	Requested units	Cross matched units	Transfused units	Returned units	Ratio C/T	Transfused to beds ratio
2010	158453	45014(28.4%)	15544(34.5%)	168(0.37%)	2.91	15.5
2011	151940	44708(29.4%)	15455(34.6%)	0	2.9	15.4
2012	145872	43080(29.5%)	14340(33.3%)	0	3.01	14.3
total	456265	132802(29%)	45339(34%)	168(0.1%)	-	-

Table 3. Distribution of requested, cross matched, transfused, returned packed cell units in hospital C- general private during 2010-2012

	Requested units	Cross matched units	Transfused units	Returned units	Ratio C/T	Transfused to beds ratio
2010	2142	2142(100%)	1135(53%)	17(0.8%)	1.9	7.57
2011	2421	2421(100%)	1491(61.9%)	32(1.3%)	1.64	9.94
2012	2192	2190(99.9%)	1284(58.6%)	49(2.2%)	1.84	8.6
total	6755	6753(99.9%)	3910(57.9%)	98(1.4%)	-	-

Table 4. Distribution of requested, cross matched, transfused, returned packed cell units in hospital D-private pediatric hematologic oncologic during2010-2012

	Requested units	Cross matched units	Transfused units	Returned units	Ratio C/T	Transfused to beds ratio
2010	1876	1867(99.5%)	1824(97.7%)	15(0.8%)	1.02	18.24
2011	2054	2054(100%)	2013(98%)	18(0.8%)	1.04	21.03
2012	2208	2208(100%)	2189(99%)	19(0.8%)	1.05	21.03
total	6138	6129(99.8%)	6026(96%)	52(0.8%)	-	-

Distribution of blood groups and Rh according to requested units are follow as Table 5.

Table 5. Distribution of Blood groups and Rh according to requested units of four hospitals

Group	Percent
O$^+$	33.2
A$^+$	29.6
B$^+$	20.9
AB$^+$	7.1
O$^-$	3.3
A$^-$	3.1
B$^-$	2.1
AB$^-$	0.7

4. DISCUSSION

Blood and its products play a great role in saving lives during emergency and elective operations. With great advances in medical sciences, the demand and utilization of blood has grown tremendously but the supply has remained constant [8]. A study on blood utilization was published by Friedman and his associates in 1973, his conclusion was that 1-2.5 figure in cross matched units to the transfusion units (C/T) ratio is a sufficient ratio for utilization. It is also stated in this study that TI (transfusion index) ratio would provide a good method to assess the efficiency of the number of transfusions (TI =Transfusion/Cross matched) [9].

Numerous other studies carried out on the same subject have reached the same conclusion as the Friedman study, which states consumption is always greater than supply [10,11]. In a comprehensive study in India of the 1,145 units of cross matched blood units, 23.14% were transfused and the other 76.86% were not used at all [12].

The results of a more detailed study carried out in Nigeria during a three months period on 986 patients are as follow:

Trauma department C/T = 2.74, emergency department C/T = 2.61, general surgery = 3.11. The percentage of unused blood units for emergency department was 63.10 %, general surgery 71.19% and trauma department 62.99%. In total, the ratio of C/T in this hospital is reported at 2.90 (cross matched =1608, transfused =555) [13].

Although our study is not as detailed as above mentioned cases and it only includes four hospitals that do not perform antibody screenings and the C/T ratio for all hospitals is 2.38. The expiration date of stored red blood cell products in our country is 35 days. Our study was carried out within a 3 years period on all four hospitals: Hospital A, C/T =1.86, Hospital B C/T=2.94, Hospital C C/T=1.79, Hospital D C/T=1.04. We had educated hemovigilance in 2012 and there is difference between years as shown Tables 1, 2, 3.

In Germany the quantity of blood infusions varies greatly among hospitals and the same trend is present in this study. Blood usage is varied among different hospitals and the ratio of blood infusion to hospital bed is as follow: Hospital A: 19.7, Hospital B:15.1, Hospital C: 8.7,Hospital D: 19.6. The above variation depends on care provided to patients and hospitals' specialization.

Blood loss varies in elective surgery patients but cancer and heart surgeries usually have a high quantity of blood consumption. Heart surgeries consume 20% of available blood. One study illustrates that cross match to transfusion ratio for the cardiac team is 2.48 [14]. But at hospital A in our survey which specializes in cardiac the C/T ratio is 1.86. Hospital D specializes in pediatric hematology oncology and C/T ratio is 1.04.

Hospital B is a 1,000 bed general hospital with cardiac and oncology departments in which C/T ratio is 2.94. The number of beds and departments can have a direct effect on the C/T ratio. The quantity of blood used depends on the number of beds and fields of specialization present at the hospital.

Numerous studies have shown that by utilizing a variety of tables (MSBOS); it is possible to reduce the number of requests and it is conceivable to reach an effective and economical solution for this problem through the use of such tables. Although our study is only descriptive and is not as detailed as the above mentioned cases and it only includes four hospitals and the average C/T ratio for the four hospitals is 2.38. There is a need to expand our teaching program, Antibody screening, do further research, gather more details and use the mentioned MSBOS tables in order to reach a more efficient method to prevent unnecessary demands.

Table 5 demonstrates blood type requests of the four hospitals in our survey which is similar to the country as a whole. Requests for A+, B+, AB +and O+ blood types shown in our study are 29.6%, 20.9%, 7.1% ,3.3% respectively. In Pourfathollah and associates study on Iranian blood donors during a one year period; of the total quantity donated 30.25% was blood type A and 37.62% was Blood O and 24.36% was blood type B and 7.77% was blood type AB [15].

5. CONCLUSION

One of four hospitals in our survey which specializes in cardiac the C/T ratio is 1.86 and the ratio of blood infusion to hospital bed is 19.7. Another hospital specializes in pediatric hematology oncology and C/T ratio is 1.04 (the ratio of blood infusion to hospital bed=19.6). A 1,000 bed general hospital with cardiac and oncology departments in which C/T ratio is 2.94. Only 42% of blood cross matched units was utilized. The number of beds and departments can have a direct effect on the C/T ratio. The quantity of blood used depends on the number of beds and fields of specialization present at the hospital.

Suitable usage of blood depends on reviewing ordering schedules. There is a need to expand ab-sceening test and our hemovigilance teaching program. Use of MSBOS helps to achieve a more efficient blood utilization and should be engaged in our locality to prevent unnecessary demands.

CONSENT

This study is not against the public interest, that the release of information is allowed by legislation.

ETHICAL APPROVAL

The authors have obtained all necessary ethical approval from suitable Institutional Committee.

COMPETING INTERESTS

Authors have declared that no competing interests exist.

REFERENCES

1. Carson JL, Grossman BJ, Kleinman S, Tinmouth AT, Marques MB, Fung MK, et al. Red blood cell transfusion: A clinical practice guideline from the AABB*. Ann Intern Med. 2012;157(1):49–58.

2. Aggarwal S SV. Attitudes and problems related to voluntary blood donation in India. Ann Trop Med Public Health. 2012; 5:50–2.

3. Communion G. M-CA. An audit of appropriate use of blood products in adult patients in a Venezuelan general university hospital. Int J Qual Health Care. 1999;11(5):391–5.

4. Smallwood JA. Use of blood in elective general surgery: an area of wasted resources. Br Med J (Clin Res Ed). 1983; (12) (286) (6368):868–870.

5. Result of type: Document Guidelines for Patient Blood Management and Blood Utilization [Internet].
Available:https://www.aabb.org/resources/marketplace/Documents/113410_sam.pdf

6. Saladino AJ. ND. Quality indicators of blood utilization: Three College of American Pathologists Q-Probes studies of 12,288,404 red blood cell units in 1639 hospitals. Arch Pathol Lab Med. 2002; 2(126):150–6.

7. Sabeen Afzal. A comparison of public and private hospital on rational use of blood in Islamabad. J Pak Med Assoc. 2013; 1(63):85–9.

8. HO O, BO B. Blood utilization in elective surgical procedur. Tropical health sciences J. 2006;13:15-17.

9. Friedman BA, Oberman HA, Schadwick AR, Kingon KI. The maximum surgical blood order schedule and surgical blood use in the United States. Transfusion J. 1976;16(4):380-387.

10. Enosolease ME, Imarengiaye G, Awodu AO. Donor blood procurement and

utilization at university of Benin teaching hospital. Benin city. Afr J Reprod Health. 2004;8:59-63.

11. Basnet RB, Lamichhane D, Scharma VK. A study of Blood requisitions and transfusion practice in surgery at Bir hospital. PMJN. 2009;9:14-19.

12. Vibhute M, Klamath SK, Shetty A. Blood utilization in elective general surgery cases: Requirements, ordering and transfusion practice. Post Graduate Medicine J. 2000;46(1):7-13.

13. Abubakr U. Musa, Mohammed A. Ndakotsu, Abdul-Aziz Hassan, et al. Pattern of blood transfusion request and

utilization at a Nigerian university teaching hospital. Sahel medical J. 2014;17(1):19-22

14. Vrotso S, Gonzalez B, Goldszer RC, Rosen G, Lapietra A, Howard L. Improving blood transfusion practice by educational emphasis of the blood utilization. Trasfus Clin Biol. 2015;22(1):1-4.

15. Pourfathollah AA, Oody A, Honarkaran N. Geographical distribution of ABO and Rh(D) blood groups among Iranian blood donors in the year 1361(1982) as compared with that of yaer 1380(2001). SCI Iran Blood Transfusion Organ. 2003; 1(1):11-17.

19

Hypertension in Children with Sickle Cell Disease: A Comparative Study from Port Harcourt, Nigeria

I. O. George[1*], P. N. Tabansi[1] and C. N. Onyearugha[2]

[1]*Department of Paediatrics, University of Port Harcourt Teaching Hospital, Nigeria.*
[2]*Department of Paediatrics, Abia State University Teaching Hospital, Nigeria.*

Authors' contributions

This work was carried out in collaboration between all authors. Author IOG designed the study, wrote the protocol, and wrote the first draft of the manuscript. Authors PNT and CNO managed the literature searches, analyses of the study. All authors read and approved the final manuscript.

Editor(s):
(1) Shinichiro Takahashi, Kitasato University School of Allied Health Sciences, Japan.
Reviewers:
(1) Mario Bernardo-Filho, Universidade do Estado do Rio de Janeiro, Brazil.
(2) Anonymous, Serbia.

ABSTRACT

Background: Sickle cell anaemia is a chronic anaemia that is characterized by episodes of severe bone pain from blood vessels occlusion by sickled red blood cells when deoxygenated, and eventual end organ affectation and multi-organ failure. The aim of this study was to compare the arterial blood pressures of children with sickle cell anaemia in steady state with those of age- and sex-matched healthy controls and to identify those with hypertension.

Materials and Methods: This cross-sectional descriptive study was conducted in the Outpatient Paediatric Haematology Clinic of University of Port Harcourt Teaching Hospital from January to March 2015. Blood pressure, weight and height were measured and a specific form was used to record data.

Results: There were a total of 50 children with sickle cell anaemia in stable state during the study period. Of these, 31 were male while 19 were females giving a Male: Female ratio of 1.6:1. All the patients had HbSS genotype. Most of them 22(44%) were between the ages of 5 and 10 years. The mean packed cell volume was 22.79±4.34. Majority of the patients had packed cell volume between 16 and 30. Most 41(82%) of them were underweight. The prevalence of hypertensive is 22%. Majority (82%) of them had low Body Mass Index.

Conclusion: There is no significant difference in the systolic blood pressure of children with sickle

Corresponding author: E-mail: geonosdemed@yahoo.com

cell anaemia compared to age and sex matched controls. Hypertension appears to be frequently undiagnosed by paediatric clinicians. Early, appropriate diagnosis is important so as to establish effective treatment for abnormal blood pressure.

Keywords: Blood pressure; children; sickle cell anaemia; body mass index; Nigeria.

1. INTRODUCTION

Sickle-cell disease is a genetic disorder of growing public health importance worldwide [1]. More than 300 000 homozygous neonates with sickle-cell anaemia are born every year, with three-quarters born in sub-Saharan Africa [2]. It is a chronic anemia that is characterized by episodes of severe bone pain from blood vessels occlusion by sickled red blood cells when deoxygenated, and eventual end organ affectation and multi-organ failure [1].

Hypertension in children may be secondary to another disease process or it may be essential hypertension. Secondary hypertension is more common in children than in adults, and common causes of hypertension in children include renal disease, coarctation of the aorta, and endocrine disease [3]. However, the majority of children and adolescents with mild to moderate hypertension have primary hypertension in which a cause is not identifiable. Hypertension in children has been shown to correlate with family history of hypertension, low birth weight, and excess weight [2,4,5]. Several studies [6,7] have shown that blood pressure is generally lower than normal in individuals with sickle cell anemia compared to age and sex matched controls. The exact mechanism of this lower blood pressure is unknown but factors such as salt losing sickle cell nephropathy have been implicated [7].

Hypertension is known to be more prevalent among people of the black race, who also frequently carry the sickle cell gene [2]. Sickle cell disease (SCD) is associated with high morbidity from recurrent episodes of vaso-occlusive and anaemic crises. Mortality most times occurs during acute crises and may be secondary to various organ failures including the kidneys. Kidney disorders are often associated with hypertension.

Comparative data on the blood pressure values of this subgroup with the normal population is scarce and mainly in the adult population of sicklers. Nevertheless, information on prevalence of hypertension among children with sickle cell anaemia in our environment is limited. This study thus seeks to determine the blood pressure levels of children with sickle cell disease and compare them with those of normal reference values. This will identify children with hypertension and its resultant morbidity such as stroke.

2. MATERIALS AND METHODS

This cross-sectional descriptive study was conducted in the Outpatient Paediatric Haematology Clinic of University of Port Harcourt Teaching Hospital (UPTH) from January to March 2015. This study enrolled all patients with SCD (haemoglobinopathy HbSS and HbSC) aged 6months to 16 years, who were seen in the outpatient service during the study. Exclusion criteria included recent (within 2 weeks) hospitalization and/or episode of acute chest pain, pain crises, febrile illness or blood transfusion.

Blood pressure (BP), weight and height were measured and a specific form was used to record data. Three BP measurements were made for each patient at three different times, always by the same author, and all care was taken to minimize anxiety and fear of the procedures. Measurements were made using a mercury sphygmomanometer with appropriate cuffs. Systolic (SBP) and diastolic BP (DBP) were defined as normal when below the value of the 95th percentile for age, sex and height. Hypertension was defined as BP greater than the 95th percentile for age, sex and height percentile [8].

Weights would then be assessed using a Seca weighing scale, with the child completely undressed. Weights will be measured in kilograms, to the nearest 0.1 kg (100 grams). Seca weighing scale was used to measure weight, and a wooden vertical stadiometer was used for height; the horizontal rod was adjusted to rest on the top of the head at a right angle with the vertical ruler. Anthropometric measurements were made with the patient barefooted and wearing as little clothing as possible. Nutritional status according to Body Mass Index (BMI) was classified using the growth charts issued by the World Health Organization (WHO).

Ethical approval was obtained from the Ethical Committee of the UPTH.

Means, standard deviation, frequencies and percentages, correlation and analyses will be done in order to predict the significant values with p value of 0.05.

3. RESULTS

There were a total of 50 children with sickle cell disease in stable state during the study period. Of these 31 were male while 19 were females giving a Male: Female ratio of 1.6:1. All the patients had HbSS genotype. There were more children 22(44%) between 5-10years as shown on (Table 1). The mean packed cell volume was 22.48±4.1 (range 15-32) (Table 2). The

frequency distribution of their packed cell volume (PCV) is as shown on (Table 3). Majority of the patients had PCV between 16 and 30. Most 41(82%) of them were underweight (Table 4). The prevalence of hypertension was 22%. (Table 5) shows frequency distribution table of their BMI and suggested that majority (82%) of them were underweight.

Table 1. Age distribution of 50 children with SCA

Age	Frequency	Percentage
<5	13	26
5-10	22	44
>10	15	30
Total	50	100

Table 2. Age, gender, blood pressure and anthropometric data

Parameters	SCA Mean(SD)	Control	P-value
Age (years)	8.23(4.54)		
Gender [frequency (%)]			
Male	31(62%)		
Female	19(38%)		
Total	50		
Packed cell volume	22.48(4.1)		
Weight(kg)	27.75(13.75)		
Height (m^2)	1.27(0.29)		
Body mass index(kg/ m^2)	16.04(3.67)		
Systolic blood pressure	92.90(9.04)	98.08(10.73)	>0.05
Diastolic blood pressure	54.90(9.82)	62.64(7.57)	>0.05

Table 3. Packed cell volume distribution of children with SCA

PCV	Frequency	Percentage
≤15	2	4.0
16-20	16	32.0
21-25	20	40.0
26-30	10	20.0
≥31	2	4.0

Table 4. BMI distribution of children with SCA

BMI	Frequency	Percentage
<19	41	82.0
19-25	7	14.0
>25	2	4.0

Table 5. Correlation of clinico-laboratory parameters with the mean blood pressure in sickle cell anaemia patients

Factors	Mean(SD) Hypertensive	Mean(SD) Non hypertensive	P-value
Frequency (%)	11(22.0%)	39(78.0%)	
Age in years	6.56(4.16)	8.70(4.57)	>0.05
Packed cell volume	21.36(3.0)	22.79(4.34)	>0.05
Weight in kg	24.59(12.01)	28.64(14.22)	>0.05
Height in meters	1.22(0.29)	1.28(0.29)	>0.05
Body Mass Index	16.03(3.56)	16.04(2.75)	>0.05

4. DISCUSSION

Systolic and diastolic blood pressures in sickle cell anaemia patients from this study were lower than the control and were not significantly different from that of the controls. Moreso, lower blood pressure (BP) has been documented in children and adults with SCD [9-11]. The reasons for lower BP in sickle cell disease population are unclear but it may be partly attributed to the occurrence of increased renal tubular sodium and water excretion thus promoting lower arterial pressures [12-14]. Other reports however are of the opinion that the lower BP is due to a lower weight and increased vasodilation in adults and children with SCD [15,16]. With increasing age especially after adolescence, kidney function may deteriorate relatively faster in persons with SCD resulting in hypertension [16].

Children with SCD have classically been thought to have low normal blood pressures. In a study of 85 children, Aygun et al. [17] identified no hypertensive patients. In addition, in a Saudi Arabian cohort of 69 children with SCD aged 1– 16 years old, blood pressure measurements were within normal range [18]. However, in the present study, 22% of patients had elevated blood pressures. Furthermore, a cohort study of thirty-eight children with SCD, based on in-clinic blood pressure screening showed prevalence of hypertension as 10.3% [19]. Another study found that BP was abnormal (hypertension and pre-hypertension) in 14.3% of the patients [20]. These findings coupled with our data suggest that hypertension may be under diagnosed in children with SCD when using standard clinic based assessments.

Most of the children with this condition in this study were underweight (low BMI). Studies have found an association between hypertension and BMI [20-23]. This may be due to the fact that patients with SCD have changes in plasma renin, endothelin and nitric oxide metabolites because of vaso-occlusion and those changes affect the balance between vasodilatation and vasoconstriction, which is not seen in undernourished children [23]. We did not confirm such association in our study.

5. CONCLUSION

There is no significant difference in the systolic blood pressure of children with sickle cell anaemia compared to age and sex matched controls. However, hypertension is well-defined, prevalent, asymptomatic, chronic conditions in children with sickle cell anaemia. Based on the data in this study, this condition appears to be frequently undiagnosed by paediatric clinicians. Early, appropriate diagnosis is important so as to establish effective treatment for abnormal blood pressure.

CONSENT

All authors declare that 'written informed consent was obtained from the patient (or other approved parties) for publication of this study.

ACKNOWLEGEMENTS

I thank Omieibi I. George and Sopiriye I. George for their valuable contributions.

COMPETING INTERESTS

Authors have declared that no competing interests exist.

REFERENCES

1. George IO, Opara PI. Sickle cell anaemia: A survey of associated morbidities in Nigerian children. African Journal of Haematology and Oncology. 2011;2(2): 187-190.

2. Grosse SD, Isaac O, Hani KA, Djesika DA, Frederic BP, Thomas, NW. Sickle cell disease in Africa: A neglected cause of early childhood mortality. American Journal of Preventive Medicine. 2011;41(6):398-405.

3. Falkner Bonita. Hypertension in children and adolescents: Epidemiology and natural history. Pediatric Nephrology. 2010;25(7): 1219-1224.

4. Silva Ana Carolina Pio da, Alberto Augusto Alves Rosa. Blood pressure and obesity of children and adolescents association with body mass index and waist circumference. Archivos latinoamericanos de nutrición. Caracas. 2006;56(3):244-250.

5. Iampolsky Marcelo Nunes, Fabíola Isabel S. de Souza, Roseli Oselka S. Sarni. Influence of body mass index and abdominal circumference on children's systemic blood pressure. Revista Paulista de Pediatria. 2010;28(2):181-187.

6. Uzsoy NK. Cardiovascular findings in patients with sickle cell anemia. Am J. Cardiol. 1964;13:320-328.

7. Radel EG, Kochen JA, Finberg L. Hyponatraemia in sickle cell disease. A renal salt losing state. J Paediatr. 1976; 88:800–805.

8. National High Blood Pressure Education Program Working Group on High Blood Pressure in Children and Adolescents. The fourth report on the diagnosis, evaluation, and treatment of high blood pressure in children and adolescents. Pediatrics. 2004; 114(2):(sup l4th report):555-576.

9. Pegelow CH, Colangelo Steinberg M, Wright EC, Smith J, Phillips G, et al. Natural history of blood pressure in sickle cell disease: Risks for stroke and death associated with relative hypertensionin sickle cell anemia. Am J Med. 1997;102 (2):171-7.

10. Johnson CS, Giorgio AJ. Arterial blood pressure in adults with sickle cell disease. Arch Intern Med. 1981;141(7):891-3.

11. De Jong PE, Landman H, Van Eps LW. Blood pressure in sickle cell disease. Arch Intern Med. 1982;142(6):1239-40.

12. Grell GA, Alleyne GA, Serjeant GR. Blood pressure in adults with homozygous sickle cell disease. Lancet. 1981;2(8256):1166.

13. The fourth report on the diagnosis, evaluation and treatment of high blood pressure in children and adolescents. Pediatrics. 2004;114(2 Suppl 4th Report): 555-76.

14. De la Sierra A, Segura J, Banegas JR, Gorostidi M, De la Cruz JJ, Armario P, et al. Clinical features of 8295 patients with resistant hypertension classified on the basis of ambulatory blood pressure monitoring. Hypertension. 2011;57(5):898-902.

15. Aderibigbe A, Omotoso AB, Awobusuyi JO, Akande TM. Arterial blood pressure in adult Nigerian sickle cell anaemia patients. West Afr J Med. 1999;18(2):114-8.

16. Rodgers GP, Walker EC, Podgor MJ. Is "relative" hypertension a risk factor for vaso-occlusive complicationsin sickle cell disease? Am J Med Sci. 1993;305(3):150-6.

17. Aygun B, Mortier NA, Smeltzer MP, Hankins JS, Ware RE. Glomerular hyperfiltration and albuminuria in children with sickle cell anemia. Pediatr Nephrol; 2011.

18. Imuetinyan BA-I, Okoeguale MI, Egberue GO. Microalbuminuria in children with sickle cell anemia. Saudi J Kidney Dis Transpl. 2011;22(4):733-8.

19. Shatat IF, Jakson SM, Blue AE, Johnson MA, Orak JK, Kalpatthi R. Masked hypertension is prevalent in children with sickle cell disease: A midwest pediatric nephrology consortium study. Pediatr Nephrol. 2012;28:115-120.

20. Ho CH, João TAC, Josefina APB. Blood pressure in children with sickle cell disease. Rev Paul Pediatr. 2012;30(1):87-92.

21. Sorof JM, Lai D, Turner J, Poffenbarger T, Portman RJ. Overweight, ethnicity and the prevalence of hypertension in school-aged children. Pediatrics. 2004;113:475-82.

22. Hatch FE, Crowe LR, Miles DE, Young JP, Portner ME. Altered vascular reactivity in sickle hemoglobinopathy. A possible protective factor from hypertension. Am J Hypertens. 1989;2:2-8.

23. Sarni RO, Souza FI, Pitta TS, Fernandez AP, Hix S, Fonseca FA. Low birth weight: Influence on blood pressure, body composition and anthropometric indexes. Arq Med ABC. 2005;30:76-82.

20

Laboratory Accuracy of Some Human Immunodeficiency Virus Screening Methods in a Nigerian Blood Bank: Is it time for Universal Adoption of Enzyme-linked Immuno-Sorbent Assay Methodologies as the Minimum Testing Paradigm?

Orkuma Joseph Aondowase[1*], Gomerep Simji Samuel[2], Egesie Julie Ochaka[3], Orkuma Jenifer Hembadoon[4], Mbaave Tsavyange Peter[5] and Onoja Anthony Michael[1]

[1]Department of Hematology, College of Health Sciences, Benue State University, Makurdi Benue State, Nigeria.
[2]Department of Internal Medicine, Faculty of Medical Sciences, University of Jos, Plateau State, Nigeria.
[3]Department of Hematology and Blood Transfusion, Faculty of Medical Sciences, University of Jos, Plateau State, Nigeria.
[4]Department of Laboratory, College Clinic, Federal School of Forestry, Jos-Plateau state, Nigeria.
[5]Department of Internal Medicine, College of Health Sciences, Benue State University, Makurdi Benue State, Nigeria.

Authors' contributions

This work was carried out in collaboration between all authors. Author OJA conceptualized, carried the research, and produced the manuscript for scientific publication. Author GSS reviewed the work and provided statistical analysis. Author EJO provided statistical analysis. Author OJH analyzed the samples, and reviewed literature. Author MTP reviewed the methodology and analyzed the study for scientific publication. Author OAM analyzed the laboratory methods and revised the manuscript for a scientific publication. All authors read and approved the final manuscript.

Editor(s):
(1) Shinichiro Takahashi, Kitasato University School of Allied Health Sciences, Japan.
Reviewers:
(1) Celso Eduardo Olivier, Department of Allergy and Immunology, Instituto Alergoimuno de Americana, Brazil.
(2) Gerald Mboowa, Department of Medical Microbiology, College of Health Sciences, Makerere University, Buganda.

Corresponding author: E-mail: orkumajoseph@yahoo.com

ABSTRACT

Aim: To compare the prevalence rates, relevant indices of laboratory accuracy and proportion of false negative test results for some WHO recommended methodologies used for HIV screening amongst blood donor sata hospital-based blood bank in Nigeria.

Study Design: A cross-sectional.

Place and Duration: Blood bank unit of Jos University Teaching Hospital (JUTH) and the Nigerian National Blood Transfusion Service (NBTS) North Central Zonal Office, Jos between May and August 2008.

Methodology: Four hundred and forty blood donors (379 males and 61 females; aged 18-55 years) predominantly family replacement blood donors who met the minimum criteria to donate blood in Nigeria were included. Blood collection, serum processing, testing and interpretation of results were carried out using standard methods and manufacturers' instruction. Serum was tested with a rapid test (Determine™ HIV- 1/2) and an EIA [Dia Pro HIV 1/2/0 ELISA] method. The samples were further tested with a 4th generation ELISA [GENSCREEN®PLUS HIV Ag- Ab ELISA].

Results: The prevalence of HIV in blood donors differed with the test method and assay as follows; Determine TM HIV 1/ 2 (3.6%), Dia Pro HIV 1/2/0 ELISA (5.5%) and GENSCREEN®PLUS HIV Ag- Ab ELISA (9.3) respectively.

Determine TM HIV-1/ 2gave a sensitivity of 0.39 (95% CI 0.24-0.55), specificity 1.00,95% CI 0.99-1.00), false negative [FN] (61%), positive predictive value [PPV] 1.00 95% CI 0.79-1.00), and a negative predictive value [NPV] 0.94, 95% CI 0.91-0.96 when compared with GENSCREEN®PLUS HIV Ag-Ab ELISA method. P<0.001.

Dia Pro HIV 1/2/0 ELISA gave a sensitivity of 0.54, 95% CI.37-0.69, specificity 0.995, 95% CI 0.99-1.00, FN(46.3%), PPV (0.9295% CI 0.73-0.99 and a NPV (0.95, 95% CI0.93-0.97) when compared with GENSCREEN®PLUS HIV Ag-Ab ELISA method. P<0.001.

Determine TM HIV 1/2 had a sensitivity of 0.67 95% CI 0.45-0.84, specificity of 1.00; 95% CI 0.99-1.00, FN (33.3%), PPV (1.00 95% CI 0.79-1.00 and a NPV 0.98, 95% CI 0.96-0.99 when compared with Dia Pro HIV 1/2/0 ELISA method. P<0.001.

Conclusion: The prevalence of HIV in blood donors is method dependent with GENSCREEN®PLUS HIV Ag-Ab ELISA higher than Dia Pro HIV 1/2/0 and Determine TM HIV 1/ 2. Dia Pro HIV 1/2/0 is more accurate and has fewer FN test results than Determine TM HIV 1/ 2. There is a need to discourage rapid testing as a major testing algorithm amongst hospital-based blood banks. Instead, ELISA methods should be adopted as the minimum testing paradigm. However, further testing with Nucleic Acid Amplification Testing (NAT) is recommended to validate reliability of this study.

Keywords: Blood donors; HIV infection; prevalence; hospital-based blood bank; laboratory accuracy; blood transfusion; Nigeria.

1. INTRODUCTION

Adequate interception of Human Immunodeficiency Virus (HIV) contaminated blood donations through responsible and responsive testing is feasible and remains the most cost-effective HIV prevention strategy required to protect blood supplies against HIV infection [1]. Unfortunately, inadequate screening for transfusion transmissible HIV (TT-HIV) continues to plague many resource-poor settings like some hospital-based blood banks in Nigeria [2].

The various testing methods currently available for screening blood donations target different parts of the virus ranging from gene sequence,

gene products or measure the hosts' immune response against the virus with respect to the antibodies produced either as an Enzyme–Linked Immuno-sorbent Assay (ELISA) or non-ELISA based methodology [3]. The HIV Nucleic Acid Amplification Testing (NAT) for instance, has emerged a superior testing technology for virus detection and in safeguarding blood supplies. Understandably, NAT is used in developed economies to safeguard donor blood and tissues from HIV contamination thereby reducing the risk of TT-HIV remarkably in many countries like Germany, France and USA. [2,4]. However, NAT is expensive, technically demanding with enormous logistic challenges and not universally available to safeguard blood supplies in many resource-poor settings and particularly where there is a lack of political will and commitment on the part of their leaders. Similarly, the enzyme immunoassays (EIA) which have undergone quality improvement from first generation to fourth generation by utilizing recombinant antigens and synthetic peptides as well as the antigen-antibody sandwich technology making it very usefully in securing blood donations against HIV infections. Even though ELISA methods are universally available to increase the sensitivity of HIV detection in a cost effective manner, the challenges of erratic power supply, paucity of skilled manpower and strict quality control measures required limits its usage. Yet, some resource-poor countries have demonstrated that, its application is achievable and have even gone a step further in developing indigenous ELISAs with sensitivity to HIV strains inherent in their localities [5]. The development of rapid HIV antibody serologic test methods for emergency diagnosis and surveillance, have emerged in popularity in protecting blood supplies especially in resource-poor settings because of its ease of performance, visually read results and in not requiring any sophisticated equipment's or other ancillary challenges associated with ELISA testing methods [6]. In many countries like Nigeria, rapid tests are convenient and acceptable for HIV screening of blood donations against HIV infection at hospital-based blood transfusion services [7]. The World Health Organization (WHO) has also recommended that, the screening for HIV in donated blood should be performed using a highly sensitive and specific anti-HIV-1 anti-HIV-2 immunoassay or a combined HIV antigen-antibody immunoassay (EIA/CLIA) capable of detecting subtypes specific to the country or region. In its absence, a highly sensitive and specific anti-HIV-1 anti-HIV-2 rapid assay could be used in laboratories with small throughput, remote areas or emergency situations [8]. This recommendation is probably in a bid to get all donations test HIV-negative before transfusion worldwide irrespective of the financial strength of the nation. However, it is imperative that, tests employed for screening in a particular area should detect the prevalent strains of the virus. Therefore, irrespective of which methodology is employed, accurate testing to eliminate false negative screening remains a top priority since, blood recipients of false negative blood donations have more than 95% risk of acquiring TT-HIV infection [9]. Many potential causes of false-negative HIV screening of blood donation may exist including; the diagnostic window in the pre-seroconversion phase, genetic variability, atypical seroconversions, a delayed or absent immune response in the very early or advanced stages of infection and laboratory reporting errors. Studies however, indicate that, about 90% of false-negative results are observed in the pre-seroconversion phase during primary HIV infection (i.e. diagnostic window) [10]. There are indications that, in many of resource-poor settings of Africa, TT-HIV resulting from inadequate blood screening accounts for the second largest mode of HIV transmission [1] Imperatively, increased application of appropriate HIV testing methods in blood donation is undoubtedly a panacea to universal access to prevention of TT-HIV in blood supplies in resource-limited settings like the hospital based blood banks in Nigeria. This is more relevant now that the support for HIV activities to many resource-poor economies is dwindling. In recent past, many hospital-based blood banks in Nigeria benefited from foreign donor support agencies through the provision of rapid test kits for TT-HIV prevention (when available) and provided training of hospital staff on blood safety among other assistance. However, with the global economic crisis spreading wild, Nigeria has witnessed an unprecedented reduction in support for HIV prevention. This development has called for more prudent allocation and management of meagre resources in a truly cost-effective manner. Quintessentially, more strategies and measures to improve the effectiveness of the routine screening of blood donors and the safety of the blood components against HIV have to be individualized and localized as appropriate.

Therefore, we sought to evaluate two HIV screening methods (one rapid test and one ELISA method) in a population of Nigerian blood donors at a tertiary hospital-based blood bank with a view to accessing their laboratory accuracies in HIV detection as well as identify the presence or absence of false negative donations in this resource poor setting by using a combined HIV antigen-antibody ELISA (GENSCREEN®PLUS HIV Ag-Ab ELISA) used at the Nigerian National Blood Transfusion service (NBTS) and shown by Chatteriee et al. [11] to produce results concordant with individual donor nucleic acid testing (ID-NAT), for validation of the specimen. Furthermore the prevalence rate with the different assays was sought.

2. MATERIALS AND METHODS

The laboratory performances of one simple/rapid test (Determine™ HIV- 1/2) and one EIA [Dia Pro HIV 1/2/0 ELISA] methodologies were accessed among 440 (379 males and 61 females) predominantly family replacements blood donors aged between 18 and 55 years at the blood bank unit of Jos University Teaching Hospital (JUTH) between May and August 2008. Blood donors who met the inclusion criteria i.e. fulfilled the conditions to donate blood in Nigeria, [12] and gave an informed written consent were consecutively enrolled, while those who did not meet the minimum criteria to donate blood and or declined to give an informed consent were excluded from the study. A questionnaire was administered by trained research assistants to identify donors' bio-data and their relevant characteristics. Ethical approval was obtained from the ethical committee of Jos University Teaching Hospital (JUTH) and all ethical standards were adhered to. Ten (10) milliliters of venous blood was collected from ante-cubital vein of all the blood donors using a large bore needle under aseptic conditions. Haemostasis was secured and the collected blood emptied into a clean evacuated tube without an anticoagulant. Care was taken to ensure that, all validation specimens were of adequate volume and of high quality by being properly collected and processed while also avoiding hemolysis and practices that would encourage fungal or bacterial contamination/growth. Freshly collected specimen were preferably tested within 24 hours of collection using Determine™ HIV- 1/2 while aliquot samples for ELISA testing were stored at -20°C and for periods not longer than one month and processed batched together. In general, the process of serum extraction and storage was carried out using the WHO recommended methods [13].

The serum collected was screened for HIV antibodies using Determine™ HIV 1/2 sourced from ABBOTT JAPAN CO. LTD, Minato-Ku, Tokyo-Japan. Thereafter, the sera were also serially tested at the Nigerian NBTS North Central Zonal Office, Jos with Dia Pro HIV 1/2/0 EIA sourced from diagnostic Bioprobes Sx/Italy and GENSCREEN®PLUS HIV Ag- Ab ELISA sourced from BIO-RAD laboratories, 3 Bd Raymond Poincaré, Marnes La Couquette-France. All procedures were carried out following the manufacturers' recommendations. The interpretation of the HIV Enzyme Immunoassay (EIA) sero-status as positive or negative was judged based on the manufacturer's instructions of recommended cut-off values and in line with the relevant controls included in the respective assays.

2.1 Statistical Analysis

Analysis of proportions of false negative results, sensitivity, specificity, positive and Negative predictive values as well as comparison of variables was carried out using the Graph Pad Prism 5 Statistical Package. A P-value ≤ 0.05 was taken as level of significance for interpretation of data using Fishers Exact Test.

3. RESULTS

This study found that, Determine™ HIV 1/2 test method gave a sensitivity of 39.02%, specificity (100%), proportion of False Negative (61%), PPV (100%), and a NPV (94.1%) when compared with GENSCREEN®PLUS HIV Ag-Ab ELISA method. (Table 2).

On the other hand, Dia Pro HIV 1/2/0 ELISA gave a sensitivity of 53.5%, specificity (99.5%), proportion of False Negative (46.3%), PPV (99.5%), and a NPV (95.4%) when compared with GENSCREEN®PLUS HIV Ag-Ab ELISA method (Table 2).

Similarly, the Determine TM HIV 1/2 test method had a sensitivity of 67%, specificity (100%), proportion of False Negative (33.3%), PPV(100%), and a NPV(98%) when compared with Dia Pro HIV 1/2/0 ELISA method. Dia Pro HIV 1/2/0 Positive (Table 2).

The prevalence of HIV amongst blood donors was different depending on the screening method employed. (Table 1).

Table 1. Prevalence of HIV among blood donors-using three different methods

	Positive	Negative	Prevalence (%)
Determine™ HIV- 1/ 2	16	424	3.6
Dia Pro HIV 1/2/0	24	416	5.5
GENSCREEN®PLUS HIV AG-AB ELISA	41	399	9.3

Table 2. A comparison of relevant indices of laboratory accuracy and proportion of false negative results for the two screening methods in different combinations amongst blood donors

	Determine™ HIV-1/ 2versus HIV Dia Pro HIV 1/2/0	Determine™ HIV- 1/ 2versus genscreen ®PLUS HIV Ag-Ab ELISA	HIV Dia Pro HIV1/2/0 versus genscreen ®PLUS HIV Ag-Ab ELISA
p-value	<0.001	<0.001	<0.001
Alpha value	<0.05	<0.05	<0.05
Statistical significance	Yes	Yes	Yes
Sensitivity	0.67	0.39	0.54
95% CI	0.45-0.84	0.24-0.55	0.37-0.69
Specificity	1.00	1.00	0.995
95% CI	0.99-1.00	0.991-1.00	0.999
PPV	1.00	1.00	0.92
95% CI	0.79-1.00	0.79-1.00	0.73-0.99
NPV	0.98	0.94	0.95
95% CI	0.96-0.99	0.91-0.96	0.93-0.97
Relative risk	53	16.98	20.7
95% CI	27-105	11.59-2481	12.73-3165
Odds ratio	1617	517	229.8
95% CI	89-29241	30.13-8871	50.3-1050
Proportion of false negative (%)	33.3	61	46.3

KEY PPV=Positive Predictive Value; NPV=Negative Predictive Value; CI=Confidence Interval

4. DISCUSSION

Since the laboratory accuracy of a HIV screening test method can be described in terms of the degree to which people with and those without HIV infection are correctly categorized(i.e. sensitivity and the specificity), [14] and in view of the WHO recommendation that a sensitivity of ≥99% and a specificity of ≥98% is required for accurate HIV testing methods, [15] the findings in our study show an overall low laboratory performance of Determine™ HIV- 1/2 (Rapid Test) and Dia Pro HIV 1/2/0 ELISA (3rd Generation ELISA) over GENSCREEN®PLUS HIV Ag- Ab ELISA. (4th Generation ELISA). Similarly, the proportion of false negative test results were higher with Determine™ HIV- 1/ 2andDia Pro HIV 1/2/0 ELISA when compared with GENSCREEN®PLUS HIV Ag- Ab ELISA. (Table 2) Also, the proportion of false negative test results with Determine™ HIV- 1/2 were more when compared with Dia Pro HIV 1/2/0 ELISA. These findings suggest an overall low performance of Determine™ HIV- 1/2 and Dia Pro HIV 1/2/0 ELISA compared to GENSCREEN®PLUS HIV Ag- Ab ELISA amongst blood donors in a hospital-based blood bank; an implication of ELISA superiority over Rapid test method (Table 2).

Generally, even though studies evaluating HIV screening kits/methods in the context of blood

donations screening at hospital-based blood banks in Nigeria to the knowledge of the authors are scarce, Determine™ HIV- 1/2 tests was validated and recommended for HIV diagnosis by the Federal Ministry of Health in Nigeria [7,16]. Additionally, this validation recommended serial testing rather than parallel testing as a tool to improving accuracy and cost effectiveness in HIV diagnosis. It also recommended rapid testing for securing blood donations against HIV infection [16]. A serial HIV testing algorithm requires testing to be carried out on all specimens using a single assay and those found to be positive are then retested with a second assay. In the serial algorithm, discordant results are considered indeterminate and retesting with a third, tiebreaker test may be required [17]. Understandably, this approach differs in the blood bank whose desire is to provide safe blood rather than make diagnosis. For instance, while a single result of HIV screening test carried out on a blood donation may suffice in deciding whether a blood unit or component for transfusion is to be release or not, (even though an initial reactive result may be repeated) a single test alone is not sufficient to determine infection or subsequent action and often involves additional testing over a period of time either to pursue the diagnosis or follow up or monitor disease progression [8,18]. Therefore, the application of serial testing method in the hospital-based blood bank may have no economic gains but rather add unnecessary costs to procuring a unit of blood for transfusion. Besides, it may promote waste of man-hours in waiting by potential blood donors. This act is capable of deterring many of these donors who are predominantly family replacements from becoming voluntary non-remunerated blood donors through education and mobilization as this is desirable if Nigeria must achieve the WHO target of 100% voluntary blood donation by 2020.

While some studies have documented that some rapid tests performs comparably to standard ELISA and western blot in patients with established HIV infection as well as in cohorts of newly infected patients tested at regular intervals during the seroconversion period,(14) others have reported on the low sensitivity of Determine HIV -1/2. [18-20]. Some studies have also reported that, certain types of rapid HIV tests are producing false-negative results [21]. A study conducted by the South African government revealed rapid HIV testing sensitivities that averaged 68.7% in Cape Town's local clinics and thus, failed to detect HIV in nearly one third of patients who had the virus [22]. In another study [23], of nine hundred ninety-four participants who had either negative or discordant rapid test results, eleven (1.1%) had acute HIV infection and an additional twenty (2.0%) had chronic HIV infection (false negative rapid test). A large South African study proved that the actual sensitivity of HIV test kits used outside of the laboratory was on average 93.5% and even with additional training and quality control improvement increased to only 95.1% [24]. While in Cameroon, the same rapid testing algorithm that produced a specificity of 98.8% had a sensitivity of 94.7%, resulting in 6 out of every 100 people receiving a negative diagnosis when they are in fact HIV-positive (15). False negatives are a threat not only to public health prevention strategy but also to the health and well-being of the individual. A false negative result, despite being incorrect in some cases, may prevent patients from seeking out other testing opportunities, taking the necessary precautions to prevent the transmission of HIV and receiving the timely care and treatment that they require [25]. In spite of these, the Nigerian government in 2011 carried out another evaluation of HIV kits [16] and excluded Determine and the ELISA based HIV assays including Dia Pro HIV1/2/0.Yet, there are concerns of sub-standard test kits circulating in the Nigerian market [18].

The prevalence of HIV amongst blood donorsin our study showed marked differences depending on the accuracy of a test method. (Table 1). In Nigeria, whereas the NBTS will logically report the prevalence based on the combined antigen-antibody test assays employed in screening at their few regional centres nationwide, studies at many hospital-based blood banks will utilize what is available and acceptable i.e. rapid test or antibody ELISA. These discrepant results may be utilized for planning, budgeting, intervention, funding, prevention and blood bank management erroneously and may not truly reflect the situation nationally. The HIV prevalence of blood donors in blood banks ought to be lower when compared with the general population, commercial sex workers, drivers, etc. by virtue of the strict adherence to deferral criterion in this setting. Therefore, a high prevalence rate detected with GENSCREEN®PLUS HIV Ag- Ab ELISA may signify a weak deferral system in which, high risk donors erroneously skip being deferred either because of insufficient tool for deferral of blood donors or insincerity of blood donors in truthfully reporting high risk behaviours before blood donation only to be detected by a more sensitive test. Therefore, for a true representation of blood safety activities in the country, national figures from the different geopolitical zones must be harmonized with a single testing methodology. This will allow for prudent management of lean blood bank budgets, aid evaluation and implementation of pre-donation screening questionnaires/interventions to intercept or defer high risk donors who knowingly or unknowingly may taint blood supplies. It will also help preserve unnecessary HIV screening and prevent donations in the window period, enable adequate planning and budgetary allocation for blood safety drives. Besides, it will help the country effectively monitor disease progression, incidence and development of resistance to treatment where applicable in a cost-effective manner. These are only achievable through adoption of appropriate methodology like ELISA testing method for HIV screening at hospital-based blood banks in Nigeria pending the universal application of NAT testing of blood supplies. In a survey of blood transfusion practice in Nigeria, [26] it was reported that, even though many hospital-based blood banks have ELISA plates and readers capable of being used for HIV screening, many lack requisite trained personnel's to effectively put them to use. With the emergence of HIV treatment in most hospitals, some hospitals now have access to function an alternate power supply which hitherto was a major impediment. Therefore, there is an urgent need to step down training from the NBTS, non-governmental organizations (NGO) and other hospitals and philanthropist with requisite knowledge on ELISA techniques in order to put these machines and equipment's into use for the overall health and safety of the country's blood supplies. When this is done, support for blood safety by partner NGOs will shift from supply of rapid kits to ELISA reagents in various hospitals. Beyond this, blood banks in immediate localities could also collaborate financially and technically in order to provide safe blood for their hospitals and communities in a cost-effective manner for the overall interest of the nation.

5. CONCLUSION

This study has shown that, the prevalence of HIV in blood donors in a Nigerian Hospital-based blood bank is largely method dependent and ELISAs perform better than Rapid test method. Even amongst ELISAs, the GENSCREEN®PLUS HIV Ag-Ab ELISA (4th generation) showed a higher prevalence than Dia Pro HIV1/2/0 (3rd Generation ELISA). Also, ELISA methodology showed more statistically significant indices of laboratory accuracy when compared with rapid tests. Therefore, the continued employment of rapid test to secure blood donations against HIV should be reconsidered instead; the Nigerian government should strive to establish NAT testing in the country. In the interim, the 4th generation ELISAs should be adopted as the minimum testing paradigm in order to secure blood donations against HIV infection at hospital-based blood banks.

ACKNOWLEDGEMENTS

We are most grateful to all the blood donors who participated in the study. We also appreciate the management of JUTH and the staff of Haematology and Blood Transfusion Department of the hospital for the co-operation and assistance we received from them in the course of this work. Profound gratitude is also expressed to the staff of the National Blood Transfusion service (NBTS) Jos Zonal Centre especially DrDamulak, Mr Kurt, MrRumji and MrDanladi for their valuable assistance in the laboratory analysis of samples. We are also grateful to Professor A O Ejele, Dr Joseph Emmanuel, Professor Banwat and Mr Monday Badung for their useful suggestions in the course of this work.

COMPETING INTERESTS

Authors have declared that no competing interests exist.

REFERENCES

1. Dhingra N. Making safe blood available in Africa. 27 June 2006.

    Available:http://www.who.int/bloodsafety/makingsafebloodavailableinafricastatement.pdf

2. Orkuma JA, Egesie JO, Banwat EB, Ejele AO, Orkuma JH. Hospital-based Human Immunodeficiency Virus antibody screening of blood donors in Nigeria: How adequate? Int J Infect Trop Dis. 2014;1(2):77-86.

3. UNAIDS/WHO Policy Statement on HIV Testing.

    Available:http://www.who.int/rpc/research_ethics/hivtestingpolicy_en_pdf.pdf

4. Novack L, Galai N, Yaari A, Orgel M, Shinar E, Sarov B. Use of seroconversion panels to estimate delay in detection of Anti-Human Immunodeficiency Virus antibodies by enzyme-linked immunosorbent assay of pooled compared to singleton serum samples. Journal of Clinical Microbiology. 2006;44(8):2909–2913.

5. Munene E, Songok E, Nyamongo JA, Langat DK, Otysula M. Evaluation of HIV ELISA Diagnostic Kit developed at the Institute of Primate Research, Nairobi, Kenya. African Journal of Health Sciences. 2002;9:117-122.

6. Constantine NT. Serologic tests for the retroviruses: Approaching a decade of evolution. AIDS. 1993;7:1–13.

7. Federal Min of Health Abuja FCT. Laboratory Based HIV Rapid Test Validation Phase 1 April; 2007.

    Availablet:http://pubs.futuresgroup.com/3531ENHANSElab.pdf (Accessed 2nd January.2015).

8. WHO. Screening of transfusion transmissible infections: In screening donated blood for transfusion-transmissible infections.

    Available:www.who.int/bloodsafety/ScreeningDonatedBloodforTransfusion.pdf

(Accessed 5th April, 2014).

9. The international newsletter on AIDS prevention and care: Blood Safety; AIDS Action. 1996;34:1-10

10. Busch MP, Kleinman SH, Jackson B, Stramer SL, Hewlett J, Preston S. Committee report. Nucleic acid amplification testing of blood donors for transfusion-transmitted infectious diseases: Report of the Inter-organizational Task Force on Nucleic Acid Amplification Testing of Blood Donors. Transfusion. 2000;40(2):143–159.

11. Chatteriee K, Coshic P, borgohain M, Premchand, Thapliyal RM, Chakroborty S and Sunders S. Individual donor nucleic testing for blood safety against HIV-1 and Hepatitis B and C viruses in a tertiary hospital. Natl Med J India. 2012;25(4):207-9.

12. FMOH. Blood donation criteria. In: Operational guidelines for blood transfusion practice in Nigeria. National Blood Transfusion Service, Federal Ministry of Health Abuja. 2007;18-23.

13. World Health Organization Regional Office for Africa, Centers for Disease Control and Prevention and Association of Public Health Laboratories: Guidelines for Appropriate Evaluations of HIV Testing Technologies in Africa. Centers for Disease Control and Prevention, Atlanta, GA; 2003.

Available:www.afro.who.int/index.php?option=com_docman&task

14. HIV diagnosis: A guide for selecting rapid diagnostic test (RDT) kits.

Available:http://www.unicef.org/supply/files/hiv_diagnosis_a_guide_for_selecting_rdt_jan08.pdf

15. Aghokeng AF, Mpoudi-Ngole E, Henriette Dimodi H, Atem-Tambe A, Tongo M, Butel C, Delaporte E, Peeters M. Inaccurate Diagnosis of HIV-1 Groupe M and O is a Key Challenge for Ongoing Universal Access to Antiretroviral Treatment and HIV Prevention in Cameroon. PLOS One. 4.11PLoS One. 2009;4(11):e7702. Published online Nov 6, 2009.

DOI:10.1371/journal.pone.0007702PMCID: PMC2768789.

16. Federal ministry of health Abuja FCT. Evaluation of the performance of nine HIV rapid test kits (RTKs) for the development of an interim national HIV testing algorithm in Nigeria: Laboratory based Phase I Study.

Available:http://pag.aids2012.org/EPoster Handler.axd?aid=14755

(Accessed 2nd January, 2015).

17. HIV diagnosis: A guide for selecting rapid diagnostic test (RDT) kits.

Available:http://www.unicef.org/supply/files/hiv_diagnosis_a_guide_for_selecting_rdt_jan08.pdf

18. Orkuma JA, Egesie JO, Banwat EB, Ejele AO, Orkuma JH, Bako IA. HIV screening in blood donors: Rapid diagnostic test versus enhanced ELISA. Niger J Med. 2014; 23(3):192-200.

19. Nkwocha GC, Adesina OA, Arowojolu AO, Bamgboye EA, Adewole IF, Ilesanmi AO. Sensitivity, specificity and predictive values of determine™ HIV-1/2, rapid HIV Screening kit for detection of HIV antibodies among booked antenatal women in University College Hospital, Ibadan. 2012;1:461.

DOI:10.4172/scientificreports.461.

20. Dessie A, Abera B, Walle F, Wolday D, Tammene W. Evaluation of determine HIV-1/2 rapid diagnostic test by 4th generation ELISA using blood donors' serum at Felege Hiwot Referral Hospital, northwest Ethiopia. Ethiop Med J. 2008;46(1):1-5.

21. Piwowar-Manning E, Tustin N, Sikateyo P, Kamwendo D, Chipungu C, Maharaj R, Mushanyu J, Richardson BA, Hillier S, Jackson JB. Validation of rapid HIV antibody tests in Five African Countries. J Int Assoc Physicians AIDS Care (Chic). 2010;9(3):170–172.

22. Wolpaw BJ, Mathews C, Chopra M, Hardie D, de Azevedo V. Jennings Kand Lurie MN. The failure of routine rapid HIV testing: A case study of improving low sensitivity in the field. BMC Health Services Research. 2010;10:73.

DOI:10.1186/1472-6963-10-73.

Available:http://www.biomedcentral.com/1472-6963/10/73

23. Bassett IV, Chetty S, Giddy J, Reddy S, Karen Bishop K, Lu Z, Losina E, Freedberg KA, Walensky RP. Screening for acute HIV infection in South Africa: Finding acute and chronic disease. HIV Med. 2011;12(1):46-53. DOI:10.1111/j.1468-1293.2010.00850.x

24.   Award winning rapid test device to deliver improved HIV testing in Africa. Available:http://atomodiagnostics.com/press-releases/award-winning-rapid-test-device-to-deliver-improved-hiv-testing-in-africa/

25.   Challenges and Failures of HIV Screening with Rapid Tests.

Available:http://www.uniteforsight.org/health-screenings/hiv accessed 12th January 2012.

26.   Federal Ministry of Health Abuja FCT/NBTS. Survey of blood transfusion practice in Nigeria.

21

Effect of *Calpurnia aurea* Seed Extract on HAART Induced Haematotoxicity in Albino Wistar Rats

Haile Nega Mulata[1], Natesan Gnanasekaran[1*], Umeta Melaku[1] and Seifu Daniel[1]

[1]*Department of Medical Biochemistry, School of Medicine, College of Health Sciences, Addis Ababa University, Ethiopia.*

Authors' contributions

This work was carried out in collaboration between all authors. Author HNM designed the study, analyses of the study performed the automated hematology auto analyzer (Sysmex KX-2IN) and statistical analyses of data. Author NG wrote the protocol, and wrote the first draft of the manuscript, managed the literature searches and provided the DPPH and TLC plates for antioxidant assay. Authors UM and SD supported the protocol writing and revised the manuscript. All authors read and approved the final manuscript.

Editor(s):
(1) Dharmesh Chandra Sharma, Incharge Blood Component & Aphaeresis Unit, G. R. Medical College, Gwalior, India.
Reviewers:
(1) Anonymous, Brazil.
(2) Aurea Regina Telles Pupulin, Department of Basic Sciences of Health-State University of Maringa, Brazil.

ABSTRACT

Aim: To investigate the effect of *Calpurnia aurea* seeds extract on highly active antiretroviral therapy (HAART), first phase regimens (Lamivudine + Efavirenz + Zidovudine) induced heamtotoxicity in rats.

Study Design: Thirty adult healthy male albino wistar rats of weighing about 140-150 gms were used in the present study. They were divided into five groups six each. Group- I distilled water only; Group- II HAART drugs only; Group- III HAART drugs + 100 mg/kg of CASE (CASE: *Calpurnia aurea* Seed Extract); Group- IV HAART drugs + 200 mg/kg of CASE and Group- V HAART drugs + 300 mg/kg of CASE were administered orally for 35 day.

Methodology: Matured dried seeds of *Calpurnia aurea* were collected, powdered and extracted using 70% ethanol. Preliminary phytochemical screening and in-vitro antioxidant properties of extract were done. The HAART and different doses of the *Calpurnia aurea* seed extract were administered orally for thirty-five days. On 35th day, the rats were fasted overnight and the blood sample was collected by cardiac puncture after sacrificed the rats by cervical dislocation.

Results: HAART did not alter the total WBC (P=0.56, 7340±500 vs 7080±1381) and platelets count (P=0.76, 751000±56059 vs 742200±11921) but significantly alter the total RBC (P=0.001, 7008000±559521 vs 8832000±142211), HCT (P=0.001, 46.56±3 vs 64.75±1) and haemoglobin (P=0.001 12.90±1.12 vs 15.42±0.49) the affected parameters were restored by CASE in dose dependent meaner. However the CASE significantly reduced the platelets counts in the experimental rats.

Conclusion: This report shows that CASE is an effective counter measure for the toxic haematopoietic effects of HAART. This is may be because of CASE contains phytochemicals such as tannins, flavonoids, terpenoids etc which attenuate the HAART induced hematopoietic cell death in the periphery and bone marrow or it may be promote hematopoietic functions by regulating erythropoietin. Furthermore CASE oral administration reduces the platelet count not in the dose dependant manner. The molecular mechanism of action of the drug needs further clarification.

Keywords: Calpurnia aurea; HAART; haematotoxicity; CASE; antioxidant.

1. INTRODUCTION

Antiretroviral drugs are pills for handling of infection by retroviruses, primarily human immunodeficiency virus (HIV). The *United States* of America, Food and Drug Administration (FDA) have been approved 24 antiretroviral drugs [1]. Among the 24 drugs the following drugs are available in Ethiopia since 2004: nucleoside reverse transcriptase inhibitors (*NRTIs*) (zidovudine, stavudine, lamivudine, abacavir, tenofovir and didanosine) and nucleotide reverse transcriptase inhibitors (NtRTIs) (nevirapine and efavirenz) and protease inhibitors (ritonavir and lopinavir) [2]. When numerous such drugs, typically three or more than three drugs, are taken in combination is known as highly active antiretroviral therapy, or HAART. The normal guidelines for management of HIV infection recommend the combination of three antiretroviral agents, either three reverse transcriptase inhibitors (RTIs) or two RTIs plus one protease inhibitor [3,4]. In resource-limited settings, combination HAART consisting of 2 RTIs [either zidovudine (AZT) or stavudine (d4T) along with lamivudine (3TC)] and 1 non-nucleoside reverse transcriptase inhibitor (NNRTI) [either nevirapine (NVP) or efavirenz (EFV)] are frequently used. AZT, a nucleoside reverse transcriptase inhibitor (NRTI) is one of the earliest antiretroviral agents used as a combination in some of the HAART regimens for the treatment of HIV /AIDS, and it was the first drug which was approved by the US FDA for use in HIV/AIDS. The last fifteen years observation HAART has been the most important marked reduction in HIV infection related morbidity and mortality and also answerable for a wide range of toxicities and life-threatening side-effects [5].

AZT is used in the first line drug combination as stavudine is more frequently associated with mitochondrial toxicity. Its use, however, is associated with haematological toxicity particularly bone marrow aplasia leading to varying degrees of cytopenias especially anemia in some patients. The mechanism of this anemia is attributed to 50-70 per cent inhibition of proliferation of blood cell progenitor cells [6,7] in a time-and dose-dependent fashion. Further, laboratory studies have also shown that AZT exhibits cytotoxicity to the myeloid and erythroid precursors in the bone marrow at drug concentrations close to those associated with the optimal antiviral effect *in vitro*. This haematological toxicity is observed in most of the patients within 3-6 months and is reversible. Female gender has been found to be a risk factor for anemia in some studies. This adverse effect of anemia from AZT limits its use in some patients. AZT has also been reported to produce pure red cell aplasia (PRCA) [8,9]. Previous studies have shown that the incidence of anemia is high in patients either acquired immunodeficiency syndrome (AIDS) or human immunodeficiency virus (HIV) infection [10,11]. HIV infection is associated with anaemia consistently adverse outcomes such as infections and neurologic weakening and progression to AIDS [11]. Earlier studies have found that the occurrence of anemia increases with progression of HIV infection. A number of other etiologic factors may also be concerned in the development of HIV-associated anemia, including, impaired erythropoietin production, blood loss from intestinal opportunistic disease, immunological myelosuppression, and micronutrient deficiencies [12]. HIV infected patients mortality was associated with low haemoglobin levels even reduce the viral load and increased CD4 cell count [11,13-15].

Research has shown that oral ingestion of plant medicinal compounds or drugs can alter the normal range of haematological parameters. These alterations could either be positive or negative [16,17]. Literature survey brings to light the different kinds of medicinal plant phytocheicals promote haematopoiesis and prevent the anaemia for some examples *Hibiscus cannabinus, Telfairia occidentalis, Ageratum conyzoides, Brillantasia nitens* Lindau and *Psidium guajava* [18-22].

Calpurnia aurea is a genus of FLOWERING PLANTS within the family of *Fabaceae*. The leaf and stem of *C. aurea* has been used for different human and animal disease [23]. In Ethiopia, traditionally, the leave of *C. aurea* is used for the treatment of syphilis, malaria, rabies, diabetes, hypertension, diarrhoea, leishmaniasis, trachoma, elephantiasis, fungal diseases and different swellings, stomach-ache, bowel, and bladder disorders [24]. Umer et al. [25] reported that the 80% methanol extract of *C. aurea* leaf revealed the presence of alkaloids, tannins, flavonoids and saponins. Hence, the present study is undertaken to investigate the anti-haematotoxic potential of hydroethanolic *C. aurea* seed extract against HAART-first phase regimen (Lamivudine + Efavirenz + Zidovudine) drugs induced haemtotoxicity in rats.

2. MATERIALS AND METHODS

2.1 Plant Materials

The *C. aurea* leaves with flower and seeds were collected from south Gondar, northern Ethiopia in June 2013. The plant has identified and authenticated by taxonomist of Ethiopian National Herbarium of Addis Ababa University and its voucher number was 001/2006.

2.2 Extraction

The seeds were washed thoroughly 2-3 times with running tap water, then shade dried and grinded in mixer. The grinded seeds were weighed 100 gm using an electronic balance and were macerated separately in 70% ethanol for 72 hours with mechanical shaking and it was filtered through Whatman No.1 filter paper. Then filtrate was evaporated using rotary evaporator and dried at 40ºC. The yield was found to be 17.62% w/v. Preliminary phytochemical tests were performed by standard phytochemical test procedures [26,27].

2.3 *In-vitro* Antioxidant Activity by Spectrophotometric Method

The DPPH radical-scavenging activity of the test extracts was examined as previously described [28]. Different concentrations (31.25-1000 µg/ml) of each extract were added, at an equal volume, to methanolic solution of DPPH (100 mM). The mixture was allowed to react at room temperature in the dark for 30 minutes. Vitamin C was used as standard controls. Three replicates were made for each test sample. After 30 minutes, the absorbance (A) was measured at 517 nm and converted into the percentage antioxidant activity. IC_{50} values denote the concentration of sample which is required to scavenge 50% of DPPH free radicals. The IC_{50} values were calculated from the linear regression curves, where the abscissa represented the concentration of the test plant extracts and the ordinate the average percent of scavenging capacity from three replicates. IC_{50} value (concentration of sample where absorbance of DPPH decreases 50% with respect to absorbance of the control) of extracts were determined [29]. The higher the antioxidant activity, the lower IC_{50} value.

2.4 Animals

Thirty adult (12 weeks' old) healthy male albino rats weighing 140-150 gms were used in the present study and housed in polypropylene cages and maintained standard laboratory conation. They were provided with standard pellet rat diet supplied by Kality Animal Nutrition Production Ltd., Addis Ababa Ethiopia, and water *ad libitum*. The research protocol was approved by the Research & Ethics Review committee (DRERC) of the department of Medical Biochemistry, Addis Ababa University with approval number SOM/BCHM/012/2013 E.C. All the animal experiments were carried out according to Committee for the Purpose of Control and Supervision of Experiments on Animals (CPCSEA) guidelines.

2.5 Extrapolation of HAART Dose

The human doses of HAART drug were extrapolated to animals by the formula; Human Equivalent Dose (HED in mg/kg) = Animal Dose (mg/kg) × (Animal Km ÷ Human Km), Where Km is a correction factor reflecting the relationship between body weight and body surface area [30]. Table 1 shows the average Km value of most frequently used laboratory animals.

Table 1. Average Km value of laboratory animals

Mouse	3
Rat	6
Guinea pig	8
Rabbit	12
Dog	20
Human adult	37

Based on the above Km value, the HAART drugs were calculated per weight of the rats. So that, the four experimental groups (II, III, IV, & V) were treated with (Lamivudine=0.53 mg/kg, Efavirenz= 0.7 mg/kg, and Zidovudine = 0.11 mg/kg) administered orally for 35 days.

2.6 Animal Grouping and Drug Dose

Group- I Normal control, given distilled water only

Group- II Positive control, given HAART drugs only

Group- III, Given HAART drugs + 100 mg/kg of CASE (CASE: *Calpurnia aurea* Seed Extract)

Group- IV, Given HAART drugs + 200 mg/kg of CASE

Group- V, Given HAART drugs + 300 mg/kg of CASE

2.7 Blood Sample Collection and Analysis

After 35 days of treatment, the rats were fasted overnight, sacrificed by cervical dislocation and blood was aseptically collected by cardiac puncture. The blood samples were taken for haematological analysis in heparinzed vials. The haematological parameters were analyzed by automated haematology auto analyser (Sysmex KX-2IN) following the manufacturer's guideline.

2.8 Statistical Analysis

The data was expressed as mean±SEM. Statistical significance between the groups were tested using one-way ANOVA followed by Dennett's post-hoc test. A P less than 0.5 were considered significant.

3. RESULTS

3.1 Phytochemical

The preliminary phytochemical analysis of 70% ethanolic extract of *C. aurea* seed showed the presence of tannins, flavonoids, terpenoids, saponins, steroids, glycosides, alkaloids compounds.

3.2 *In-vitro* Antioxidant Activity

The percentage inhibition in *C. aurea* seed extract and standard ascorbic acid (vitamin C) Vs concentration shows that the antioxidant activities of 70% ethanol extract of *C. aurea* seed and the standard vitamin C was found to be positively correlated with the % inhibition. The IC_{50} (Inhibition Concentration at 50%) value of *C. aurea* extract were calculated as 88.46 µg/ml while that of Ascorbic Acid was 51.41 µg/ml from their corresponding regression curves.

3.3 Haematological Profile

The WBC total count shows that no significant difference between HAART administered rats (group- II) as compared with the normal rats (Group- I).This finding is against the pervious finding of Kayode et al. [31] they are reported that acute administration of lamivudin and efavirenz increased total WBC count 40% and 43% respectively and Osonuga et al. [32] reported that HAART administered rats showing significant decrease WBC total count. However, the WBC count mean value shows an increase (p<0.05) in group IV and V, those receiving HAART and 200 and 300 mg/kg CASE compared with the normal rats (Group- I). Only Group- V shows statistically significant increase (p<0.05) in LYM# compared with the normal rats (Table 2).

RBC, MCV, MCH and MCHC mean values found significantly decreased (p<0.05) in HAART administered group II rats. Previous study showed that the toxic effects of antiretroviral drugs lead to anemia. These could be as a result of these drugs interfering with the progenitor cells of the bone marrow leading to suppression of their activity [33]. The affected parameters are restored by CASE in dose dependent manner. However the platelet count is not altered by HAART, but CASE receiving rats are significantly reduced the platelet count.

4. DISCUSSION

This study revealed a significant alterations total RBC, HCT and haemoglobine level in positive control (Group II) rats that the primary regime of

HAART induced anemia. Several antiretroviral drugs, most importantly zidovudine and other nucleoside reverse transcriptase inhibitors (NRTIs), are known to cause anemia in adults and children [34-37]. Maternal highly-active antiretroviral therapy containing zidovudine reduces mother-to-child HIV transmission but may increase the risk for infant anemia through breast milk [38]. Zidovudine is a well-known drug causing haematotoxicity [39,40]. Zidovudine use is yet not without adverse effect mainly bone marrow aplasia foremost to varying degrees of cytopenias (blood cell deficiencies) mostly anemia. This calls for adequate evaluation and monitoring of patients on this drug. Its major side effect; which is anemia limits its use in some patients [41]. Highly active antiretroviral drugs (zidovudine + Lamivudine) cause suppression of the bone marrow cell precursors, leading to haematotoxicity. Lamivudine induced anemia is more readily attributed to red cell aplasia (RCA). Which is an unusual disorder in which maturation occurs in the formation of erythrocytes [42].

Evaluation of haematological parameters can be used to determine the degree of harmful or helpful effects of foreign compounds as well as plant extract on blood [43]. The outcome of this study showed that the CASE shows salubrious effects on HAART induced haematotoxicity. The salubrious effects are indications that the animals recovered from haematotoxicity. In the Traditional Chinese medicine, Radix *Astragali* is commonly used as a health food supplement to reinforce the body vital energy. Previous study also showed that the *Astragali* Radix extract could improve haematopoietic functions by regulating erythropoietin (EPO) expression. EPO is an erythrocyte-specific hematopoietic growth factor produced by kidney and liver [44]. Flavonoids, including formononetin, ononin, calycosin, and calycosin-7-O-β-d-glucoside, are considered to be the major active ingredients within Radix *Astragali*. These four flavonoids can induce the expression of EPO [45]. Pervious study in *C. aurea* leaves [25] and present study in *C. aurea* seed contains flavonoids, it may be promotes the EPO synthesis and restored the HAART affected parameters.

HAART drugs amplify chemically reactive species in blood, possibly by producing more oxidized metabolites deriving from the interaction between reactive oxygen species (ROS) and infected cell biomolecules [46]. This is supported by some biochemical mechanisms, such as mitochondrial interference, following treatment with HAART-AZT [47-49]. RBCs are prone to oxidative stress being the first cells in the body because they are extremely vulnerable to oxidative injure due to the high concentration of iron in haemoglobin and oxygen the chief cradle of the oxidative process. RBCs have a rich polyunsaturated fatty acid (PUFA) chains in the plasma membrane and they are highly susceptible to oxidation [50]. This molecular mechanism taken to account for reduction of the total RBC count in positive control (Group II) rats. The CASE treated groups (IV and V) significantly increase the total RBC count may be related to its antioxidant activity. The phytochemical results confirm that the CASE contains tannins and flavonoids which are powerful antioxidant phytochemicals. Tannins do not function solely as primary antioxidants (i.e., they donate hydrogen atom or electrons), they also function as secondary antioxidants. Tannins have the ability to chelate metal ions such as Fe^{2+} and interfere with one of the reaction steps in the Fenton reaction and thereby retard oxidation [51]. The inhibition of lipid peroxidation by tannin constituents can act via the inhibition of cyclooxygenase [52]. Flavonoids act as antioxidants by 'mopping up' free radicals in cells, thereby limiting the oxidative damage. They are well known to reduce lipid-peroxidation and lipoxygenase enzyme activities. They apply these antioxidant properties as free radical scavengers, chelators of divalent cation [53,54]. Moreover, the high-level of ROS can damage the haematopoietic reconstitution capacity of haematopoietic stem cells (HSCs). Thus, the application of antioxidant intervention in the *in-vivo* mobilization of bone marrow haematopoietic stem cells may be effective against the negative effects of ROS on bone marrow haematopoietic stem cells. Antioxidant intervention may also better protect the haematopoietic reconstitution capacity of HSCs [55].

HAART did not alter the White blood cell count in the present study. However in CASE treated groups (IV and V) WBC count increase in a dose dependent manner compare with both positive (Group II) and negative control (Group I). The effect of low dose of CASE did not alter the WBC count. The phytochemical result of CASE reveals that presence of cardiac glycosides. The cardiac glycosides have an anti-inflammatory property and are attributed to cause increase in WBC count [56].

Table 2. Haematological profile of normal control, and HAART and CASE administered albino wistar rats

Haematology parameters	Group - I (Dis. Water)	Group - II (HAART)	Group – III (100 mg/kg CASE + HAART)	Group – IV (200 mg/kg CASE +HAART)	Group – V (300 mg/kg CASE +HAART)
WBC per µL	7080±1381.087[a]	7340±1500.599[a]	7360±639.218[a]	7740±1319.318[b]	9060±1556.792[c]
LYM%	71.376±1.670[a]	73.18±2.126[a]	77.38±3.717[a]	72.86±2.642[a]	76.60±2.762[b]
LYM# per µL	5300±474.342[a]	5384±521.973[a]	5580±1231.828[b]	5560±860[b]	7120±1358.823[c]
RBC per µL	8832000±14221.111[a]	7008000±55952.224[b]	7146000±158472.999[b]	7160000±28360.834[c]	7536000±25611.161[d]
HCT (PCV) %	64.75±0.633	46.56±3.793[b]	48.58±1.928[b]	51.172±1.248[c]	63.992±1.810[d]
HGB g/dL	15.42±0.498[a]	12.90±1.126[b]	13.50±0.532[b]	14.244±0.293[c]	15.80±0.192[d]
MCV per fL	73.102±0.857[a]	66.306±0.240[b]	66.42±0.788[b]	67.86±0.409[b]	72.82±0.991[c]
MCH per pg	21.66±0.309[a]	19.90±0.315[a]	19.942±0.122[a]	21.112±0.178[a]	21.28±0.185[a]
MCHC per g/dL	32.06±0.426[a]	27.244±0.227[b]	27.34±0.163[b]	31.57±0.247[c]	31.94±0.615[c]
PLT per µL	751000±56059.7895[a]	742200±119212.164[a]	507200±92496.162[b]	414000±13309.576[c]	598600±56772.881[d]
MPV per fL	7.698±0.230[a]	7.82±0.073[a]	8.06±0.112[a]	7.72±0.211[a]	7.94±0.181[a]

The significant decrease of platelet count recorded in all CASE treated groups compared with both positive (Group II) and negative control (Group I) not in dose dependent manner. These data are in agreement with the data reported by Tohti et al. [56]. These decreases might be attributed to the toxic effect of the CASE because of the fact that it contain saponins and cardiac glycosides.

5. CONCLUSION

This report shows that oral administration of CASE is an effective counter measure for the toxic hematopoietic effects of HAARTM may be CASE phytochemicals such as tannins, flavonoids, terpenoids, etc attenuate the HAART induced hematopoietic cell death in the periphery and bone marrow or it may be promotes hematopoietic functions by regulating erythropoietin. Furthermore CASE oral administration reduces the platelet count not in the dose dependant manner. The molecular mechanism of action of the drug needs further clarification.

CONSENT

It is not applicable.

ACKNOWLEDGEMENTS

Mr. Feysa Chala from EHNRI chemistry laboratories and Mr. Kissi Mudi from phyto-chemistry laboratory, Mr. Yohanis G. and Mohamed M. from biochemistry laboratory, Aster Seyoum and Mr. Tesfay Getachew from the animal laboratory for their kind assistance during laboratory works.

COMPETING INTERESTS

Authors have declared that no competing interests exist.

REFERENCES

1. Flexner C. HIV drug development: the next 25 years. Nature Reviews Drug Discovery. 2007;6(12):959-966.

2. Huruy K, Mulu A, Mengistu G, Shewa-Amare A, Akalu A, Kassu A, Torben W. Immune reconstitution inflammatory syndrome among HIV/AIDS patients during highly active antiretroviral therapy in Addis Ababa, Ethiopia. Japanese Journal of Infectious Diseases. 2008;61(3):205.

3. Dybul M, Fauci AS, Bartlett JG, Kaplan JE, Pau AK. Guidelines for using antiretroviral agents among HIV-infected adults and adolescents: The panel on clinical practices for treatment of HIV. Annals of Internal Medicine. 2002;137(5):381-433.

4. Yeni PG, Hammer SM, Carpenter CC, Cooper DA, Fischl MA, Gatell JM, Volberding PA. Antiretroviral treatment for adult HIV infection in 2002: Updated recommendations of the international AIDS society-USA panel. The Journal of the American Medical Association. 2002;288(2):222-235.

5. Calmy A, Hirschel B, Cooper DA, Carr A. A new era of antiretroviral drug toxicity. Antivir Ther. 2009;14(2):165-179.

6. Groopman JE. Zidovudine intolerance. Rev Infect Dis. 1990;12(5):S500-S506.

7. Miles SA. Hematopoietic growth factors as adjuncts to antiretroviral therapy. AIDS Res Hum Retroviruses. 1992;8:1073-1080.

8. Hassan A, Babadoko AA, Mamman AI, Ahmed SA. Zidovudine induced pure red cell aplasia: A case report. Niger J Med. 2009;18:332-333.

9. Weinkove R, Rangarajan S, Van Der Walt J, Kulasegaram R. Zidovudine-induced pure red cell aplasia presenting after 4 years of therapy. AIDS. 2005;19:2046-2047.

10. Rajesh R, Vidyasagar S, Varma DM, Mohiuddin S, Noorunnisa. Evaluation of incidence of zidovudine induced anemia in Indian human immunodeficiency virus positive patients in comparison with stavudine based highly active antiretroviral therapy. Int J Risk Saf Med. 2011;23(3):171-80.

11. Belperio PS, Rhew DC. Prevalence and outcomes of anemia in individuals with human immunodeficiency virus: A systematic review of the literature. Am J Med. 2004;16(7A):27-43.

12. Semba RD, Gray GE. Pathogenesis of anemia during human immunodeficiency virus infection. J Invest Med. 2001;49:225-39.

13. Sullivan PS, Hanson DL, Chu SY, Jones JL, Ward JW. Epidemiology of anemia in human immunodeficiency virus (HIV)-infected persons: Results from the multistate adult and adolescent spectrum

of HIV disease surveillance project. Blood. 1998;91:301-308.

14. Mocroft A, Kirk O, Barton SE, Dietrich M, Proenca R, Colebunders R. Euro SIDA study group. Anaemia is an independent predictive marker for clinical prognosis in HIV-infected patients from across Europe. Euro SIDA Study Group. AIDS. 1999;13:943-50.

15. Lundgren JD, Mocroft A. Anemia and survival in human immunodeficiency virus. Clin Infect Dis. 2003;37(4):297-303.

16. Ofuya ZM, Ebong OO. Plasma ascorbic acid levels in adult Females in Port-Harcourt, South-Eastern Nigeria. West African Journal of Pharmacology and Drug Research. 1996;12:32-36.

17. Ajagbonna OP, Onifade KI, Suleiman U. Haematological and biochemical changes in rats given extract of *Calotropis procera*. Sokoto J Vet Sci. 1999;1:36-42.

18. Agbor GA, Oben JE, Ngogang JY. Hematinic activity of *Hibiscus cannabinus*. Afr J Biotechnol. 2005;4(8):833-837.

19. Dina OA, Adedapo AA, Oyinloye OP, Saba AB. Effect of *Telfairia occidentalis* extract on experimentally induced anemia in domestic rabbits. Afr J Biomed Res. 2006;3:181-183.

20. Ita SO, Etim OE, Ben EE, Ekpo OF. Hematopoietic properties of ethanolic leaf extract of *Ageratum conyzoides* (Goat weed) in albino rats. Nigerian Journal of Physiological Sciences. 2007;22(1-2):83-87.

21. Akah PE, Okolo CE, Ezike AE. The haematinic activity of the methanol leaf extract of *Brillantasia nitens* Lindau (*Acanthaceae*) in rats. African Journal of Biotechnology. 2009;8(10):2389-2393.

22. Uboh Friday E, Iniobong E. Okon, Moses B. Ekong. Effect of aqueous extract of *Psidium guajava* leaves on liver enzymes, histological integrity and hematological indices in rats. Gastroenterology Research. 2010;3(1):32-38.

23. Asres K, David P, Polo M. Two novel minor alkaloids from Ethiopian *C. aurea*. Planta Medica. 1986;25:302-304.

24. Tadeg H, Mohammed E, Asres K, Gebre-Mariam T. Antimicrobial activities of some selected traditional Ethiopian medicinal plants used in the treatment of skin

disorders. J Ethnopharmacol. 2005;100:168-175.

25. Umer S, Tekewe A, Kebede N. Antidiarrhoeal and antimicrobial activity of *C. aurea* leaf extract. BMC Complementary and Alternative Medicine. 2013;13:21.

26. Harborne JB, Harborne AJ. Phytochemical methods: A guide to modern techniques of plant analysis. Kluwer Academic Publishers, London, UK. Elsevier Science. 1998;3:11-320.

27. Kumar KA, Narayani M, Subanthini A, Jayakumar M. Antimicrobial activity and phytochemical analysis of citrus fruit peel utilization of fruit waste. Int J Environ Sci Tech. 2011;3:5415-5421.

28. Abdel-Hameed ESS. Total phenolic contents and free radical scavenging activity of Certain Egyptian *Ficus species* leaf samples. Food Chem. 2009;114(4):1271-1277.

29. Williams RJ, Spencer JPE, Rice-Evans C. Flavonoids and isoflavonones (Phytoestrogens): Absorption, Metabolism and Bioactivity. Serial review: Free Radical Biology and Medicine. 2004;36:838-849.

30. Natural Health Research Institute. Extrapolation of Animal Dose to Human; 2008. Accessedon 19/11/2013. Available:http://www.naturalhealthresearch.org/nhri/extrapolation-of-animal-dose

31. Kayode AAA, Kayode OT, Aroyeun OA, Stephen MC. Hematologic and hepatic enzyme alterations associated with acute administration of antiretroviral drugs. Journal of Pharmacology and Toxicology. 2011;6:293-302.

32. Osonuga OA, Osonuga OI, Osonuga AA, Osonuga A. Hematologic Toxicity of Antiretroviral Drug, Zidolam (zidovudine and lamivudine) in Adult Wistar Rats Asian Journal of Medical Sciences. 2010;1:41-44.

33. Montessori V, Press N, Harris M, Akagi L, Montaner JS. Adverse effects of antiretroviral therapy for HIV infection. Canadian Medical Association Journal. 2004;170(2):229-238.

34. Moh R, Danel C, Sorho S, Sauvageot D, Anzian A, Minga A, et al. Haematological changes in adults receiving a zidovudine-containing HAART regimen in combination

with cotrimoxazole in Cote d'Ivoire. Antivir Ther. 2005;10:615-624.

35. Lahoz R, Noguera A, Rovira N, Català A, Sánchez E, Jiménez R, Fortuny C. Antiretroviral-related hematologic short-term toxicity in healthy infants: implications of the new neonatal 4-week zidovudine regimen. Pediatr Infect Dis J. 2010;29(4):376-9.

36. Majluf-Cruz A, Luna-Castanos G, Trevino-Perez S, Santoscoy M, Nieto-Cisneros L. Lamivudine-induced pure red cell aplasia. Am J Hematol. 2000;65(3):189-191.

37. John MA, Rhemtula YA, Menezes CN, Grobusch MP. Lamivudine-induced red cell aplasia. J Med Microbiol. 2008;57(8):1032-1035.

38. Dryden-Peterson S, Shapiro RL, Hughes MD, Powis K, Ogwu A, Moffat C, Moyo S, Makhema J, Essex M, Lockman S. Increased risk of severe infant anemia following exposure to maternal HAART, Botswana. J Acquir Immune Defic Syndr. 2011;56(5):428-436.

39. Moyle G, Sawyer W, Law M, Amin J, Hill A. Changes in hematologic parameters and efficacy of thymidine analogue-based, highly active antiretroviral therapy: A meta-analysis of six prospective, randomized, comparative studies. Clinical Therapeutics. 2004;26:92-97.

40. Moore DA, Benepal T, Portsmouth S, Gill J, Gazzard BG. Etiology and natural history of neutropenia in human immunodeficiency virus disease: A prospective study. Clinical Infectious Diseases. 2001;32:469-475.

41. Murray RK. Red & white blood cells. In: Harpers's biochemistry (Granner RK, Mayes PA, Rodwell VW, eds.) McGraw-Hill, USA. 2000;780-786.

42. John MAA, Rhemtula YA, Menezes CN, Grobusch MP. Lamivudine-induced red cell aplasia. Journal of Medical Microbiology. 2008;57(8):1032-1035.

43. Yakubu MT, Oladiji AT, Akanji MA. Mode of cellular toxicity of aqueous extract of Fadogia agresti (Schweinf. Ex Hiern) stem in male rat liver and kidney. Human Exp. Toxicol. 2009;28(8):469-478.

44. Zheng KY, Choi RC, Xie HQ, Cheung AW, Guo AJ, Leung KW, et al. The expression of erythropoietin triggered by Danggui Buxue Tang, a Chinese herbal decoction prepared from Radix astragali and Radix angelicae Sinensis, is mediated by the hypoxia-inducible factor in cultured HEK293T cells. Journal of Ethnopharmacology. 2010;132:259-267.

45. Ngondi JL, Oben J, Forkah DM, Etame LH, Mbanya D. The effect of different combination therapies on oxidative stress markers in HIV infected patients in Cameroon. AIDS Res Ther. 2006;3(1):19.

46. Hulgan T, Morrow J, Richard TD, Raffanti S, Morgan M, Rebeiro P, Haas D W. Oxidant stress is increased during treatment of human immunodeficiency virus infection. Clinical Infectious Diseases. 2003;37(12):1711-1717.

47. Cossarizza A, Moyle G. Antiretroviral nucleoside and nucleotide analogues and mitochondria. AIDS. 2004;18(2):137-151.

48. De la Asunción JG, Del Olmo ML, Sastre J, Millán A, Pellín A, Pallardó FV, Viña J. AZT 'treatment induces molecular and ultrastructural oxidative damage to muscle mitochondria. Prevention by antioxidant vitamins. The Journal of Clinical Investigation. 1998;102(1):4-9.

49. Bryszewska M, Zavodnik IB, Niekurzale A, Szosland K. Oxidative processes in red blood cells from normal and diabetic individuals. Biochem Mol Biol Int. 1995;37:345-54.

50. Karamac M, Kosinska A, Amarowicz R. Chelating of Fe(II), Zn(II) and Cu(II) by tannin fractions separated from hazelnuts, walnuts and almonds. Bromat Chem Toksykol. 2006;39:257-260.

51. Zhang YJ, DeWitt DL, Murugesan S, Nair MG. Novel lipi-peroxidation and cyclooxygenase-inhibitory tannins from Picrorhiza kurrora seeds. Chem Biodiver. 2004:1:426-441.

52. Chebil L, Humeau C, Falcimaigne A, Engasser J, Ghoul M. Enzymatic acylation of flavonoids. Process Biochemistry. 2006;41:2237-2251.

53. Middleton EJR, Kandaswami C, Theoharides TC. The effects of plant flavonoids on mammalian cells: Implications for inflammation, heart disease, and cancer. Pharmacological Reviews. 2000;52:673-751.

54. Hao Y, Cheng D, Ma Y, Zhou W, Wang Y. Antioxidant intervention: A new method for improving hematopoietic reconstitution

capacity of peripheral blood stem cells. Medical Hypotheses. 2011;76(3):421-423.

55. Anthai AB, Ofem OE, Ikpi DE, Ukafia S, Agiang EA. Phytochemistry and some haematological changes following oral administration of ethanolic root extract of *Gongronema latifolium* in rats. Nigerian J. Physiol. Sci. 2009;24(1):79-83.

56. Tohti I, Tursun M, Umar A, Imin H, Moore N. Aqueous extracts of *Ocimum basilicum* L. (Sweet basil) decrease platelet aggregation induced by ADP and thrombin *in vito* and rats arterio-venous shunt thrombosis *in vivo*. Thromb. Res. 2006;118(6):733-739.

22

Level of Pentraxin-3 in Patients with Acute Leukemia in Septicemia and Its Prognostic Value

Ashraf Elghandour[1], Hashem Naenaa[1], Mohamed Eldefrawy[1], Magdy Elbordeny[2] and Hadeer Mohammed[1*]

[1]Internal Medicine, Alexandria University, Egypt.
[2]Clinical Pathology, Alexandria University, Egypt.

Authors' contributions

This work was carried out in collaboration between all authors. Author AE designed the study and contributed in writing protocol and manuscript. Authors HN and M. Eldefrawy contributed in writing manuscript. Author M. Elbordeny did the laboratory work and contributed in writing manuscript. Author HM collected samples & data and contributed in writing manuscript. All authors read and approved the final manuscript.

Editor(s):
(1) Tadeusz Robak, Medical University of Lodz, Copernicus Memorial Hospital, Poland.
Reviewers:
(1) Golam Hafiz, Department of Pediatric Hematology and Oncology, Bangabandhu Sheikh Mujib Medical University, Dhaka, Bangladesh.
(2) Shigeki Taga, Department of Obstetrics and Gynecology, Japanese Red Cross Okayama Hospital, Japan.

ABSTRACT

Introduction: In acute leukemia, sepsis is potentially fatal. Pentraxin3 is a protein rapidly produced in response to primary inflammatory signals. It shows high levels in sepsis, specially associated with vascular and end-organ damage.
Aim of the Work: To measure the level of PTX3 in sepsis in patients with acute leukemia and correlate its level to higher risk of complications compared with CRP.
Study Design: Prospective study.
Place and Duration of the Study: Department of hematology, Alexandria main university hospital, from April 2012 to August 2013.
Methods: The study included 60 patients, they had routine workup for leukemia. Serum CRP and plasma PTX3 levels were measured with ELISA on days 1, 2, 3 of febrile neutropenia after chemotherapy.
Results: Male to female ratio 1:1, age ranged from 18 to 62 years (median of 40 yrs). 41 patients

---

Corresponding author: E-mail: dr.hadeerfathy@hotmail.com

suffered from acute myeloid leukemia, and 19 from acute lymphoblastic leukemia. High PTX3 levels on the 1st day of sepsis have been a strong indicator for development of complications (septic shock and mortality) (P=.001) compared to CRP (P=.032). High PTX3 level has been associated with coagulation impairment (P=.001). PTX3 showed sensitivity of 100% and specificity of 70% for prediction of bad prognosis, whereas CRP showed sensitivity of 88.5% and specificity of 60.5%.

Conclusion: PTX3 is highly recommended in diagnosis of sepsis in patients with acute leukemia during neutropenia and it shows high sensitivity and specificity in prediction of bad prognosis (septic shock, coagulation impairment and mortality) in comparison with CRP.

Keywords: Sepsis; febrile neutropenia; PTX3; CRP.

1. INTRODUCTION

Sepsis is a potentially fatal condition characterized by an inflammatory state called SIRS orsystemic inflammatory response syndrome which is induced by an infection. It is considered one of the most common causes of complications and mortality during neutropenia after chemotherapy in acute leukemia patients. [1,2].

Early detection of infection as well as early prediction of bad prognosis using serological markers can aid in early intervention and treatment of infectious condition and thus improvement of outcome of acute leukemia treatment and reduction of mortality during bone marrow aplasia [3].

Pentraxin 3 (PTX3) is a member of the pentraxin superfamily. It is a protein which is encoded by the PTX3 gene in humans. The PTX3 protein is composed of 381 amino acids, of 40,165 Da molecular weight. It has a carboxy-terminal (203 amino acid long) pentraxin domain and an amino-terminal (178 amino acid long) domain unrelated to other known proteins [4].

PTX3 is released by several types of cells, particularly by mononuclear phagocytes, dendritic cells (DCs), fibroblasts and endothelial cells in response to inflammatory signals (e.g. Toll-like receptor (TLR) engagement, TNFα, IL-1β). It then binds to the complement component C1q, the extracellular matrix component TNFα induced protein 6 and selected microorganisms. PTX3 activates the classical pathway of complement activation and facilitates pathogen recognition by macrophages and DCs. In addition to its pro-inflammatory activity, PTX3 also has been shown to play a role in protecting against severe inflammatory reactions [5-9].

PTX3 concentration in healthy individuals is lower than 2 ng/ml and increases rapidly in response to inflammation and infection [10,11]. It is expressed in a variety of cells at inflammatory sites and also stored in neutrophil-specific granules. The stored PTX3 in neutrophils is released into the extracellular space and localizes to neutrophil extracellular traps (NETs) In septic patients, specially associated with vascular damage, the circulating PTX3 concentration increases to characteristically high levels [12-15]. C-reactive protein (CRP) belongs to the group of short pentraxins. Because of its origin and induction by proinflammatory cytokines and bacterial products, PTX3 level is used to diagnose sepsis more rapidly than CRP. Also the plasma PTX3 level shows a good correlation with mortality and dysfunction of several organ systems [16-19].

2. METHODOLOGY

The study is a prospective observational analytical study, it took place at the Haematology Department in Alexandria University Main Hospital between 2012 and 2013. The study has included 60 patients with sepsis and acute leukemia patients after receiving chemotherapy, during severe neutropenia (ANC< 500).

All patients diagnosed with acute leukemia based on complete blood count, bone marrow examination and flow cytometry [20-21] will be subjected to the following during the period of neutropenia: Thorough history taking by checking all the complaints that may imply a source of infection, Thorough daily clinical examination during the period of neutropenia, Daily complete blood picture with differential blood count [20,21]. Complete sepsis work up for neutropenic fever including blood culture from peripheral lines as well as from central lines, sputum culture, urine analysis, chest radiograph, swab from any evident infected sites [22,23]. Measurement of quantitative C-reactive protein level in the serum [24] and measurement of pentraxin 3 level in plasma measured with a sandwich-type ELISA [25,26]. (Both are measured from day 1 to day 3 afterthe onset of fever with a cut-off point of 3 mg/l and 2 ng/dl respectively), Hepatic and renal function tests [27].

3. RESULTS AND DISCUSSION

Table 1 shows the demographic data of the patients. In patients with AML, M1 was found in 22%, M2 was found in 9.7%, M4 was found in 29.2% and M5 was found in 39% of patients. Most of the studied patients were AML M5.

Table 1. Demographic data of the 60 patients

Table 1 shows characters of studied cases		
Gender		
Males	28	(46.7%)
Females	32	(53.3%)
Mean age (years)		39.2±7.22
Range (years)		18-62
Type of leukemia		
AML	41	(68.3%)
B- ALL	15	(25%)
T- ALL	4	(6.7%)

There has been 16 patients developed septic shock and 12 died from 60 patients. Eight patients suffered from severe sepsis and multiorgan failure on days 6, 7, 9, 10 and 11. Two patient developed severe chest infection and intubated, died after mechanical ventilation. Two patient developed sudden arrest on day 6 & 9. Four other patients developed septic shock, but survived after treatment of sepsis and shock. For other 44 patients, correction of sepsis by antibiotics & antifungal drugs was successful.

Table 2 shows the Distribution of the studied patients regarding pentraxin 3 and CRP levels on the three days of the study. There was positive correlation between PTX3 and CRP on the three days as shown in Table 3.

In cases with severe sepsis who developed septic shock or death, PTX3 showed high levels from the 1st day, whereas CRP showed less sensitivity. Relation between bad and good prognosis regarding PTX3 and CRP level on day 1 is shown in table 4. Fig. 1 and Tables 5 and 6 show ROC curve, area under the curve and curve coordinates respectively, to represent the sensitivity and specificity of CRP and pentaraxin 3 on day 1 in cases with bad prognosis.

Table 2. Distribution of the studied patients regarding pentraxin 3 and CRP levels on the three days of the study

Pentraxin 3 (PTX3) (ng/ dl)			
Day 1 (Mean)	5.32±4.91		
Median	3.44		
Day 2 (Mean)	9.2±6.34	.003*	
Median	7.0		
Day 3 (Mean)	8.88±6.11	.020*	.22
Median	6.2		
C-reactive protein (CRP) (mg/L)			
Day 1 (Mean)	100.54±33.1		
Median	101		
Day 2 (Mean)	147.8±66.6	.0001*	
Median	140		
Day 3 (Mean)	169.33±92.42	.0001*	.107
Median	150		

There was positive correlation between PTX3 level on day 1 and INR with P value =.001. Blood culture were positive in 12 cases (20% of cases), while 48 cases (80%) were negative for organisms after 7 days of incubation. In 26 patients there was evidence of lower respiratory tract infection either by clinical examination or by chest radiographs, in other 14 patients upper respiratory tract infection was present. Cannula site infection in 4 patients, gastrointestinal infection in 12 patients and urinary tract infection in 10 patients were present. The evidence of fungal pneumonia and/or fungal oropharyngitis was present in 10 patients.

Table 3. Correlations between the PTX3 at different days and CRP

		PTX3 day 1	PTX3 day 2	PTX3 day 3
CRP day 1	Pearson Correlation	.531		
	P	.003*		
CRP day 2	Pearson Correlation		.450	
	P		.013*	
CRP day 3	Pearson Correlation			.525
	P			.003*

4. DISCUSSION

There was statistically positive correlation between PTX3 and CRP on the three days of the study. In agreement with our results, Vänskä et al. [28] held a similar study in Kuopio University which evaluated pentraxin 3 as a marker for complications of neutropenic fever in 100 hematologic patients receiving intensive chemotherapy in comparison with CRP.

High PTX3 was showed to be associated with mortality in severe sepsis and bacteremic patients [15,29,30] CRP is a widely-used short pentraxin. As an inflammatory marker, it has a limited specificity and poor diagnostic value [31,32]. In this study, there was a separate analysis for the 16 patients who developed complications (septic shock or mortality), and comparison of plasma PTX 3 level and serum CRP level on day1 revealed that: Ten patients

had plasma PTX3 level above 10 ng/ml on the 1st, 2nd and 3rd day. For the same patients, CRP levels were high in a rising manner along the 1st, 2nd and 3rd day to reach the peak on the last one.

Table 4. Relation between bad and good prognosis regarding PTX3 and CRP level on day 1

PTX3	Bad prognosis	Good prognosis
Mean	8.22	4.26
S.D.	1.39	2.01
T		3.65
P		.001*
CRP	**Bad prognosis**	**Good prognosis**
Mean	125.6	92.6
S.D.	22.6	30.2
T		.98
P		.032

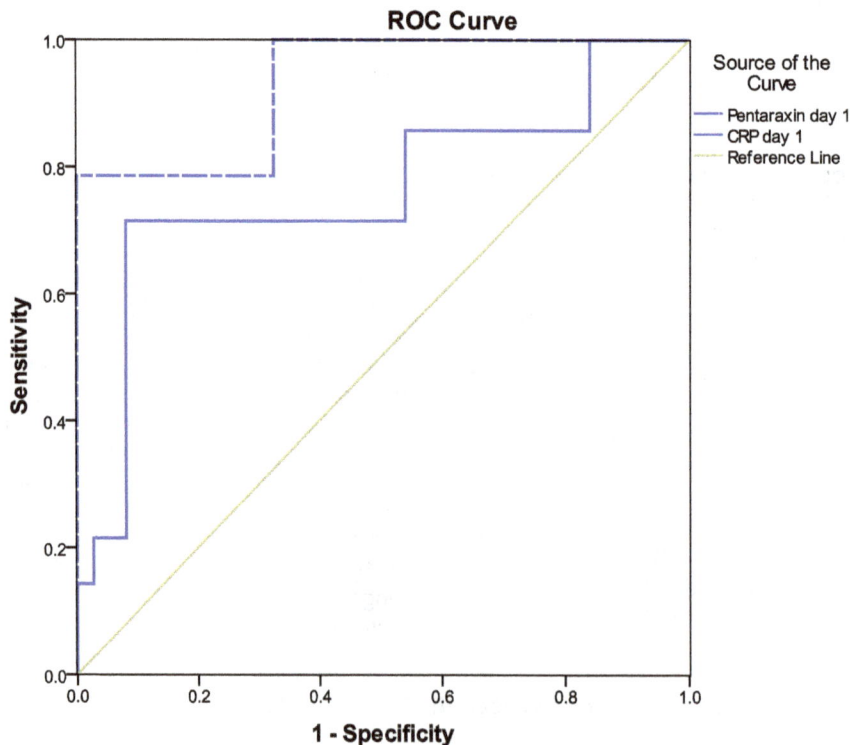

Fig. 1. ROC curve to determine the sensitivity and specificity of CRP and PTX3 on day 1 in cases with bad prognosis (septic shock and death)

Table 5. Area under the curve

Test result variable(s)	Area	Std. error(a)	Asymptotic sig.(P)	Asymptotic 95% confidence interval	
				Lower bound	Upper bound
Pentaraxin day 1	0.906	0.071	.001*	0.813	1.016
CRP day 1	0.789	0.107	.022	0.574	0.987

Table 6. Coordinates of the curve

Test result variable(s)	Positive if greater than or equal to(a)	Sensitivity %	Specificity %
Pentraxin 3 day 1	3.3500	100.0	70.0
CRP day 1	89.00	88.5	60.5

So, Peak levels of pentraxin 3 were obtained from the first day unlike CRP. Six patients had pentraxin3 level > 5 ng/ml on the first day and > 10 ng/ml on the 2nd day. In either case CRP attained arising manner reaching the maximum on the third day.

From the results mentioned above, high PTX3 on day one can predict bad prognosis with a strong statistical significance. This was agreed by, Vänskä et al. [28] who said that high PTX3 level on day 0 was associated with the development of septic shock and its level was constantly high in non-survivors. Another study at The Tampere University hospital of Finland in 2011 included 132 patients affected by bacteremia. Measuring of PTX3 level revealed that the maximum PTX3 values on days 1-4 were markedly higher in non-survivors compared with survivors [29]. Coppadoro [33] said that PTX3 remained significantly higher in nonsurvivors than in survivors over the first 5 days of sepsis, and that septic shock patients had higher PTX3 levels than patients with severe sepsis on day one. He also said that early persisting elevation of plasma pentraxin 3 is associated with coagulation impairment in severe sepsis and septic shock.

PTX3 can up-regulate tissue factor in activated monocytes, so an association between PTX3 and clotting activity in sepsis may be involved in development of DIC in these conditions [34]. In this study, 22 cases were complicated by coagulation impairment in the form of prolonged INR and/or PTT. There was statistically positive correlation between PTX3 level on day one and INR value. It is worth saying that the coagulation defect in these cases may be affected by impairment in liver functions in some of them due to severe sepsis and Multiorgan failure. However, in some cases impairment of liver functions occurred without concurrent coagulation defect.

A number of cases [16] showed decrease in the levels of both CRP and pentraxin 3 level after the first (12 cases) or second day (4 cases), all of them showed improvement of fever within hours after treatment which indicated a good response to antibiotic therapy. This proves that early interventions and appropriate antimicrobial treatment can be lifesaving. This requires early diagnosis and risk determination which can be provided by the use of pentraxin 3 which is highly sensitive.

Respiratory tract infection was the most common cause of infection during sepsis. With increased incidence of lower than upper respiratory tract infection. Rodrigues et al. [35] said that chest infection is the most common source of infection in neutropenic fever. The evidence of fungal infection was determined in 10 patients either clinically (oropharyngeal) or by chest CT. Four of them were complicated by severe sepsis and septic shock and showed very high levels of Pentraxin 3 (>10 ng/ml). It is worth mentioning that these cases were treated from septic shock.

A study in mice made by Gaziano et al. [36] showed that PTX3 induced a curative response in mice with invasive aspergillosis either alone or in combination with antifungal agents. Prophylactic PTX3, either locally or systemically, was effective but it did not show direct activity on fungal cells. Therefore, the effect of PTX3 appears to rely on its ability to increase protective T-helper1-dependent resistance. So, the results showed the following: 1) complete resistance to infection and reinfection in mice treated with PTX3 alone. 2) the protective effect of PTX3 was found similar or superior to that observed with liposomal or deoxycholate amphotericin B, respectively. 3) protection was associated with accelerated recovery of phagocytes and T-helper-1 lymphocytes in lung. 4) PTX3 potentiated the therapeutic effect of suboptimal doses of antifungal drugs. These data suggest the potential therapeutic use of PTX3 either alone or in combination to antifungal therapy in Aspergillus fumigatus infections [36].

5. CONCLUSION

PTX3 is a highly sensitive marker for detection of sepsis with high prognostic value. High PTX3 levels indicate septic shock, coagulation impairment and multiple organ failure with high sensitivity and specificity. It is recommended to perform further studies to confirm the therapeutic value of PTX3 in treatment of fungal infection and production of drugs approved for human use.

CONSENT

All authors declare that written informed consent was obtained from the patient (or other approved parties) for publication of this results.

ETHICAL APPROVAL

All authors hereby declare that all experiments have been examined and approved by the appropriate ethics committee and have therefore been performed in accordance with the ethical standards laid down in the 1964 Declaration of Helsinki. Research was agreed by the ethical committee on March 2012 (IRB 0101978)

COMPETING INTERESTS

Authors have declared that no competing interests exist.

REFERENCES

1. Bone RC, Balk RA, Cerra FB, Dellinger RP, Fein AM, Knaus WA, et al. Definitions for sepsis and organ failure and guidelines for the use of innovative therapies in sepsis. The ACCP/SCCM Consensus Conference Committee. American College of Chest Physicians/Society of Critical Care Medicine; 1992. Chest. 2009; 136(5):28.

2. Levy M, Fink M, Marshall J, Abraham E, Angus D, Cook D, et al. 2001 SCCM/ESICM/ACCP/ATS/SIS International Sepsis Definitions Conference. Intensive Care Med. 2003;29(4):530-8.

3. Kumar A, Haery C, Paladugu B, Kumar A, Symeoneides S, Taiberg L, et al. The duration of hypotension before the Initiation of antibiotic treatment Is a critical determinant of survival in a murine Model of escherichia coli septic shock: Association with serum lactate and inflammatory cytokine levels. Journal of Infectious Diseases. 2006;193(2):251-8.

4. Agrawal A, Singh PP, Bottazzi B, Garlanda C, Mantovani A. Pattern Recognition by Pentraxins. Advances in experimental medicine and biology. 2009;653:98-116.

5. Bottazzi B, Vouret-Craviari V, Bastone A, De Gioia L, Matteucci C, Peri G, et al. Multimer formation and ligand recognition by the long pentraxin PTX3. Similarities and differences with the short pentraxins C-reactive protein and serum amyloid P component. J Biol Chem. 1997;272:32817-23.

6. Diniz SN, Nomizo R, Cisalpino PS, Teixeira MM, Brown GD, Mantovani A, et al. PTX3 function as an opsonin for the dectin-1-dependent internalization of zymosan by macrophages. Journal of Leukocyte Biology. 2004;75(4):649-56.

7. Emsley J, White HE, O' Hara BP, Oliva G, Srinivasan N, Tickle IJ, et al. Structure of pentameric human serum amyloid P component. Nature. 1994;367(6461):338-45.

8. Garlanda C, Bottazzi B, Bastone A, Mantovani A. Pentraxins at the crossroads between innate immunity, inflammation, matrix deposition, and female fertility. Annual review of immunology. 2005;23:337-66.

9. Nauta AJ, Bottazi B, Mantovani A, Salvatori G, Kishore U, Schwaeble WJ, et al. Biochemical and functional characterization of the interaction between pentraxin 3 and C1q. Eur J Immunol. 2003; 33:465-73.

10. Bottazzi B, Garlanda C, Cotena A, Moalli F, Jaillon S, Deban L, et al. The long pentraxin PTX3 as a prototypic humoral pattern recognition receptor: interplay with cellular innate immunity. Immunological Reviews. 2009;227(1):9-18.

11. Yamasaki K, Kurimura M, Kasai T, Sagara M, Kodama T, Inoue K. Determination of physiological plasma pentraxin 3 (PTX3) levels in healthy populations. Clinical Chemistry and Laboratory Medicine : CCLM / FESCC. 2009;47(4):471-7.

12. Brinkmann V RU, Goosmann C, Fauler B, Uhlemann Y, Weiss DS. Neutrophil extracellular traps kill bacteria. Science. 2004;303:1532-5.

13. Jaillon S, Peri G, Delneste Y, Frémaux I, Doni A, Moalli F, et al. The humoral pattern recognition receptor PTX3 is stored in neutrophil granules and localizes in extracellular traps. Exp med. 2007;204:793-804.

14. Martin GS MD, Eaton S, Moss M. The epidemiology of sepsis in the united states from 1979 through 2000. N Engl J Med. 2003;348:1546-54.

15. Mauri T, Bellani G, Patroniti N, Coppadoro A, Peri G, Cuccovillo I, et al. Persisting high levels of plasma pentraxin 3 over the first days after severe sepsis and septic shock onset are associated with mortality. Intensive Care Med. 2010;36(4):621-9.

16. Åkerfeldt T, Larsson A. Pentraxin 3 Increase is much less pronounced than C-reactive protein increase after surgical procedures. Inflammation. 2011;34(5):367-70.

17. Black S, Kushner I, D. S. C-reactive protein. J Biol Chem. 2004;279:48487-90.

18. Deban L, Jaillon S, Garlanda C, Bottazzi B, Mantovani A. Pentraxins in innate immunity: lessons from PTX3. Cell and Tissue Research. 2011;343(1):237-49.

19. Pierrakos C, Vincent JL. Sepsis biomarkers: a review. Critical Care (London, England). 2010;14(1):R15.

20. Bain B. complete blood count. In: Lewis S, Bain B, Bates I, (eds). Practical haematology Dacie and Lewis. 10th ed. New York: Charchilllivingstone, 2006;5:80-110.

21. Newland J. The peripheral blood smear. In: Goldman L, Ausiello D, (eds). Cecil Medicine. 23rd ed. Philadelphia, Pa: Saunders Elsevier. 2007;161.

22. Lee A, Mirrett S, Reller LB, Weinstein MP. Detection of bloodstream infections in adults: how many blood cultures are needed? J Clin Microbiol. 2007;45:3546-8.

23. Carlet J. Rapid diagnostic methods in the detection of sepsis. Infect Dis Clin North Am. 1999;13:483-94.

24. Fischbach FA. Manual of laboratory and diagnostic tests. 7th ed, Lippincott: Williams &Wilkins. 2004;(2)317-99.

25. Peri G. PTX3, A prototypical long pentraxin, is a early indicator of acute myocardial infarction in humans. Circulation. 2000;102: 636.

26. Lequin R. Enzyme immunoassay (EIA)/enzyme-linked immunosorbent assay (ELISA). Clin Chem. 2005;5:2415-8.

27. Pincus MR, Abraham NZ. Interpreting laboratory results. In: Mc Pherson RA, Pincus MR, eds. Henry's Clinical Diagnosis and Management by Laboratory Methods. 21st ed. Philadelphia, Pa: Saunders Elsevier. 2006;54:720-4.

28. Vänskä M, Koivula I, Hämäläinen S, Pulkki K, Nousiainen T, Jantunen E, et al. High pentraxin 3 level predicts septic shock and bacteremia at the onset of febrile neutropenia after intensive chemotherapy of hematologic patients. Haematologica. 2011;96(9):1385-9.

29. Huttunen R, Hurme M, Aittoniemi J, Huhtala H, Vuento R, Laine J, et al. High plasma level of long pentraxin 3 (PTX3) is associated with fatal disease in bacteremic patients: A prospective cohort study. Plos One. 2011;6(3):17653.

30. Silvestre J, Póvoa P, Coelho L, Almeida E, Moreira P, Fernandes A, et al. Is C-reactive protein a good prognostic marker in septic patients? Intensive Care Med. 2009;35(5):909-13.

31. Clyne B, JS O. The C-reactive protein. J Emerg Med. 1999;17:1019-25.

32. Póvoa P, Coelho L, Almeida E, Fernandes A, Mealha R, Moreira P, et al. C-reactive protein as a marker of infection in critically ill patients. Clinical Microbiology and Infection. 2005;11(2):101-8.

33. Coppadoro A, Mauri T, Bellani G, Patroniti N, Cugno M, Grassi A, et al. Early persisting elevation of plasma pentraxin 3 is associated with mortality and with coagulation impairment in severe sepsis and septic shock. Critical Care. 2010;14(Suppl 1):1-2.

34. Napoleone E, Di Santo A, Peri G, Mantovani A, de Gaetano G, Donati MB, et al. The long pentraxin PTX3 up-regulates tissue factor in activated monocytes: another link between inflammation and clotting activation. Journal of Leukocyte Biology. 2004;76(1):203-9.

35. Rodrigues RS, Marchiori E, Bozza FA, Pitrowsky MT, Velasco E, Soares M, et al. Chest computed tomography findings in severe influenza pneumonia occurring in neutropenic cancer patients. Clinics. 2012;67(4):313-8.

36. Gaziano R, Bozza S, Bellocchio S, Perruccio K, Montagnoli C, Pitzurra L, et al. Anti-aspergillus fumigatus efficacy of pentraxin 3 alone and in combination with antifungals. Antimicrobial Agents and Chemotherapy. 2004;48(11):4414-21.

Haematological Parameters of Adult and Paediatric Subjects with Sickle Cell Disease in Steady State, in Benin City, Nigeria

O. E. Iheanacho[1*]

[1]*Department of Haematology and Blood Transfusion, University of Benin Teaching Hospital, Benin City, Nigeria.*

Author's contribution

The sole author designed, analyzed and interpreted and prepared the manuscript.

Editor(s):
(1) Ricardo Forastiero, Department of Hematology, Favaloro University, Argentina.
Reviewers:
(1) Shubhangi V. Agale, Department of Pathology, Grant Govt Medical College, Byculla, Mumbai, India.
(2) Yakubu Abdulrahaman, Haematology Department, Usmanu Danfodiyo University, Sokoto, Nigeria.

ABSTRACT

Background: Sickle cell disease (SCD) remains a major health burden in Sub-Saharan Africa and the management requires regular monitoring of the patients. The monitoring includes routine assessment of haematological parameters and any deviation can best be appreciated when steady state values are previously known. This study evaluated the patients with SCD in steady state to determine certain haematological parameters (particularly the full blood count values).

Methods: This is a cross-sectional study. One hundred and forty-three (known) SCD subjects in steady state and thirty controls (HB phenotype AA) had their full blood count parameters evaluated using haematology auto analyser – white blood cell (WBC), granulocyte (GRA) and platelet (PLT) counts as well as haemoglobin concentration (HB), mean cell volume (MCV) and mean cell haemoglobin (MCH). The participants were regrouped into adult and paediatric groups and their results analysed accordingly.

Results: The adult SCD patients had their mean haematological values as follows: HB 7.7±2.5 g/L, MCV 77.5±19.3 fl, MCH 25.1±6.5 pg, WBC 12.0±5.9x10^9 /L and PLT 306.6±169.3x10^9 /L. Their paediatric counterparts had the following mean values: HB 6.9±1.3 g/L, MCV 77.4±11.0 fl, MCH 24.6±3.7 pg, WBC 16.0±6.9x10^9 /L and PLT 329.1±101.9x10^9 /L. The adult patients had

---

Corresponding author: E-mail: donnoocho@yahoo.com

significantly higher HB (p<0.05) and lower WBC (p<0.05) than the paediatric patients.
Conclusion: This study has therefore provided some steady state haematological values of both paediatric and adult SCD patients in our locality and could be useful in establishing reference values.

Keywords: Sickle cell disease; steady state; haematological parameters; adult and paediatric.

1. INTRODUCTION

Sickle cell disease (SCD) is an inherited chronic condition that arises from a point mutation in the DNA coding for the synthesis of b-globin chain. It results in the production of sickle haemoglobin which has a high tendency to polymerise and deform red cells, leading to chronic haemolysis [1]. Sickle cell disease is primarily a red cell disorder but significant changes are observed in other haematological parameters such as white cells and platelets which play important roles in pathophysiology of the disease and in prediction of outcome [2]. The SCD patients experience alternating periods of apparent good health (steady state) and acute exacerbation of symptoms (crisis) as well as development of chronic complications. The haematological parameters in these periods vary but at the same time provide evidence-based management information for diagnosis, treatment, monitoring and prognostication. Although the haematological parameters of SCD patients vary significantly from those of normal HbAA individuals, these patients are able to adapt to their steady state haematological values and remain apparently healthy. The importance of some of the steady state haematological values such as Haemoglobin (HB) concentration, white blood cell (WBC) and platelet (PLT) counts in prediction of clinical severity as well as management of SCD has been documented [3,4]. Lower steady state HB is associated with higher risk of stroke [5] whereas higher values are reported to have higher rates of severe pain [6]. Furthermore, red cell transfusions beyond the steady state HB may increase blood viscosity [7] with attendant consequences such as worsening of vaso-occlusion and osteonecrosis. High WBC count (above 11×10^9 /L) [4] is associated with SCD complications including cerebrovascular accidents.[5] Some researchers have also shown that lowering the WBC count through the use of drugs such as Hydroxyurea improves the clinical outcome of these patients [8]. Other parameters for assessment include the red cell indices such as MCV, MCH and mean cell haemoglobin concentration (MCHC) which are useful in detecting co-existing causes of anaemia in the patients. Over the years several modalities of

treatment of SCD such as blood transfusion, haematinics and hydroxyurea have been used and these modify the haematological parameters of these patients. Knowledge of the steady state haematological values in these patients becomes an important asset for the managing physician.

Several works [4,9,10] on related topic have been carried out in our locality but many did not study the adult and paediatric groups separately, despite the fact that some of the haematological parameters vary normally with age. Moreover the most recent similar study 9 in our immediate environment was carried out about a decade ago. Meanwhile there has been some improvement in access to medical care, socioeconomic development and education over the years; [1,12] a phenomenon which may impact the haematological values in patients with SCD [13]. The aim of this study therefore, is to determine the haematological parameters in paediatric and adult patients with SCD (in our locality) who are in steady state, as well as to compare these values with those of normal HbAA controls. This could provide reference values for the management of these patients and also reveal any deviation from earlier reports as a result of changes in treatment and socioeconomic factors on the parameters.

2. METHODOLOGY

This is a cross-sectional (case-control) study on sickle cell disease patients (in steady state) who attend clinics at the University of Benin Teaching Hospital (UBTH) and the Sickle Cell Centre in Benin City, Edo state, Nigeria. The controls were recruited from healthy staff and children of the staff of the hospital, whose HB phenotypes were AA. Steady state was defined by the absence of clinical event in the preceding three weeks as well as blood transfusion in the preceding three months [14]. Subjects who are up to eighteen years of age were taken as adults and others included in the paediatric age group. Haemoglobin phenotypes of subjects had been previously determined by cellulose acetate haemoglobin electrophoresis at pH 8.6, using tris-buffer. Subjects who had conditions that could alter the haematological values were excluded. These conditions include: transfusion in the preceding three months, pregnancy and renal failure.

The study was approved by the hospital ethics and research committee and informed consent obtained from the study participants and/or parents (where applicable).

2.1 Procedure

For each subject, the venepuncture site was carefully cleaned with methylated spirit and two and a half millilitres (2.5 ml) of venous blood collected (into commercially prepared ethylene di-amine tetra-acetic acid, EDTA, bottle) from the ante-cubital vein using plastic syringe. Full blood count: haematocrit, haemoglobin concentration and total white cell and platelet counts were obtained from the EDTA sample, using automated blood cell counter (PCE-210N, Erma Inc, Tokyo, Japan; 2012. A three-part haematology autoanalyzer that measures blood cells using the principle of electric resistance, and colorimetry for haemoglobin). The procedure was done in the main haematology laboratory, UBTH. Well mixed blood sample was aspirated, by letting the equipment sampling probe into the blood sample and then pressing the start button. Approximately 20 ul of blood was aspirated by the auto analyzer; after about 30 seconds the results of the full blood count parameters were displayed and subsequently printed out. The parameters collated included: white blood cell (WBC), granulocyte (GRA), platelet (PLT) counts, haemoglobin (HB) concentration, mean cell volume (MCV) and mean cell haemoglobin (MCH).

2.2 Statistical Analysis

Data were analyzed using SPSS version 16.0 (Statistical Package for Social Sciences). The means, ranges and standard deviations (S.D) of the haematological values in the patients and in controls were calculated. Values in the patients were compared with values in controls using the student t-test. The p-value <0.05 was considered to be statistically significant.

3. RESULTS

A total of 143 cases and 30 controls were enrolled. The cases consisted of 73 (51.0%) males and 70 (49.0%) females, while controls were made up of 17 (56.7%) males and 13 (43.3%) females. There were 75 (52.4%) adult and 68 (47.6%) paediatric cases as well as 15 (50%) adult and 15 (50%) paediatric controls. The mean ages for the adult and paediatric SCD subjects were 27.9±9.1 and 8.5±4.4, respectively (as shown in Table 1).

The haematological values in SCD subjects and controls are shown in Tables 2 and 3. The SCD subjects had significantly higher mean WBC, GRA and PLT counts but lower HB than their respective controls ($p<0.05$). The adult SCD patients had their mean haematological values as follows: Haemoglobin concentration (HB) 7.7 ±2.5g/L, mean cell volume (MCV) 77.5±19.3 fl, mean cell haemoglobin (MCH) 25.1±6.5 pg, white blood cell count (WBC) 12.0±5.9x10^9 /L, granulocyte count (GRA) 7.3±4.4x10^9 /L and platelet count (PLT) 306.6±169.3x10^9 /L. Their paediatric counterparts had the following mean values: HB 6.9±1.3 g/L, MCV 77.4±11.0 fl, MCH 24.6±3.7pg, WBC 16.0±6.9x10^9 /L, GRA 8.7±5.2x10^9 /L and PLT 329.1±101.9x10^9 /L.

The haematological values in adult and paediatric subjects were compared in Table 4. The adult patients had significantly higher HB ($p<0.05$) and lower WBC ($p<0.05$) than the paediatric patients. The comparison of the haematological parameters in male and female subjects is depicted in Tables 5 and 6. This revealed no statistically significant difference between males and females ($p>0.05$), for all the values tested.

Table 1. Demographic parameters of SCD subjects and controls

Adult	Subjects (n=75)	Control (n=15)
Sex	Frequency (%)	Frequency (%)
Male	38 (50.7%)	9 (60%)
Female	37 (49.3%)	6 (40%)
Mean age (years ±2SD)	27.9±9.1	28.2±6.6
Paediatric	**Subjects (n=68)**	**Control (n=15)**
Sex	Frequency (%)	Frequency (%)
Male	35 (51.5%)	8 (53.3%)
Female	33 (48.5%)	7 (46.7%)
Mean age (years ±2SD)	8.5±4.4	9.4±4.1

Table 2. Haematological parameters of adult SCD subjects and controls

Variable	Subjects (n=75)	Control (n=15)	p-value
WBC (x10^9 /L ±2SD)	12.0±5.9	5.6±1.5	<0.001
GRA (x10^9 /L ±2SD)	7.3±4.4	2.8±1.0	0.001
HB (g/dl ±2SD)	7.7±2.5	14.1±1.8	<0.001
MCV (fl ±2SD)	77.5±19.3	80.2±6.5	0.595
MCH (pg ±2SD)	25.1±6.5	27.7±2.5	0.135
PLT (x10^9 /L ±2SD)	306.6±169.3	199.2±58.6	0.018

KEY: WBC- white blood cell count; GRA-granulocyte count; PLT-platelet count; HB-haemoglobin concentration; MCV-mean cell volume; MCH-mean cell haemoglobin

Table 3. Haematological parameters of paediatric SCD subjects and controls

Variable	Subjects (n=68)	Control (n=15)	p-value
WBC (x10^9 /L ±2SD)	16.0±6.9	5.5±1.1	<0.001
GRA (x10^9 /L ±2SD)	8.7±5.2	2.7±0.8	<0.001
HB (g/dl ±2SD)	6.9±1.3	12.7±0.7	<0.001
MCV (fl ±2SD)	77.4±11.0	73.7±4.2	0.204
MCH (pg ±2SD)	24.6±3.7	25.6±2.2	0.315
PLT (x10^9 /L ±2SD)	329.1±101.9	249.9±52.0	0.005

Table 4. Comparison of the haematological parameters of adult and paediatric SCD subjects

Variable	Adult (n=75)	Paediatric (n=68)	p-value
WBC (x10^9 /L ±2SD)	12.0±5.9	16.0±6.9	**<0.001**
GRA (x10^9 /L ±2SD)	7.3±4.9	8.7±5.2	0.105
HB (g/dl ±2SD)	7.7±2.5	6.9±1.3	**0.027**
MCV (fl ±2SD)	77.5±19.3	77.4±11.0	0.990
MCH (pg ±2SD)	25.1±6.5	24.6±3.7	0.548
PLT (x10^9 /L ±2SD)	306.6±169.3	329.1±101.9	0.345

Table 5. Haematological parameters of adult male and female SCD subjects

Variable	Male (n=38)	Female (37)	p-value
WBC (x10^9 /L ±2SD)	13.1±5.9	10.9±5.8	0.111
GRA (x10^9 /L ±2SD)	8.1±4.8	6.6±4.9	0.198
HB (g/dl ±2SD)	7.8±2.6	7.6±2.6	0.710
MCV (fl ±2SD)	74.1±2.1	80.0±1.8	0.130
MCH (pg ±2SD)	24.0±7.0	26.2±5.8	0.142
PLT (x10^9 /L ±2SD)	324.4±190.1	288.3±145.3	0.359

Table 6. Haematological parameters of paediatric male and female SCD subjects

Variable	Male (n=35)	Female (33)	p-value
WBC (x10^9 /L ±2SD)	16.1±6.7	15.8±7.3	0.884
GRA (x10^9 /L ±2SD)	9.7±6.0	7.7±3.9	0.128
HB (g/dl ±2SD)	7.0±1.0	6.9±1.5	0.723
MCV (fl ±2SD)	75.5±1.1	79.5±1.1	0.136
MCH (pg ±2SD)	24.3±3.8	24.8±3.7	0.565
PLT (x10^9 /L ±2SD)	330.5±109.1	327.6±95.2	0.908

4. DISCUSSION

Haematological parameters in SCD patients have been widely studied in our locality but the need to establish paediatric values as distinct from adult values has not been appreciated despite the effect of age on some of the haematological values. This work was therefore carried out in an attempt to fill in the gap. A review of the sex and age distribution in this study revealed that males were only slightly more than females in both paediatric and adult groups; just as there was no significant difference in their mean ages. It is worthy of note that the mean age for the adult cases is higher compared to 23.69±10.94 years reported by Omoti [9] several years ago. Akinbami [10] in a more recent study in Lagos had a mean age of 23.79±7.81 years in a work that also lumped both adult and paediatric cases together.

The SCD patients have chronic haemolysis, [1] low erythropoietin response [15] and shortened red cell survival which explains the low HB observed in the SCD subjects of this study. However, a more detailed analysis revealed a higher mean HB in the adult subjects; in line with previous finding that haemoglobin concentration increases with age. [16] The mean HB for the paediatric patients (6.9±1.3 g/dl) was in agreement with Akodu's [17] work in Lagos and close to that observed by Abbas [18] in Sudanese children. On the other hand, the adult patients had a mean HB which corresponded with mean HB of 7.54±2.26 g/L observed by Omoti, [9] in a work whose subjects were predominantly adults (mean age of 23.69 years). Despite the low HB level, the patients enjoy apparent good health as they have adapted to this anaemic state. Nevertheless it has been reported that SCD patients with lower steady state HB may have higher risk of complications such as stroke [5].

The findings of low MCV and MCH in SCD patients by other researchers [9,10] were similarly observed in the SCD patients; although the differences were not statistically significant when compared to controls. The mean MCV and MCH values in the paediatric patients were lower than 84 ±16fl reported by Abbas [18] in his study population. These observations may reflect a background iron deficiency in the SCD patients in our environment; although iron deficiency anaemia is expected to be uncommon due to chronic haemolysis with increased iron turnover and higher rate of blood transfusion in SCD patients. This present study also observed low MCV and MCH in both paediatric groups (SCD and control); a phenomenon which may be related to increased iron demand for growth in children. Akodu [17] reported identical values in their SCD group whereas their control group had lower values. Adeyemo [19] in another related research in Lagos noted low MCV and MCH, but equally revealed a high frequency of HB variants (such as beta thalassaemia trait) co-existing with

SCD in their study population. Thalassaemia is a known cause of low MCV and MCH; hence the need to screen and determine its contribution to the observed values.

The WBC and GRA counts for the adult SCD patients were comparable to the findings in a previous study [9] whereas their paediatric counterparts had a higher mean count. A similar study on Sudanese children showed a much higher mean WBC ($21.7±10.3\times10^9$/l) [18]. The higher values of WBC and GRA counts for the SCD patients (with respect to their control group) is consequent upon the persistent low grade inflammation and a shift of granulocytes from the marginated to the circulating compartment [20]. The observation of a higher mean WBC and GRA counts in the paediatric SCD subjects may require further investigation to ascertain if it is due to subclinical infection since the children are known to have higher incidence of infections [21]. However hydroxyurea, a drug with the capacity to lower WBC count [22], is administered more on adult SCD patients in our environment and may affect the WBC values in these patients. Nonetheless, high WBC is associated with poor clinical phenotype in SCD [4,5,23], thus such patients may benefit from hydroxyurea therapy [22].

The mean platelet count of the SCD patients were higher than those of their control group as expected, due to the decrease or absent splenic sequestration of platelets [24]. The increase in erythropoietin (which has structural homology with thrombopoietin [25,26] as a result of anaemia in SCD patients may also contribute to the high platelet count observed in the SCD subjects (compared to controls). The observation was in agreement with several other reports [9,10,18]. The value for the paediatric patients was equally comparable to the 319.2 x 10^9/L reported by Abbas [18]. Their adult counterparts had relatively lower mean platelet count (although the difference was not statistically significant); an observation which conforms with normal finding of decreasing platelet count with increase in age [27] as a result of decreasing thrombopoietin levels [28]. Furthermore, the greater frequency of hydroxyurea administration in our adult SCD patients may contribute to this observation. Hydroxyurea has been reported to lower platelet count in SCD patients [22].

5. CONCLUSION

This study has therefore provided some steady state haematological values of both paediatric and adult SCD patients in our locality and could be useful in establishing reference values. The low MCV and MCH in SCD patients require further investigation in order not to miss a growing iron deficiency in a group of patients known to be otherwise prone to iron overload.

ACKNOWLEDGEMENTS

The author is grateful to Prof OA Awodu, Dr B Nwogoh and Mrs JN Iheanacho for their support in data management and vetting.

COMPETING INTERESTS

Author has declared that no competing interests exist.

REFERENCES

1. Ashutosh L, Elliot PV. Sickle cell disease. In: Postgraduate Haematology. 5th Ed. Hoffbrand AV, Catovsky D, Tuddenham EGD (Eds), Blackwell. 2005;104-118.
2. Okpala I. The intriguing contribution of white blood cells to sickle cell disease: A red cell disorder. Blood Rev. 2004;18:65-73.
3. Okpala I. Leukocyte adhesion and the pathophysiology of sickle cell disease. Curr Opin Hematol. 2006;13:40-44.
4. Emmanuelchide O, Charle O, Uchenna O. Hematological parameters in association with outcomes in sickle cell anemia patients. Indian J Med Sci. 2011;65:393-398.
5. Ohene-Frempong K, Weiner SJ, Sleeper LA, et al. Cerebrovascular accident in sickle cell disease: Rates and risk factors. Blood. 1998;288-294.
6. Platt OS, Thorington BD, Brambilla DJ, et al. Pain in sickle cell disease: Rates and risk factors. N Engl J Med. 1991;325:11-16.
7. Kaul DK, Fabry M, Windisch P, et al. Erythrocytes in sickle cell anaemia are heterogenous in their rheological and haemodynamic characteristics. J Clin Invest. 1983;72:22-31.
8. Zimmerman SA, Schultz WH, Davis JS, et al. Sustained long-term hematologic efficacy of hydroxyurea at maximum tolerated dose in children with sickle cell disease. Blood. 2004;103(6):2039-2045.
9. Omoti CE. Haematological values in sickle cell anaemia in steady state and during vaso-occlusive crisis in Benin City, Nigeria. Ann Afr Med. 2005;4(2):62-67.
10. Akinbami A, Dosunmu A, Adediran A, et al. Haematological values in homozygous sickle cell disease in steady state and haemoglobin phenotypes AA control in Lagos, Nigeria. BMC Res Notes. 2012;5: 396.
11. Koko J, Dufillot D, M'Ba-Meyo J, et al. Mortality of children with sickle cell disease in a pediatric department in Central Africa. Archives de Pédiatrie. 1998;5:965–969.
12. Athale UH, Chintu C. Clinical analysis of mortality in hospitalized Zambian children with sickle cell anaemia. East African Medical Journal. 1994;71:388–391.
13. Izuora AN, Njokanma OF, Animasahun BA, et al. The influence of socioeconomic status on the hemoglobin level and anthropometry of sickle cell anemia patients in steady state at the Lagos University Teaching Hospital. Niger J Clin Pract. 2011;14:422-7.
14. Akinola NO, Stevens SME, Franklin IM, Nash GB, Stuart J. Subclinical ischaemic episodes during the steady state of sickle cell anaemia. J Clin Pathol. 1992;45:902-906.
15. Sherwood JB, Goldwesser E, Chilcoat R, et al. Sickle cell anaemia patients have low erythropoietin levels for their degree of anaemia. Blood. 1987;67:46-49.
16. Ershler WB, Sheng S, McKelvey J, et al. Serum erythropoietin and aging: A longitudinal analysis. J Am Geriatr Soc. 2005;53:1360-1365.
17. Akodu SO, Njokanma OF, Adeolukehinde O. Erythrocyte indices in pre-school Nigerian children with sickle cell anaemia in steady state. Int J Hematol Oncol Stem Cell Res. 2015;9(1):5-9.
18. Abbas M. Haematological parameters in Sudanese children with sickle cell disease. Am J Res Com. 2014;2(2):20-32.
19. Adeyemo T, Ojewunmi O, Oyetunji A. Evaluation of high performance liquid chromatography (HPLC) pattern and prevalence of beta-thalassaemia trait among sickle cell disease patients in Lagos, Nigeria. Pan Afr Med J. 2014;18: 71.
20. West MS, Wethers D, Smith J, et al. Laboratory profile of sickle cell disease: A cross-sectional analysis. The cooperative study of Sickle Cell Disease. J Clin Epidemiol. 1992;45(8):893-909.

21. Leikin SL, Gallagher D, Kinney TR, et al. Mortality in children and adolescents with sickle cell disease. Cooperative Study of Sickle Cell Disease. Pediatrics. 1989; 84(3):500-508.

22. Silva-Pinto AC, Angulo IL, Brunetta DM, et al. Clinical and hematological effects of hydroxyurea therapy in sickle cell patients: a single-center experience in Brazil. Sao Paulo Med J. 2013;131(4):238-243.

23. Olatunji PO, Davies SC. The predictive value of white cell count in assessing clinical severity of sickle cell anaemia in Afro-Caribbeans patients. Afr J Med Sci. 2000;29(1):27-30.

24. Freedman ML, Karpatkin S. Elevated platelet count and megathrombocytes number in sickle cell anaemia. Blood. 1975;46(4):579-582.

25. Bartley TD, Bogenberger J, Hunt P, et al. Identification and cloning of a megakaryocyte growth and development factor, that is a ligand for the cytokine receptor Mpl. Cell. 1994;77(7):1117-1124.

26. de Sauvage FJ, Hass PE, Spencer SD, et al. Stimulation of magakaryocytopoiesis and thrombopoiesis by the c-Mpl ligand. Nature. 1994;369(6481):533-538.

27. Buckley MF, James JW, Brown DE, et al. A novel approach to the assessment of variation in the human platelet count. Thromb Haemost. 2000;83:480-484.

28. Ishiguro A, Nakahata T, Matsubara K, et al. Age-related changes in thrombopoietin in children: Reference interval for serum thrombopoietin levels. Br J Haematol. 1999;106:884-888.

Cerebrovascular Disease in Children with Sickle Cell Disease: Is There Any Need for Iron Therapy?

I. O. George[1*] and A. I. Frank-Briggs[1]

[1]Department of Paediatrics, University of Port Harcourt Teaching Hospital, Nigeria.

Authors' contributions

This work was carried out in collaboration between both authors. Author IOG designed the study, wrote the protocol, and wrote the first draft of the manuscript. Authors IOG and AIF managed the literature searches, analyses of the study. Both authors read and approved the final manuscript.

Editor(s):
(1) Ricardo Forastiero, Department of Hematology, Favaloro University, Argentina.
Reviewers:
(1) Anonymous, Ain Shams University, Egypt.
(2) Anonymous, University of Benin Teaching Hospital, Nigeria.
(3) Adrià Arboix, Department of Neurology, University of Barcelona, Spain.

ABSTRACT

Background: Iron deficiency is a common problem affecting children world-wide. It has been recognized to have an association with stroke. The aim of this study was to evaluate the prevalence of iron deficiency anaemia among children with sickle cell anaemia with cerebrovascular accident and the need for iron therapy.

Materials and Methods: All cases of cerebrovascular disease in children with sickle cell anaemia presenting in the department of Paediatrics of the University of Teaching Hospital were prospectively investigated for serum ferritin, haemoglobin, and MCV, MCHC and blood film.

Results: A total of 152 children with sickle cell disease were seen during this period. One hundred and forty nine had HbSS genotype while 3 had HbSC genotype. Cerebrovascular disease was diagnosed in 7 patients giving a prevalence rate of 4.6%. Of these, 2(28.6%) had low serum ferritin levels (P=0.09) with hypochromia and microcytosis.

Conclusion: Iron deficiency anaemia is not uncommon among sickle cell patients with cerebrovascular disease. There is need for elaborate iron study in these patients so as to identify at risk cases and institute prompt treatment.

Keywords: Cerebrovascular disease; sickle cell anaemia; iron deficiency.

*Corresponding author: E-mail: geonosdemed@yahoo.com

1. INTRODUCTION

Sickle cell disease (SCD) is one of the commonest but preventable inherited diseases [1]. It affects all races of the world; it affects the people of tropical Africa, Mediterranean Sea, Middle East and South India [1]. It has contributed considerably to the high childhood mortality rate.

Nigeria has an estimated population of 150 million with annual growth rate of 3.2%. The current figure of people in Nigeria with this disease is not known since the majority born in rural community do not survive childhood and for lack of proper statistics. However, estimates of about 2.3% of the Nigerian population suffer from sickle cell disorder and about 25% of Nigerians are healthy carriers of the abnormal haemoglobin gene [2].

Clinically evident cerebrovascular disease (CVD) is a devastating complication of sickle cell anaemia (SCA) that affects from 6 to 12 percent of patients [3-5]. Cerebrovascular diseases are very rare in persons with Hb SC disease. In children under age 10 years, the most common cause of CVD is cerebral infarction. Ischemic stroke typically presents with signs and symptoms of hemiparesis or monoparesis, hemianesthesia, visual field deficits, aphasia, cranial nerve palsies, or acute change in behaviour. Although recovery occasionally is complete, intellectual, motor, and sensory impairments are typical sequelae. Intracranial haemorrhage becomes increasingly more common with advancing age. In haemorrhagic CVD, more generalized phenomena such as coma, headache, and seizures occur. Recurrent CVD causes progressively greater impairment and increased likelihood of mortality. Factors such as low haemoglobin levels, increased systolic blood pressure, transient ischaemic attack, acute chest syndrome and male gender are linked to a higher risk of silent cerebral infarcts (SCIs), or silent strokes, in children with SCA [3].

Despite the reasonable speculation that a decrease in haemoglobin might possibly compromise the oxygen-carrying ability of the blood flow and subsequently increase the risk of cerebrovascular or cardiovascular diseases, the relationship between the iron deficiency anaemia (IDA) and the stroke was seldom studied [6]. In 1983, Alexander et al. [7] first reported that a patient developing a right hemiparesis and aphasia was found to have underlying IDA and marked thrombocytosis [7]. A few years later, another brain infarction cases were reported and thought to have resulted from the thrombocytosis secondary to the IDA [8,9]. Despite these peculiar cases, the relative importance of IDA seems to have been overlooked as most researchers have chosen to focus on sickle cell anaemia. Even after the publication of Framingham study [10] which seemingly implicated haematocrit as an important risk factor for some cardiovascular diseases, the possible relationships between the IDA and the stroke were still yet to be investigated through a large scaled study [11]. Given this, the study aims to evaluate the association of IDA and CVD in children with sickle cell disease.

2. MATERIALS AND METHODS

This was a prospective study of all children with sickle cell disease who presented in the Department of Paediatrics of the University of Port Harcourt Teaching Hospital (UPTH) with cerebrovascular disease from February 2014 to February 2015. Information obtained from the patients such as age, gender, age at diagnosis of sickle cell disease, episodes of cerebrovascular disease, mode of treatment, CT scan findings, full blood count, film report, serum ferritin, mean corpuscular volume (MCV) and mean corpuscular haemoglobin concentration (MCHC) were entered and analysed with SPSS version 22.0.

Haematologic test were performed using Abbott Cell Dyn Ruby analyzer (Abbott Diagnotic, Abbott, IL, USA).The ferritin test was performed by using the Chemiluminescent Microparticle Immunoassay (CMIA) method.

Diagnosis of sickle cell disease was made by haemoglobin electrophoresis. Cerebrovascular disease (CVD) was defined as sudden loss of speech, weakness, or paralysis of one side of the body. Confirmation of CVD was made by brain CT scan.

Iron-deficiency anemia was defined as a packed cell volume level of <33%, mean corpuscular volume <85fL, and serum ferritin level <7ng/ml.

Differences among clinical outcomes were analyzed by the Student's t test. A p-value<0.05 was considered statistically significant.

Ethical approval was from the Ethical Committee of UPTH.

3. RESULTS

A total of 152 children with sickle cell disease were seen during the study period (See Table 1). There were 83(54.6%) males and 69(45.4%) females. One hundred and forty nine (98.0%) had HbSS genotype while 3(2.0%) had HbSC genotype. Patient ages varied from 0.8 to 16 years with a mean of 7.34±3.56 years. CVD was diagnosed in 7 patients giving a prevalence rate of 4.6%. The mean age at diagnosis of cerebrovascular disease was 6.7±2.4 years. Of the 7 patients who had stroke, 2 had more than one episode of stroke, giving a 28.6% recurrence rate. None of children below 2 years had a stroke. The highest cases of CVD were seen between the ages of 2 and 10 years. The neuro-logical symptoms observed were weakness of limbs 5(71.4%), Speech disturbances 4(42.9%) Seizure 3(42.9%), Coma 2(28.6%), confusion 1(14.3%).Computed Tomography (in 4 of the 7 children) showed cortical infarction (n=3) and Right middle cerebral artery infarction (n=1), Left middle cerebral infarction (n=1). None of children with CVD received antiplatelet therapy. Serum ferritin level was low in 2(28.6%) [P=<0.05] patients. The Mean packed cell volume (PCV) of the study group was 17±1.5 (range 15-20). PCV was below 21% in all the cases of CVD.

4. DISCUSSION

Children less than 2 years of age had the lowest incidence of CVD suggesting that there may be a protective mechanism functioning in early life or that, in SCD, the pathology responsible for CVD develops over time. However, we found the incidence of CVD to be higher in the 2 to 10 years of age. This finding suggests that a subset of patients may have additional risk factors for early stroke.

Children who have suffered a CVD in the past have a high risk of having another stroke. SCD children have a 67 percent risk of recurrence with

CVD recurring up to nine months apart [12].The recurrence rate for CVD in this study was 28.6%. This is much lower than had been recorded in previous studies [13,14].This was because our patients were already on preventive transfusion program and hydroxyuria which explains the lower recurrence rate noted.

Anaemia in SCD is a reflection of overall severity of SCD. Haematologic disorders are the most frequent cause of ischaemic stroke of unusual cause [15]. Most of children with CVD in our study had severe anaemia. Severe anaemia may create an added risk for CVD. It has been suggested that the increased cerebral blood flow and flow velocity associated with chronic anaemia cause flow disturbances that may lead to cerebrovascular damage [16].

Table 1. Age Distribution of 152 Children with Sickle Cell Disease

Age(Years)	Frequency	Percentage
<1	9	6.0
1-<5	54	35.5
5-<10	66	43.4
>10	23	15.1

Table 2. Age Distribution of the 7 SCA with CVD

Age(Years)	Frequency	Percentage
<2	0	0
2-<5	2	28.6
5-<10	4	57.1
>10	1	14.3

SCA=Sickle Cell Anaemia; CVD=Cerebrovascular Disease

Table 3. PCV of the 7 SCA Children with CVD

PCV	Frequency	Percentage
10-<15	1	14.3
15-<20	5	71.4
21-25	1	14.3

Table 4. Haematological Parameters of Children with CVD

Factors	Mean value (SD) without iron deficiency	Mean value(SD) with iron deficiency	P-value
Serum ferritin (ng/ml)	13.2(3.4)	3.2(2.1)	<0.05
MCV (fl)	89(2.3)	75(1.4)	<0.05
MCHC (%)	35(3.1)	29(1.3)	>0.05
MCH (pcg)	21.3	21.3(2.4)	>0.05
Microcytosis (no.)	0	2	
Hypochromia (no.)	0	2	

MCV=Mean Corpuscular Volume; MCHC=Mean Corpuscular Haemoglobin Concentration; MCH= Mean Corpuscular Haemoglobin

Iron deficiency anaemia (IDA) is the most common cause of anaemia, affecting roughly two billion people worldwide [14]. It can cause low energy, weakness, frequent infections, dizziness, and can affect appetite, cognitive and motor development in the young [14]. Though normally not thought of as a life threatening condition, a number of studies have found that iron deficiency anemia may increase risk of ischaemic CVD [10]. We found a 28.6% prevalence rate of iron deficiency among our patients with cerebrovascular disease. Three mechanisms to explain an association between IDA and childhood ischemic stroke have been suggested: a hyper-coagulable state directly related to iron deficiency and/or anemia; thrombocytosis secondary to IDA; and anaemic hypoxia, whereby a mismatch between oxygen supply and end-artery oxygen demand leads to ischemia and infarction [17]. Several reports have already indirectly suggested iron deficiency anaemia as a risk factor for CVD [18-20]. Mount et al. report a series of four young children with ischemic stroke underlying with significant IDA [21]. Remarkably, several reports have revealed that in children populations the IDA seems to contribute to the development of the stroke [22-24]. Maguire et al. conducted the first case-control study to investigate whether IDA is associated with stroke in young children [25].The authors found that children with IDA accounted for more than half of all stroke cases in children without an underlying medical illness, which suggests that IDA is a significant risk factor for stroke in otherwise healthy young children.

5. CONCLUSION

Iron deficiency anaemia is not uncommon among sickle cell patients with cerebrovascular disease. There is need for elaborate iron study in these patients so as to identify at risk cases and institute prompt treatment. Supplementation therapy for iron deficiency may be an important strategy to prevent cerebrovascular disease.

CONSENT

A written consent was obtained from parents.

COMPETING INTERESTS

Authors have declared that no competing interests exist.

REFERENCES

1. Oludare, Gabriel O, Matthew C Ogili. Knowledge, attitude and practice of premarital counseling for sickle cell disease among Youth in Yaba, Nigeria. Afr J Reprod Health. 2013;17(4):175-182.

2. Ademola SA. Management of sickle cell disease: A Review for Physician Education in Nigeria (Sub-Saharan Africa). Anemia. 2015;2015:Article ID-791498:21. DOI:10.1155/2015/791498

3. George IO, Frank-Briggs AI. Stroke in Nigerian children with sickle cell anaemia. Journal of Public Health and Epidemiology. 2011;3(9):407-409.

4. Oniyangi O, Ahmed P, Otuneye OT, Okon J, Aikhionbare HA, Olatunji OO, Akano AA. Strokes in children with sickle cell disease at National Hospital Abuja Nigeria. Niger J of Paed. 2013;40(2):158-164.4040.

5. Ohene-Frempong, K, Weiner SJ, Sleeper LA, Miller ST, Embury S, Moohr JW. Cerebrovascular accidents in sickle cell disease: Rates and risk factors. Blood. 1998;91(1):288-294.

6. Chang YL, Hung SH, Ling W, Lin HC, Li HC, Chung SD. Association between ischemic stroke and iron-deficiency anemia: A population-based study. Plos One. 2013;8(12):82952.

7. Alexander MB. Iron deficiency anemia, thrombocytosis, and cerebrovascular accident. South Med J. 1983;76:662-663.

8. Ganesan V, Prengler M, Mc Shane M, Wade AM, Kirkham FJ. Investigation of risk factors in children with arterial ischemic stroke. Ann Neurol. 2003;53:167-173.

9. Nikolsky E, Aymong ED, Halkin A, Grines CL, Cox DA, et al. Impact of anemia in patients with acute myocardial infarction undergoing primary percutaneous coronary intervention: Analysis from the controlled abciximab and device investigation to lower late angioplasty complications (CADILLAC). Trial J Am Coll Cardiol. 2004; 44:547-553.

10. Kannel, WB., Gordon T, WOLF, PA, Mc Namara P. Hemoglobin and the risk of cerebral infarction: The framingham study. Stroke. 1972;3(4):409-420.

11. Gagnon DR, Zhang TJ, Brand FN, Kannel WB. Hematocrit and the risk of cardiovascular disease-the Framingham study: A 34-year follow-up. Am Heart J. 1994;27:674-682.

12. Kwiatkowski JL, Zimmerman RA, Pollock AN, et al. Silent infarcts in young children with sickle cell disease. Br J Haematol. 2009;146:300-305.

13. Lagunju I A, Brown B J. Adverse neurological outcomes in Nigerian children with sickle cell disease. Int J Hematol. 2012;96:710-718.

14. Yazdanbakhsh K, Ware RE, Noizat-Pirenne F. Red blood cell alloimmunization in sickle cell disease: Pathophysiology, risk factors, and transfusion management. Blood. 2012; 120(3):528-537.

15. Arboix A, Bechich S, Oliveres M, García-Eroles L, Massons J, Targa C. Ischemic stroke of unusual cause: Clinical features, etiology and outcome. Eur J Neurol. 2001;8(2):133-9.

16. Prohovnik I, Pavlakis SG, Piomelli S, Bello J, Mohr JP, Hilal S, De Vivo DC. Cerebral hyperemia, stroke and transfusion in sickle cell disease. Neurology. 1989;39:344.

17. Hartfield DS, Lowry NJ, Keene DL, Yager JY. Iron deficiency: A cause of stroke in infants and children. Pediatr Neurol. 1997; 16:50-53.

18. Baptist EC, Castillo SF. Cow's milk-induced iron deficiency anemia as a cause of childhood stroke. Clin Pediatr (Phila). 2002; 41:533-535.

19. Dubyk MD, Card RT, Whiting SJ, Boyle CA, Zlotkin SH, et al. Iron deficiency anemia prevalence at first stroke or transient ischemic attack. Can J Neurol Sci. 2012;39: 189-195.

20. Nicastro N, Schnider A, Leemann B. Iron-deficiency anemia as a rare cause of cerebral venous thrombosis and pulmonary embolism. Case Rep Med. 2012;497814. DOI:10.1155/2012/497814

21. Munot P, De Vile C, Hemingway C, Gunny R, Ganesan V. Severe iron deficiency anaemia and ischaemic stroke in children. Arch Dis Child. 2011;96:276-279.

22. Saxena K, Ranalli M, Khan N, Blanchong C, Kahwash SB. Fatal stroke in a child with severe iron deficiency anemia and multiple hereditary risk factors for thrombosis. Clin Pediatr (Phila). 2005;44:175-180.

23. Basak R, Chowdhury A, Fatmi L, Saha N, Mollah A, et al. Stroke in the young: Relationship with iron deficiency anemia and thrombocytosis. Mymensingh Med J. 2008;17:74-77.

24. Mehta PJ, Chapman S, Jayam-Trouth A, Kurukumbi M. Acute ischemic stroke secondary to iron deficiency anemia: A case report. Case Rep Neurol Med. 2012; 487080.

25. Maguire JL, De Veber G, Parkin PC. Association between iron-deficiency anemia and stroke in young children. Pediatrics. 2007;120:1053-1057.

25

Blood Coagulation Tests and Platelets Counts in Diabetic Rats Treated with *Ficus sur*, *Jatropha tanjorensis*, *Mucuna pruriens* and *Chromolaena odorata* Leaf Extracts

Ijioma Solomon Nnah[1*]

[1]*Department of Veterinary Physiology, Pharmacology, Biochemistry and Animal Health, College of Veterinary Medicine, Michael Okpara University of Agriculture, Umudike, Nigeria.*

Author's contribution

The sole author designed, analyzed and interpreted and prepared the manuscript.

<u>*Editor(s):*</u>
(1) Dharmesh Chandra Sharma, Incharge Blood Component & Aphaeresis Unit, G. R. Medical College, Gwalior, India.
<u>*Reviewers:*</u>
(1) Anonymous, Turkey.
(2) Julio Sergio Marchini, Ribeirao Preto School of Medicine, Sao Paulo university, Brazil.

ABSTRACT

Aim: This study was designed to study the effects of leaves extracts of four indigenous Nigerian medicinal plants namely- *Ficus sur, Jatropha tanjorensis, Mucuna pruriens* and *Chromolaena odorata* on platelets counts and blood coagulation tests (bleeding and clotting times) in alloxan induced diabetic rats with a view to further assess their safety in the management of diabetes mellitus.
Design: Animal experiments were carried out on whole animals in the Physiology Laboratory of the College of Veterinary Medicine, Michael Okpara University of Agriculture, Umudike, Nigeria.
Methodology: Forty five diabetic rats were divided into 9 groups of 5 rats each (groups 2-9), while group 1 comprised of 5 normal rats. Treatment was assigned to each group with a specified extract and dosed. At the end of treatment period bleeding and clotting times as well as platelets counts was determined for each animal.
Results: All doses of the extracts significantly (P<.05) lowered the observed elevated platelets counts in the diabetic rats with 150 mg/kg of *Ficus sur, Jatropha tanjorensis, Mucuna pruriens* and *Chromolaena odorata* lowering elevated platelets by 48.50, 47.26, 62.15 and 32.54% respectively.

*Corresponding author: E-mail: ijiomasolo@yahoo.co.uk

Same dose increased bleeding time by 460.6, 431.8, 430.3 and 213% respectively. Clotting time was also raised by 86.8, 63.57, 48.06, and 43.41 respectively.

Conclusion: The results show that the leaf extracts of *Ficus sur, Jatropha tanjorensis,* and *Mucuna pruriens* contain principles with anti-haemostatic and fibrinolytic and could be of value in the prevention of blood coagulation diseases often associated with diabetes mellitus but leaves that of *Chromolaena odorata* for further evaluation.

Keywords: Bleeding time; Chromolaena odorata; clotting time; Ficus sur; Jatropha tanjorensis; Mucuna pruriens; platelets.

1. INTRODUCTION

Hematological parameters have been associated with health indices and are of diagnostic significance in routine clinical evaluation of the state of health [1]. Coagulation tests such as bleeding time and clotting time have over the years been used to assess platelet functions. These two parameters, although considered by many as obsolete provides enough information about platelets activation and function and may serve as a means of accessing clinical conditions such as disseminated intravascular coagulation, Von willebrand disease, thrombocytopenia, end stage liver failure and uremia. Diabetes mellitus is a metabolic and endocrine system disorder characterised by hyperglycaemia resulting from defects in insulin secretion or insulin action or both. It is reported that chronic disruption of membrane fluidity, protein denaturation, lipid peroxidation, alteration in platelets functions coupled with hyperglycaemia are associated with long term damage, dysfunction and eventually the failure of organs especially the eyes, kidneys, nerve, heart and blood vessels among diabetics [2], and that about 80% of people with diabetes mellitus die a thrombotic death due to enhanced activation of platelets and clotting factors [3].

Several green leafy vegetables and weeds abound in tropical Africa that could be used in the management of hematological abnormalities [1]. These medicinal plants in addition to their healing potentials give clues in towards the development of new agents whose physiological and pharmacological dynamics can be properly harnessed for the promotion of the health of man and other animals. Little wonder, it was reported that the primary aim of sourcing for plants drug through any of the known strategies is mainly to detect the active ingredients in plants that exert definite pharmacological effects in the body, since the results of such investigations would most often serve as a lead for the biological evaluation of these plants and to new drug discovery [4]. *Ficus sur, Jatropha tanjorensis,*

Mucuna pruriens and *Chromolaena odorata* are among plants under study whose hypoglycaemic activities have been reported [5,6,7].

Ficus sur commonly called wild fig is a medium sized tree of 6-9 meters high with large alternate and spirally arranged leaves with regularly serrated margins. The leaves have found relevance in traditional medicine in the treatment of diarrhoea, anaemia, wounds, stomach problems, infertility, peptic ulcer and gonorrhea. *Jatropha tanjorensis,* belonging to family *Euphorbiaceae,* is a common weed of field crops in the higher rainfall forest zones of West Africa. In Nigeria, it is commonly called hospital too far or catholic vegetable. The leaves are commonly consumed vegetable in many parts of southern Nigeria [8], where it is considered a natural remedy against diabetes mellitus. Extracts from the leaves of the plant have also been used to treat malaria infection and hypertension in some parts of Nigeria [8,9]. The leaves were initially and popularly consumed in Nigeria as soups and as a tonic with the claim that it increases blood volume and hence employed in anemia treatment. *Mucuna pruriens* is a tropical legume known as velvet bean or cowitch. It is found in Africa, India and the Caribbean. The plant is notorious for the extreme itchiness it produces on contact, particularly with the young foliage and seed pods. The plant is an annual climbing shrub with long vines that can reach over 15m in length. When the plant is young, it is almost completely covered with fuzzy hairs, but when older, it is almost completely free of hairs. The leaves are tripinnate, ovate, reverse ovate, rhombus shaped or widely ovate. *Mucuna pruriens* bears white, lavender or purple flowers. Its seeds pods are about 10cm long and are covered in loose, orange hairs that cause a severe itch if they come in contact with the skin. The chemical compounds responsible for the itch are a protein, mucunain and serotonin. The seeds are shiny black or brown drift seeds [10]. The plant's extract have been long used in tribal communities to treat snakebites, edema, intestinal worms, diabetes, high blood pressure, high cholesterol, intestinal gas, muscle pain, rheumatism, abortions, cancer, catarrh, cholera, cough, diarrhea, dysentery, impotency, kidney stones, menstrual disorder, nervousness, scorpion stings, sterility, tuberculosis, asthma, burns, cancer, cholera, coughs, cuts, diarrhea, dog bites, insanity, menstrual problem, mumps, paralysis, ringworm, sores, syphilis, tumors, and as a diuretic agent [10]. *Chromolaena odorata* on the other hand, is a rapidly growing perennial herb with multi-stemmed shrub and grows up to 2.5 m tall in open areas. Available literature reveals that the plant contains carcinogenic pyrrolizidine alkaloid and can cause toxicity and allergic reactions in cattle. However there is report that the extract from the leaves is used traditionally to treat skin wounds [11].

This study was designed to investigate the effects of these four indigenous Nigerian medicinal plants on bleeding times, clotting time and platelets counts in alloxan induced diabetic rats with a view to complementing their reported usefulness in the management of diabetes mellitus.

2. MATERIALS AND METHODS

2.1 Collection and Preparation of Plant Extracts

Fresh leaves of *Ficus sur*, *Mucuna pruriens*and *Chromolaena odorata* were collected from a farm settlement in Isiegbu - Ozuitem, Bende Local Government Area of Abia State while *Jatropha tanjorensis* was collected from Owerri-Aba in Ugwunagbo Local Government Area of Abia State in the month of March, 2014. The leaves of were dried under shade for seven days, after which they were pulverished to fine powder using a manual blender. Thirty five (35) grams of each powdered sample was introduced into the extraction chamber of the soxhlet extractor and extraction was done using ethanol as a solvent. Temperature was maintained at 70°C through-out the extraction period of 48 hours. At the end of the period, the extract was dried in a laboratory oven at 40°C to obtain dried extracts of each sample.

2.2 Animals

Fifty albino rats (130-160g), obtained from the Animal house unit of the Department of Physiology and Pharmacology, Michael Okpara University of Agriculture, Umudike were used for the study. All animals were fed with standard animal feed and water *ad libitum* and handled in accordance with the NIH guidelines for Care and Use of Laboratory Animals (Pub. No.85-23, Revised 1985), as expressed by Akah et al. [12].

2.3 Induction Diabetes

Sixty five rats of both sexes weighting 140-180g were made diabetic by a single intraperitoneal injection of alloxan monohydrate (Sigma Chemical Co., USA) 10% (W/V) in normal saline at a dose of 160 mg/kg body weight. 8 days later blood was obtained from the tails of each rat and tested for glucose level to confirm the development of diabetes using a glucose meter (Roche Co.Germany). The rats with fasting glucose levels above 190 mg/dL were considered diabetic. Forty five of the diabetic rats were used for the study while five normal rats constituted the normal control group.

2.4 Bleeding and clotting times

The animals were grouped and assigned daily oral treatments as indicated below:

Group 1: Normal control which received normal saline
Group 2: Untreated diabetic rats (diabetic control)
Group 3: Diabetic rats treated with 150 mg/kg *Ficus sur.*
Group 4: Diabetic rats treated with 300 mg/kg *Ficus sur.*
Group 5: Diabetic rats treated with 150 mg/kg *Jatropha tanjorensis.*
Group 6: Diabetic rats treated with 300 mg/kg *Jatropha tanjorensis.*
Group 7: Diabetic rats treated with 150 mg/kg *Mucuna pruriens.*
Group 8: Diabetic rats treated with 300 mg/kg *Mucuna pruriens.*
Group 9: Diabetic rats treated with 150 mg/kg *Chromolaena odorata.*
Group 10: Diabetic rats treated with 300 mg/kg *Chromolaena odorata.*

The rats were kept in Aluminum cages and allowed access to feed and water while ensuring that highest level of hygiene was maintained. Treatments were done daily via the oral route and lasted for 21 days. At the end of the period, bleeding time was determined for each animal using Duke's method while clotting time was determine by Ivy's method as reported by Ibu and Adeniyi [13]. For bleeding time, the tip of the tail of each rat was cut to cause bleeding. A stopwatch was started as soon as animal began to bleed. A blotting paper was used to wipe off blood every 15 seconds. As soon as bleeding ceased the stopwatch was stopped and the time recorded as bleeding time for that particular animal. For the clotting time, a drop of blood from the tail of each rat was placed on a clean glass slide and a stopwatch was started at the same time. A pin was passed across the drop of blood once every 15 seconds. As soon as threads of fibrin were noticed, the stopwatch was stopped and the time recorded as the clotting time for that particular rat. Percentage increase in bleeding and clotting times were calculated using the formula:

% Increase = [(Time in test - Time in diabetic control)/ (Time in diabetic control) x (100/1)]

2.5 Platelets Counts

After 21 days of treatment, the rats in all groups were sacrificed on the 22nd day and blood samples collected by cardiac puncture for platelets counts using an Automated Haematology Analyser, following standard procedures stipulated by the producer, Mindray Company, China. Percentage reductions in platelets counts were calculated using the formula:

% Reduction = $\dfrac{A - B}{A}$ X 100

Where

A = Counts in diabetic control
B = Counts in test

3. RESULTS

3.1 Effects of Plant Extracts on Platelet Counts in Alloxan Induced Diabetic Rats

The diabetic control rats showed significantly ($p< 0.05$) elevated platelets counts when compared to the normal control rats at the end of 21 days (Table 1). All doses of *F. sur, J. tanjorensis, M. pruriens* and *C. odorata* significantly ($p< 0.05$) lowered these elevated platelets values in all treated diabetic rats with 150mg/kg body weight of *M. pruriens* achieving the highest platelets lowering effect of 62.15% (Table 1).

3.2 Effects of Plant Extracts on Bleeding and Clotting Times in Alloxan Induced Diabetic Rats

All doses of *F. sur, J. tanjorensis,* and *M. pruriens* significantly ($p< 0.05$) increased bleeding times in the treated diabetic rats except 300 mg/kg *C. odorata* which did not significantly affect same (Table 2). The clotting time was also significantly increased by all doses of the extracts except 300 mg/kg *C. odorata* which increased same by only 6.20% (Table 3).

Table 1. Effects of extracts on platelets counts in alloxan induced diabetic rats

Group	Treatment (mg/kg)	Platelets counts X 10^9/L	% Reduction in platelets counts
1.	Normal control	909± 227.5	
2.	Diabetic control	1611.8±102.8	
3.	150 *F. sur*	830±30.7*	48.50
4.	300 *F. sur*	694.3±160.9*	56.92
5.	150 *J. tanjorensis*	850±95.3*	47.26
6.	300 *J. tanjorensis*	744±82.9*	53.84
7.	150 *M. pruriens*	610±488.5*	62.15
8.	300 *M. pruriens*	737.7±16.2*	54.23
9.	150 *C. odorata*	1087.3±265.5*	32.54
10.	300 *C. odorata*	909±32.96*	43.60

*P< 0.05 versus diabetic control

Table 2. Effects of extracts on bleeding time in alloxan induced diabetic rats

Group	Treatment (mg/kg)	Bleeding time (Min)	% Increase in bleeding time
1.	Normal control	4.76±0.10	
2.	Diabetic control	1.32±0.19	
3.	150 *F. sur*	7.40±0.25*	460.61
4.	300 *F. sur*	11.54±0.59*	774.24
5.	150 *J. tanjorensis*	7.02±0.25*	431.82
6.	300 *J. tanjorensis*	7.70±0.79*	483.33
7.	150 *M. pruriens*	7.0±0.73*	430.30
8.	300 *M. pruriens*	8.90±0.31*	574.24
9.	150 *C. odorata*	4.14±0.24*	213.64
10.	300 *C. odorata*	1.11±0.42	-15.90

*P< 0.05 versus diabetic control

Table 3. Effects of plants extracts on clotting time in alloxan induced diabetic rats

Group	Treatment (mg/kg)	Clotting time (Min.)	% Increase in clotting time
1.	Normal control	2.0 ±0.18	
2.	Diabetic control	1.29±0.09	
3.	150 *F. sur*	2.41±0.13*	86.82
4.	300 *F. sur*	2.32±0.14*	79.84
5.	150 *J. tanjorensis*	2.11±0.18*	63.57
6.	300 *J. tanjorensis*	1.98±0.24*	53.49
7.	150 *M. pruriens*	1.91±0.19*	48.06
8.	300 *M. pruriens*	2.42±0.21*	87.60
9.	150 *C. odorata*	1.85±0.21*	43.41
10.	300 *C. odorata*	1.37±0.04	6.20

*P<0.05 versus diabetic control

4. DISCUSSION

The results of this indicate increase in platelets counts which may have accounted for the lowered bleeding and clotting times observed in the diabetic rats and tends to agree with existing literature reports. It is reported that platelets hyperactivity in patients with hyperglycaemia resulting from a dysregulated signaling pathways that lead to an increased tendency to activate and aggregate response to a given stimulus [14]. Platelets activation therefore triggers thrombus formation, microcapillary embolization and facilitates the development of other cardiovascular diseases. Akingbami et al. [15] added that diabetes mellitus is characterized by enhanced platelets activation and coagulation proteins and reduced fibrinolytic activity which usually precede the development of cardiovascular complications. The increased platelets counts in the diabetic rats may have been responsible for the observed decrease in bleeding and clotting times and may increase the risk of intravascular blood clotting and associated diseases [16,3].

The significant (p<0.05) reduction in platelets counts and corresponding elevations in bleeding and clotting times in all diabetic rats treated with leaf extracts of *Ficus sur, Jatropha tanjorensis, and Mucuna pruriens* suggest that the extracts contain strong principles with anti-hemostatic and fibrinolytic properties in addition to their hypoglycaemic properties reported by [5,6,7]. The extracts may have achieved these effects by stimulating decrease in formation and activation of blood platelets, a process which usually does not favor the blood clotting and shown by increased bleeding and clotting times. *C. odorata* ethanol leaf extract, reported to have hypoglycaemic activity which could be of value in the management of diabetes mellitus [6,17], its use in diabetes requires further evaluation as the extract was observed not to significantly affect bleeding and clotting times in the treated diabetic rats and has been reported to have haemostatic and fibrinolytic activity in experimental rats [18]. This may be the reason for the use of *C. odorata* leaf extract to promote wound healing and to stop bleeding [11].

The results obtained agree with Houghton and Skari [19], on the use of *Mucuna pruriens* extract to prolong bleeding and clotting times and justifies the use of *Ficus sur, Jatropha tanjorensis* and *Mucuna pruriens* in bleeding disorders associated with diabetes mellitus.

5. CONCLUSION

The results of this study have shown that ethanol leaf extracts of *Ficus sur, Jatropha tanjorensis and Mucuna pruriens,* can be used to remedy the abnormal platelets, bleeding and clotting times values observed in diabetic rats and justify the use of these agents in diabetes management as their effects may be useful in the management of thrombosis and other blood coagulation problems associated with the condition, but leaves the use of *Chromolaena odorata* for the same purpose to be further evaluated.

CONSENT

Not applicable.

ETHICAL APPROVAL

Not applicable.

COMPETING INTERESTS

Author has declared that no competing interests exist.

REFERENCES

1. Saliu JA, Elekofehinti OO, Komolafe K, Oboh G. Effects of some green leafy vegetables on the Hematological parameters of Diabetic Rats. J. Nat. Prod. Plant Resource. 2012;2(4).
2. Sunday EA. Evaluation of the Hypoglycaemic, Hypolipidemic and Antioxidant effets of methanolic extract of "Ata-Ofa" polyherbal Tea (A- poly herbal) in Alloxan-induced Diabetic rats. Drug Invention Toady. 2011;3(11):270-276.
3. Carr ME. Diabetes mellitus; a hypercoagulable state. J. Diabetes Complications. 2001;15(1):44-54.
4. Ojieh AE, Adegor EC, Lawrence EO. Preliminary phytochemical screening, analgesic and anti-inflammatory properties of *Celosia isertii*. European Journal of Medicinal Plants. Science domain International. 2013;3(3):369-380.
5. Akomas SC, Okafor AI, Ijioma SN. Glucose level, haematological parameters

and lipid profile in *Ficus sur* treated diabetic rats. Comprehensive Journal of Agriculture and Biological Sciences. 2014;2(1):5-11.
6. Ijioma SN, Okafor AI, Ndukuba PI, Nwankwo AA, Akomas SC. Hypoglycaemic, haematologic and lipid profile effects of *Chromolaena odorata* ethanol leaf extract in alloxan induced diabetic rats. Annals of Biological Sciences. 2014;2(3):27-32.
7. Ijioma SN, Okafor AI, Ndukuba PI, Akomas SC. Hypoglycaemic, hematologic and hypolipidemic activity of Jatropha tanjorensis ethanol leaf extract in alloxan induced diabetic rats. Annals of Biological Research. 2014;5(9):15-19.
8. Orhue EG, Idu M, Atamari JE, Ebite LE. Hematological and histopathological studies of *Jatropha tanjorensis* leaves in Rabbits. Asian Journal of Biological Sciences. 2008;1(2):84-89.
9. Omobuwajo OR, Alade GO, Akanmu MA, Obuotor EM, Osasan SA. Microscopic and toxicity studies on the leaves of *Jatropha tanjorensis*. African Journal of Pharmacy and Pharmacology. 2011;5(1):12-17.
10. Deka M, Kalita JC. Preliminary phytochemical analysis and acute oral toxicity study of *Mucuna pruriens* LINN in Albino Mice. International Research Journal of Pharmacy. 2012;3(2).
11. Hataichanok P, Xiaobo Z, Jason L, Kyung-Won M, Wandee G, Seung JB. Hemostatic and wound healing properties of *Chromolaena odorata* Leaf Extract. Hindawi Journal of Dermitology. 2013;Article I.D 168269.
12. Akah PA, Alemji JA, Salawu OA, Okoye TC, Offiah NV. Effects of *Vernonia amygdalina* on biochemical and hematological parameters in diabetic rats. Asian Journal of Medical Sciences. 2009;1(3):108-113.
13. Ibu JO, Adeniyi KO. A Manual of Practical Physiology, Published by Jos University Press, Jos. 1989;126.
14. Nicholas K, Jeffrey JR, Antonios K, John RR. Platelets function in patients with Diabetes Mellitus: from a theoretical to a practical perspective. International Journal of Endocrinology. 2011; ID742719.
15. Akingbami A, Dada AO, John OS, Ushanaiki O, Adediran A, Odesanya M, Ogbara A, Uche E, Okunoye O, Arogundade O, Aile K. Mean platelets volume and platelets counts in type 2

diabetes mellitus patients on treatment and non diabetes mellitus controls in Lagos, Nigeria. The pan African Medical Journal. 2014;18:42.

16.   Ceriello A. Coagulation activation in diabetes mellitus: The role of hyperglycaemia and therapeutic prospects. Diabetologia. 1993;36(11):1119-1125.

17.   Onkaramurthy M, Veerapur VP, Thippeswamy BS, Reddy TN, Rayappa H, Badami S. Anti-diabetic activity of *Chromolaena odorata*. J. Ethnopharmacol. 2013;145(1):363-372.

18.   Akomas SC, Ijioma SN. Bleeding and clotting time effect of ethanolic extracts of *Chromolaena odorata* versus *Ocimum gratissimum* treated albino rats. Comprehensive Journal of Medical Sciences. 2014;2(1):9-13.

19.   Houghton PJ, Skari KP. The effect on blood clotting of some west African plants used against snake bite. J. Ethno-pharmacol. 1994;44(2):99-108.

26

Assessment of Some Fibrinolytic Parameters during Pregnancy in Northern Nigeria

Imoru Momodu[1*] and Olutayo Ifedayo Ajayi[2]

[1]*Department of Haematology, Aminu Kano Teaching Hospital/Bayero University, P.M.B. 3452, Kano, Kano State, Nigeria.*
[2]*Department of Physiology, School of Basic Medical Sciences, University of Benin, P.M.B. 1154, Benin-City, Nigeria.*

Authors' contributions

This work was developed in collaboration by the both authors. Author IM designed the study, wrote the protocol, managed the literature searches and analysed the data while author OIA contributed to the literature searches and the analysis of the data. Both authors read and approved the final manuscript.

<u>*Editor(s):*</u>
(1) Dharmesh Chandra Sharma, Incharge Blood Component & Aphaeresis Unit, G. R. Medical College, Gwalior, India.
<u>*Reviewers:*</u>
(1) Yaşam Kemal Akpak, Ankara Mevki Military Hospital, Turkey.
(2) Celso Eduardo Olivier, Instituto Alergoimuno de Americana, Brazil.
(3) Margaret Markiewicz, Medical University of South Carolina, USA.

ABSTRACT

Aim: The study was undertaken to assess the fibrinolytic activity during pregnancy and to determine the effects of maternal age, gestation period and parity on fibrinolytic parameters in Northern Nigeria.
Materials and Methods: 150 pregnant and 100 non-pregnant women, aged 17-40 years, were recruited for the research in Aminu Kano Teaching Hospital, Kano between August 2010 and October 2011. Blood samples collected were analysed for the plasma levels of fibrinogen, d-dimer and Fibrin Degradation Products (FDP) using standard laboratory methods.
Results: Pregnant women had significantly higher values of fibrinogen concentration, d-dimer and FDP of 3.46 ± 0.35 g/L, 0.78 ± 0.82 μg/mL and 10.17 ± 15.08 μg/mL respectively compared to 3.12 ± 0.3g/L, 0.45 ± 0.78 μg/mL and 2.8 ± 7.63 μg/mL, in non-pregnant women ($P<0.05$). D-dimer values for the first, second and third trimesters showed statistically significant differences ($P<0.05$) while fibrinogen levels showed no significant effects within the gestation period ($P>0.05$). Maternal

Corresponding author: E-mail: imorumomodu67@yahoo.com

age and parity had no significant influences on fibrinogen concentration, d-dimer and FDP levels (*P*>0.05).

Conclusion: Changes in fibrinolytic parameters in this study are associated with increased levels of fibrinogen, d-dimer and FDP during pregnancy, irrespective of maternal age and parity, and these changes can be linked to increased fibrinolytic activity during pregnancy. It is recommended that plasma fibrinogen, d-dimer and FDP levels be determined during pregnancy to prevent the risk of thrombosis that the pregnant women are prone to.

Keywords: Assessment; fibrinolytic parameters; pregnancy; Northern Nigeria.

1. INTRODUCTION

Fibrinolysis is a normal body process where fibrin clot, the product of coagulation, is broken down by plasmin at various sites leading to the production of circulating fragments or soluble fibrin degradation products (FDP) that are cleared by other proteinases or by kidney and liver [1-3].

Normal pregnancy is associated with changes in all aspects of haemostasis, including increase in concentrations of most clotting factors such as coagulation factors V, VII, VIII, IX, X, XII, fibrinogen and von-Willebrand factor and decreasing concentrations of some of the natural anticoagulants with diminishing fibrinolytic activity [4-6]. These changes have been associated with increased risk of thromboembolism during pregnancy and puerperium [4].

Increased fibrinogen concentration during pregnancy documented by previous authors [6-8] has been associated with increase in fibrinogen synthesis due to its utilization in the utero-placental circulation or as a result of hormonal changes such as increasing progesterone levels [6] while increased d-dimer level observed by earlier authors [9-11] has been associated with increased fibrinolysis following fibrin formation, increased coagulation activation and thrombin generation or combination of both [12-14].

The study of some fibrinolytic parameters (fibrinogen, d-dimer and FDP) during pregnancy was necessitated to further clarify the general concept of reduced fibrinolytic activity during pregnancy that is in dispute by earlier authors [15-18].

2. MATERIALS AND METHODS

This study was conducted on two-hundred and fifty apparently healthy subjects (150 pregnant and 100 non-pregnant women), aged 17-40 years in Aminu Kano Teaching Hospital (AKTH),

Kano between August 2010 and October 2011. Ethical approval and consent were obtained from AKTH and the subjects respectively. Pregnant and non-pregnant women with histories of recurrent miscarriages, liver disease, renal disease, diabetes and hypertension, and non-pregnant women on oral contraceptives were excluded from the study.

A venous blood sample (4.5 mL) collected from each subject was mixed with 0.5ml of 3.2% trisodium citrate solution in a plain container. Blood samples in the citrated containers were centrifuged at 2500 rpm for 15 minutes and the plasma separated into plastic containers for the determination of fibrinogen, d-dimer and FDP.

Plasma fibrinogen concentration was determined by modified Clauss method (Catalogue number 050-500 and manufactured by PZ Cormay, Poland). D-dimer and FDP were performed according to the manufacturer's instructions using Latex agglutination kits of catalogue numbers 150-700 and 00541 respectively manufactured from PZ, Poland and Diagnostica stago, France respectively.

2.1 Statistical Analysis

The mean values and standard deviations of the parameters in pregnant and non-pregnant women were assessed using Student's t-test while differences with regard to gestational age, maternal age and parity were analyzed using one-way analysis of variance (ANOVA). The differences were considered significant when the p values were ≤ 0.05.

3. RESULTS

3.1 Fibrinolytic Parameters in Pregnant Women

The fibrinolytic parameters (fibrinogen, d-dimer and FDP) were estimated in pregnant and non-pregnant women. The mean values of plasma fibrinogen, d-dimer and FDP in pregnant and non-pregnant women are shown (Table 1). Pregnant women were found to show significantly higher values of fibrinogen concentration, d-dimer and FDP compared to non-pregnant women (p< .05).

3.2 Changes of Fibrinolytic Parameters with Gestation Period

Mean values of plasma fibrinogen, d-dimer and FDP for first, second and third trimesters are shown (Table 2). Values of fibrinogen concentration and FDP for the first, second and third trimesters showed no significant differences (p> .05) while d-dimer values increased significantly with increasing gestation period (p< .05).

3.3 Influences of Maternal Age on Fibrinolytic Parameters

Effects of maternal age on fibrinogen concentration, d-dimer and FDP are displayed (Table 3). The varied mean values of fibrinogen concentration, d-dimer and FDP for different age groups (17-22 years, 23-28 years, 29-34 years and 35-40 years) showed no significant differences (p> .05).

3.4 Effects of Parity on Fibrinolytic Parameters during Pregnancy

Effects of 0, 1-2 and ≥3 parity on fibrinogen concentration, d-dimer and FDP are shown (Table 4). The different mean values of fibrinogen, d-dimer and FDP with regard to 0, 1-2 and ≥3 parity, showed no significance (p> .05).

4. DISCUSSION

It has been generally documented that there is diminished fibrinolytic activity during pregnancy but this common reports seem to be questionable [15-18].

This study has shown significantly higher value of fibrinogen concentration in pregnancy compared to non-pregnant women and this is in line with the widely documented reports fromprevious authors [6-9,19,20]. The study has further confirmed the earlier finding on increase in fibrinogen level as pregnancy progresses [10,21,22] but there was no significant change in the fibrinogen level within the gestation period which agrees with the report of Buseri et al. [19]. However, increased fibrinogen concentration during pregnancy has been linked to assisting the prevention of post-partum haemorrhage through deposition of 5-10% of the

Table 1. Fibrinolytic parameters in pregnant and non-pregnant women

Parameter	Non-pregnant women (control)	Pregnant women
Number of subjects	100	150
Fibrinogen concentration (g/L)	3.12±0.3	3.46±0.35*
D-dimer (μg/mL)	0.45±0.78	0.78±0.828*
FDP (μg/mL)	2.8±7.63	10.17±15.08*

*P <0.05, pregnant women compared to the control group

Table 2. Changes of fibrinolytic parameters with gestational age

Parameter	First trimester (n=24)	Second trimester (n=66)	Third trimester (n=60)
Fibrinogen concentration (g/L)	3.4±0.80	3.6±0.88	3.6±0.72
D-dimer (μg/mL)	0.36±0.4*	0.88±0.82	0.75±0.88
FDP (μg/mL))	4.32±8.29	11.36±19.16	10.73±10.72

*P <0.05, first trimester compared to second and third trimesters

Table 3. Effects of maternal age on fibrinolytic parameters during pregnancy

Parameter	17-22 years	23-28 years	29-34 years	35-40 years	P value
Number of subjects	24	67	48	11	
Fibrinogen concentration (g/L)	3.6±0.79	3.5±0.70	3.8±0.87	3.2±0.85	>0.05
D-dimer (μg/mL)	1.08±0.92	0.64±0.67	0.84±0.94	0.7±0.88	>0.05
FDP (μg/mL)	10.1±10.23	10.07±20.61	11.51±14.91	16..36±24.05	>0.05

Table 4. Parity influence on fibrinolytic parameters during pregnancy

Parameter	0 Parity	1-2 Parity	≥3 Parity	P value
Number of subjects	42	51	57	
Fibrinogen concentration (g/L)	3.6±0.85	3.7±0.71	3.5±0.84	>0.05
D-dimer (µg/mL)	1.12±0.79	1.30±1.02	1.10±0.91	>0.05
FDP (ug/mL)	14.29±22.98	22.83±38.07	17.59±14.36	>0.05

total circulatory fibrinogen at the placental site [23,24]. There was no parity influence on fibrinogen level during pregnancy in this study and this is consistent with the earlier report [22] but the effect of maternal age on fibrinogen concentration during pregnancy documented by the previous author [22] is in contrary to our finding in this study. However, the divergent view expressed by Durotoye et al. [22] may be associated with the wider age groups considered in their study.

Significantly increased d-dimer level during pregnancy was observed in this study and this is in agreement with the earlier findings [10,11,25-27]. This study further revealed that the d-dimer levels increased significantly in the second and third trimesters of pregnancy and these are consistent with the reports of previous authors [10,11,28-30] which showed progressive rise in the d-dimer concentrations of up to 600 ng/mL. There was no influence of maternal age on the d-dimer level during pregnancy in this study and this is in line with the report of Jeremiah et al. [30]. This observation in this study, may be associated with increased fibrinolysis from the second trimester of pregnancy probably due to increased fibrin formation to prevent thrombosis. However, elevated d-dimer level has been associated with increased fibrinolytic activity as a result of coagulation activation and thrombin generation [12-14].

The study has further confirmed earlier reports on increased fibrin degradation products during pregnancy [17,31-33]. The study further revealed that there was no effect of gestational age on FDP level. However, increased FDP level has been associated with increased fibrinolysis [33] probably to neutralize the effect of increased fibrin formation during pregnancy.

Maternal age and parity showed no significant effects on fibrinogen concentration, d-dimer and FDP levels in this study.

5. CONCLUSION

In conclusion, changes in fibrinolytic parameters in this study have been associated with increased levels of fibrinogen, d-dimer and FDP

during pregnancy, irrespective of maternal age and parity. The altered parameters in this study can be linked to increased fibrinolytic activity probably to neutralize or counterbalance increased intravascular coagulation during pregnancy to reduce thrombosis. It is recommended that plasma fibrinogen concentration, d-dimer and FDP levels be included amongst ante-natal tests to aid in monitoring pregnant women who are prone to thrombosis while innovative approach to unravel mechanism of fibrinolytic status in pregnancy should include the measurement of some parameters such as tissue plasminogen activator (tPA), plasminogen, plasminogen activator inhibitor type 1 (PAI- 1) amongst others, since tPA has been observed to primarily initiate fibrinolysis in the vascular system, and its low level in the blood with increased PAI-1 has been associated with an increased risk of arterial thrombosis [34-36].

CONSENT

We declare that written informed consent was obtained from every pregnant woman or control subject studied.

ETHICAL APPROVAL

Ethical approval was obtained from the ethical committee of Aminu Kano Teaching Hospital, Kano to carry out the research.

ACKNOWLEDGEMENT

I would like to thank the members of staff of Obstetrics and Gynaecology of Aminu Kano Teaching Hospital, Kano for their assistance in the selection of apparently healthy pregnant subjects for this research.

COMPETING INTERESTS

Authors have declared that no competing interests exist.

REFERENCES

1.   Walker JB, Neisheim ME. The molecular weights, mass distribution, chain

composition and structure of soluble fibrin degradation products released from fibrin clot perfused with plasmin. Journal of Biological Chemistry. 1999;274:5201-5212.

2. Lijnen HR. Elements of the fibrinolytic system. Ann N Y Acad Sci. 2001;936: 226-236.

3. Cesarman-Naus G, Hajjar KA. Molecular mechanism of fibrinolysis. British Journal of Haematology. 2005;129:307-321.

4. Prisco D, Ciuti G, Falciani M. Haemostatic changes in normal pregnancy. Haematologica reports. 2005;1:1-5.

5. Simioni P, Campello E. Haemostatic changes in pregnancy. Reviews in Health Care. 2013;4:3s.
Available:http://journals.edizioniseed.it/index.php/rhc/article/view/878 (Accessed 10 Nov, 2013)

6. Kametas N, Krampt E, McAuliffe F, Rampling MW, Nicolaides KH. Haemorrheological adaptation during pregnancy in a Latin American population. European Journal of Haematology. 2001; 66:305-311.

7. Salawu L, Durosinmi MA. Erythrocyte rate and plasma viscosity in health and disease. Nigerian Journal of Medicine. 2001;10:11-13.

8. Imoru M, Emeribe AO. Haemorrheologic and fibrinolytic activities in pregnant women: Influence of gestational age and parity. African Journal of Biotechnology. 2009;8:6641-6644.

9. Uchikova EH, Ledjev II. Changes in haemostasis during normal pregnancy. European Journal of Obstetrics and Gynaecology and Reproductive Biology. 2005;119:185-188.

10. Kline JA, Williams GW, Hernandez-Nino J. D-dimer concentrations in normal pregnancy: New diagnostic thresholds are needed. Clinical chemistry. 2005;51(5): 825-829.

11. Reger B, Peterfalvi A, Litter I, et al. Challenges in the evaluation of D-dimer and fibrinogen levels in pregnant women. Thromb Res. 2013;131:183-187.

12. Bellart J, Gilabert R, Fontcuberta J, Borrell M, Miralles RM, Cabero L. Fibrinolysis change in normal pregnancy. Journal of Perinatal Medicine. 1997;25:368-372.

13. Kjellberg U, Anderson NE, Rossen S, Tengborn L, Hellgren M. APC resistance and other haemostatic variables during pregnancy and puerperium. Thrombosis and Haemostasis. 1999;81:527-531.

14. Eichinger S. D-dimer testing in pregnancy. Pathophysiology of Haemostasis and Thrombosis. 2004;33:327-329.

15. Howie PW. Blood clotting and fibrinolysis in pregnancy. Postgrad Med J. 1979; 55(643):362-366.

16. Maki M, Soga K, Seki H. Fibrinolytic activity during pregnancy. Tohoku J Exp Med. 1980;132(3):349-354.

17. Stirling Y, Woolf L, North WRS, Seghatchian MJ, Meade TW. Haemostasis in normal pregnancy. Thrombosis and Haemostasis. 1984;52:176-182.

18. Holmes VA, Wallace JMW. Haemostasis in normal pregnancy: A balancing act? Biochemical society transactions. 2005;33 (2):428-432.

19. Buseri FI, Jeremiah ZA, Kalio FG. Influence of pregnancy and gestation period on some coagulation parameters among Nigerian antenatal women. Research Journal of Medical Sciences. 2008;2:275-281.

20. Szecsi PB, Lorgensen M, Klainbard A, Anderson MR, Colov NP, Stender S. Haemostatic reference intervals in pregnancy. Thrombosis and Haemostasis. 2010;103:718-727.

21. Greer IA. Haemostasis and Thrombosis in pregnancy. In: Bloom AL, Forbes CD, Thomas DP, Tuddenham EGD (editors). Haemostasis and Thrombosis (3rd ed), Churchill Livingstone, Edinburgh. 987-1015.

22. Durotoye IA, Babatunde AS, Olawumi HO, Olatunji PO, Adewuyi JO. Haemostatic parameters during pregnancy in Ilorin, Nigeria. The Tropical Journal of Health Sciences. 2012;19(2):18-22.

23. Kobayashi T, Asahina T, Machara K, Itah M, Kanayama N, Terao T. Congenital afibrinogemia with successful delivery. Gynae and Obstet Inv. 1996;42(1):66-69.

24. Hellgren M. Hemostasis during normal pregnancy and puerperium. Thrombosis and Haemostasis. 2003;29:125-130.

25. Van Wersch JWJ, Ubachs JMH. Blood coagulation and fibrinolysis during normal pregnancy. Eur J Clin Chem Clin Biochem. 1991;29:45-50.

26. Bremme K, Ostlund E, Almqvist I, Heinonen K, Blomback M. Enhanced Thrombin generation and fibrinolytic activity in normal pregnancy and the puerperium. Obstet Gynaecol. 1992;80(1): 132-137.

27. Morse M. Establishing a normal range for D-dimer levels through pregnancy to aid in the diagnosis of pulmonary embolism and deep vein thrombosis. Journal of Thrombosis Haemostasis. 2004;2:1202-1204.

28. Nolan T, Smith R, Devoe L. Maternal plasma D-dimer levels in normal and complicated pregnancies. Obstet Gynecol. 1993;81:235-238.

29. Francalanci I, Comeglio P, Allessandrello Liotta A, Cellai AP, Fedi S, Paretti E, et al. D-dimer plasma levels during normal pregnancy measured by specific ELISA. Intl J Clin Lab Res. 1997;27:65-67.

30. Jeremiah ZA, Adias TC, Opiah M, George SP, Mgbere O, Essien EJ. Elevation in D-dimer concentrations is positively correlated with gestation in normal uncomplicated pregnancy. International Journal of Women's Health. 2012;4:437-443.

31. Woodfield DG, Cole SK, Allan AGE, Cash JD. Serum fibrin degradation products throughout normal pregnancy. Brit Med J. 19684:665-8.

32. Yuasa S, Ishizawa M, Yuki Y, Minoura T, Fujita N, Takahashi H, et al. Coagulation and fibrinolysis in pregnancy. Rinsho Byori. 1992;40(12):1287-1291.

33. Higgins JR, Walshe JJ, Darling MRN, Norris L, Bonnar J. Haemostasis in the uteroplacental and peripheral circulations in normotensive and pre-eclamptic pregnancies. American Journal of Obstetrics and Gynaecology. 1998;179: 520-526.

34. Hamsten A, Walldius G, Szamosi A, Blomback M, De Faire U, Dahlen G, et al. Plasminogen activator inhibitor in plasma: Risk factor for recurrent myocardial infarction. Lancent. 1987;2:3-9.

35. Jansson JH, Nilsson TK, Olofsson BO. Tissue plasminogen activator and other risk factors as predictors of cardiovascular events in patients with severe angina pectoris. Eur Heart J. 1991;12:157-161.

36. Chandler WL, Jascur ML, Henderson PJ. Measurement forms of tPA in plasma. Clinical Chemistry. 2000;46:38-46.

27

Case Report: Portal Vein Thrombosis as a Cause of Haematemesis in a Healthy African Adolescent

F. A. Fasola[1*], A. Akere[2] and F. O. Fowodu[1]

[1]Department of Haematology, University College Hospital, Ibadan, Nigeria.
[2]Department of Medicine, University College Hospital, Ibadan, Nigeria.

Authors' contributions

This work was carried out in collaboration between all authors who managed the patient. Author FAF designed the study and wrote the first draft of the manuscript. Author FAF managed the literature searches. Authors FAF and AA participated in revising the writing up. All authors read and approved the final manuscript.

Editor(s):
(1) Dharmesh Chandra Sharma, Incharge Blood Component & Aphaeresis Unit, G. R. Medical College, Gwalior, India.
Reviewers:
(1) Nitin Gupta, Dept. of Orthopaedics, Cygnus Medicare, India.
(2) Pratibha Dhiman, Department of Hematology, Institute of Liver and Biliary Sciences, New Delhi, India.
(3) Anonymous, University of Bari, Italy.
(4) Anonymous, University of Palermo, Italy.

ABSTRACT

Introduction: Thromboembolic incidents typically occur as deep vein thrombosis of the limbs and pulmonary embolism but can also occur in unusual sites such as cerebral or sinus, mesenteric, portal, hepatic renal and retinal veins. When thromboembolism occurs in any of these unusual sites, diagnosis is often unsuspected and missed. The relatively low incidence of thrombosis in healthy children further presents a potential diagnostic dilemma. High index of suspicion is therefore required for timely diagnosis in order to prevent complications.
Presentation of Case: We report a case of a 15 year-old girl with 10 years history of recurrent haematemesis. She was managed initially as a case of upper gastrointestinal bleeding of unknown aetiology and subsequently as a case of chronic liver disease and then later, as case of bleeding diathesis. The patient had several oesophageal variceal band ligation, courses of propranolol, omeprazole, livolin and several units of blood transfused. Abdominal ultrasound, Computed Tomographic scan of abdomen and angiography revealed portal vein thrombosis with periportal collaterals. The proteins C and S levels were low. A diagnosis of portal vein thrombosis (PVT)

Corresponding author: E-mail: folukefasola@yahoo.com

secondary to Proteins C and S deficiencies was then made. Patient has been symptom free since commencement of anticoagulation but there was no recanalization of the vessels.
Conclusion: The potential role of prothrombotic risk factors and PVT should be explored in paediatric age group with gastrointestinal bleeding for early diagnosis and management to reduce complications.

Keywords: Portal vein thrombosis; protein C; protein S; anticoagulant; children.

ABBREVIATIONS

PVT – Portal vein thrombosis.

1. INTRODUCTION

The first report of portal vein thrombosis (PVT) was in 1868 [1]. Since then there has been several reports due to greater availability of diagnostic methods. Despite this, the diagnosis is often missed in clinical practice and treatment is delayed [1]. In PVT, thrombus formation occurs in the portal vein and may extend to other branches of the portal system [2]. The involved blood vessels can be partially or totally occluded resulting in portal hypertension, organization of the thrombus and tortuous collaterals [2]. The incidence in the general population is approximately 1% [2] while it is up to 26% in some risk groups [3]. In some countries the prevalence is not well defined due its rarity and initially asymptomatic nature [4].

There are differences in etiological and clinical presentations between children and adults [1]. In adults, liver cirrhosis play a leading role, hypercoagulability and intra-abdominal inflammatory conditions are the main causes of PVT not associated with cirrhosis. In children and adolescents, the main causes are direct injury of the vein and intra-abdominal infections. The natural history of PVT may range from asymptomatic to non-specific symptoms and acute massive haematemesis. In acute PVT, abdominal pain may be marked with abrupt variceal bleeding. Symptoms abate as collaterals develop and diagnosis may be missed. Patients with chronic PVT often present with clinical features of complication such as portal hypertension. Growth retardation may occur in children [1]. Diagnosis of PVT depends on imaging-studies including Doppler ultrasonography, computed tomography (CT), magnetic resonance imaging (MRI), and portography. A variety of treatment could be administered, which include anticoagulation, portal venography with infusion of streptokinase or urokinase and open surgical thrombectomy.

The prognosis of PVT depends on the aetiology. However, it is much better in children than in adults because of low incidence of malignancy and cirrhosis and a 10 year survival rate of 70% in them [1]. Portal vein thrombosis is an infrequent diagnosis in children and adolescent nevertheless it is an important cause of upper gastrointestinal (UGI) bleeding in children [5]. We hereby present a case of PVT in an adolescent.

2. PRESENTATION OF CASE

A 15 year-old girl was referred to the haematology clinic with 10 years history of recurrent haematemesis. Her body mass index was 27 kg/m^2. Patient was the only child and the father was late. Patient's first episode of haematemesis was at 5 years and was associated with abdominal pain. Thereafter, haematemesis became recurrent and were managed with ranitidine and gastric lavage. At 13 years, she had the worst episode of haematemesis, associated with haematochezia and melaena for 3 days during which she received 7 units of stored blood before being referred to our hospital for further management. This patient could not undergo endoscopy prior to presentation at our centre because, all along she was being managed at a secondary health centre where there was no endoscopic facility. At presentation at our centre, she was febrile with a temperature of 38°C. Peripheral blood film for malarial parasite was positive. Abdominal examination then revealed vague epigastric tenderness with mildly tender, soft liver and spleen, 2 and 4cm below coastal margin respectively confirmed by abdominal ultrasound. An urgent upper gastrointestinal (GI) endoscopy revealed multiple bleeding oesophageal varices occupying the entire diameter of the oesophagus. Diagnosis then was upper gastrointestinal bleeding (UGIB) from oesophageal varices secondary to portal hypertension probably due to chronic liver disease. She was managed with rabeprazole and mist magnesium trisilicate. Prothrombin time (PT) and activated partial thromboplastin time (aPTT) were 14 and 40 seconds for the patient with control result of 13 and 33 seconds respectively. The PT, INR was 1.1. Full blood count (FBC) revealed anaemia with haematocrit (hct) of 32% and platelet count of 55,000/mm3. Liver function test (LFT) result was: Total Bilirubin , 0.1mg/100ml; Conjugated bilirubin, 0.05/mg/100ml; Total protein, 7.9g/100ml; Albumin, 3.7/g/100ml; SGOT, 23u/L; SGPT, 20/u/L; ALP, 68u/L; blood urea, creatinine and electrolytes were within normal range. Oesophageal variceal band ligation was performed and platelet concentrate was transfused. She was also placed on propranolol for secondary prophylaxis. After discharge from hospital admission, FBC at follow up clinic showed hct of 44%, platelet count was 320 x 10^9/l, LFT, was normal, PT and aPTT results showed that PT,INR was 0.96 (test -13sec control 13.5), APTT (test,27 sec control,33sec). Screening for HIV, hepatitis B and C viruses were negative. Request for liver biopsy was declined. Hepatic venous pressure gradient was not done.

Because the abdominal ultrasound done did not reveal much information about the portal system, CT angiography of the portal vein was requested for as a secondary diagnostic test at 15 years during an episode of haematemesis, revealed intraluminal clots in the portal vein with its intrahepatic branches and portal hepatis as well as tortuosity of vessels in the region of the porta hepatis consistent with periportal collaterals (Fig. 1). Other test results were PC; 56% (70-140%), PS; 49% (60-140%) while antithrombin, homocysteine and fasting lipid profile were normal. Based on this, a diagnosis of portal vein thrombosis secondary to proteins C and S deficiencies was made and she was commenced on subcutaneous clexane which was later changed to dabigatran. So, our diagnosis was based on the finding of clots in the portal vein on angiography which was probably secondary to the deficiency of proteins C and S. This diagnosis is a form of non-cirrhotic portal hypertension because, the liver in this patient was normal. Abdominal Ultrasound after one year of dabigatran showed overall appearance in keeping with chronic portal vein thrombosis with development of collaterals at the portal hepatis (Fig. 2).

Follow up endoscopy showed post oesophageal variceal ligation scars. Patient has not had any episode of haematemesis since the commencement of anticoagulation. Surgical modalities of treating this condition include splenectomy, splenic artery ligation and azygoportal disconnection. But, none of these was offered to the index patient since she has responded to the medical treatment offered so far.

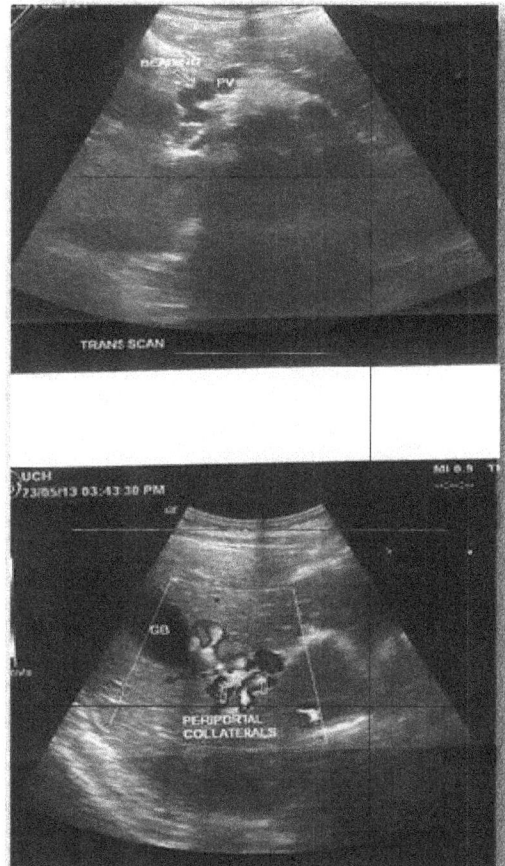

Fig. 1. Abdominal ultrasound report before anticoagulation

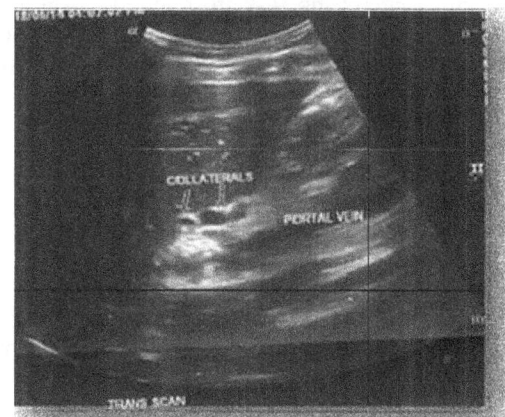

Fig. 2. Abdominal ultrasound report one year after anticoagulation

3. DISCUSSION

Thromboembolic disorder is uncommon in children and adolescent (0-18 years) [6]. This is because of age related reduction in thrombin generation and increased ability to inhibit thrombin [7]. Unlike in adults, the diagnosis of both spontaneous and risk related thromboembolic complications such as portal vein thrombosis is rare. When thromboembolic event occurs, it is often seen in hospitalized sick children with cancer, prolonged immobilization, cardiovascular surgery and venous cather insertion [8]. The observation of a thromboembolic event, diagnosed as portal vein thrombosis in our patient who was healthy is unusual. Protein C (PC) and protein S (PS) are natural anticoagulants that regulate the coagulation cascade through the selective inactivation of Factors Va and VIIIa. The principal mode of presentation of patients deficient in proteins C and S is with deep vein thrombosis and pulmonary embolism [9]. Portal vein thrombosis (PVT) as seen in our patient is uncommon. More so, this is an infrequent diagnosis in children and adolescent hence, the reason for delayed diagnosis in our patient. When acute portal vein thrombosis goes unrecognized, symptoms resolve and collateral vessels develop to progress to portal hypertension with varices which is not a desirable outcome. Clinical diagnosis is challenging due to the non-specific nature of its signs and symptoms [10]. Even though, doppler ultrasound is considered to be effective as first line diagnostic test, this was not so in our patient in whom the first doppler ultrasound performed at the age of 13 years did not detect portal vein thrombosis. This might be because the sensitivity and specificity of the test are dependent on the expertise of attending radiologist. Also, the presence of a detectable flow through a partially occluded portal vein may contribute to misdiagnosis [1].

Another source of confusion was the thrombocytopenia at presentation which was probably due to haemodilution as result of multiple blood transfusions she received or as a result of platelet consumption due to the thrombosis [10,11]. The presence of splenomegaly at the time of thrombosis might have also contributed to the thrombocytopenia [1,6]. The low suspicion of PVT in our patient could also be explained by the scarcity of reports and rarity of this condition, particularly in an African population. There is no doubt a high index of suspicion for thromboembolism is required for timely diagnosis. Bleeding oesophageal varices due to PVT in the absence of liver disease is rare with a different clinical course and management strategy [10]. A differential diagnosis to consider in this patient is noncirrhotic portal hypertension (NCPH)/idiopathic portal hypertension (IPH) which is common in developing countries. The aetiopathogenesis of NCPH/IPH includes infections, immunological abnormalities, exposure to arsenic and drugs [12]. Patients with IPH have been reported to have higher incidence of protein C and S deficiencies or factor V Leiden mutations Similar to our patient, the patients with IPH often present with more than one episode of well tolerated haematemesis but in contrast to our patient, massive splenomegaly with anemia is characteristic in IPH [12]. The association of abdominal pain with the sudden onset of upper gastrointestinal bleeding and negative viral serology may further support the diagnosis of PVT. The clinical feature of PVT could be ill-defined [11] hence, the diagnostic dilemma and eventual detection of portal vein thrombosis with low levels of PC and PS after several years of haematemesis in the index case. The age of our patient and duration of symptoms are suggestive of inherited rather than acquired aetiology of PC /PS deficiencies particularly as the LFT were normal [13]. However, the inherited aetiology could not be substantiated because family study was not carried out. But, it appears the patient had recurrent acute thrombosis on a chronic portal vein thrombosis. Acquired deficiencies of these proteins can occur with oral anticoagulants, liver disease, renal disease, disseminated intravascular coagulopathy, pregnancy and certain hormonal therapy [14]. These conditions were not evident from the clinical and laboratory findings in our patient. Hereditary thrombophilia contribute substantially to the development of VTE in the young particularly when the VTE is unprovoked [14] besides coinheritance of prothrombotic factors is not uncommon [13] and this increases the risk of primary VTE considerably. Therefore, combined deficiency of both PC and PS might be responsible for the early presentation as well as the severe symptoms observed in our patient [13,15,].

Reports on combined deficiency of PC and PS resulting in portal hypertension from PVT are few and in non-Africans [16,17]. Pooled prevalence of PC deficiency in portal vein thrombosis is 5.6% while that of PS is 2.6% [18]. The risk of recurrent VTE in children is highest in those with combined prothrombotic risk factors [19] as demonstrated in our patient by the recurrent haematemesis. The implication of this risk of recurrent thrombosis is that she will require lifelong anticoagulation. This patient was probably having acute on chronic PVT given the clinical presentation.

Rate of recanalization is poor if anticoagulant is not instituted early as observed in our patient [20]. Therapeutic options in chronic PVT are controversial and vary significantly. These include endotherapy (endoscopic band ligation or sclerotherapy) and shunt surgery [21]. Splenectomy could also be performed. Patients with chronic portal vein thrombosis with ongoing thrombotic risk factors will require treatment with long-term anticoagulation [22,3].Early diagnosis is paramount, because early treatment could encourage recanalization. Also most of the pathological changes of PVT are irreversible and prophylactic measures would minimize the risk of complications such as hepatic dysfunction and ascites.

4. CONCLUSION

This case represents an unusual scenario of recurrent haematemsis from childhood to adolescence due to portal vein thrombosis and protein C and S deficiencies in an adolescent. It also illustrates one of the consequences of delayed diagnosis and institution of anticoagulant. This report is aimed to increase physician's index of suspicioon of the potential role of prothrombotic factors in the aetiology of portal vein thrombosis in children and adolescent patients with upper GIT bleeding particularly when it becomes recurrent. It should be considered in clinical practice for early intervention.

CONSENT

Consent was obtained from patient and mother for publication of this case report.

ETHICAL APPROVAL

It is not applicable.

COMPETING INTERESTS

Authors have declared that no competing interests exist.

REFERENCES

1. Wang JT, Zhao HY, Liu YL. Portal vein thrombosis. Hepatobiliary Pancreat Dis Int. 2005,4(4):515-518.
2. Ogren M, Bergqvist D, Bjorck M, Acosta S, Eriksson H, Sternby NH. Portal vein thrombosis: Prevalence, patient characteristics and lifetime risk: A population study based on 23,796 consecutive autopsies. World J Gastroenterol. 2006;12:2115-2119.
3. Manzano-Robleda MC, Barranco-Fragoso B, Uribe M, Méndez-Sánchez N. Portal vein thrombosis: What is new? Ann Hepatol. 2015;14(1):20-7.
4. Lertpipopmetha K, Auewarakul CU. High incidence of hepatitis B infection-associated cirrhosis and hepatocellular carcinoma in the southeast Asian patients with portal vein thrombosis. BMC Gastroenterol. 2011;11:66-74. DOI:10.1186/1471-230X-11-66
5. Rajoriya N, Tripathi D. Historical overview and review of current day treatment in the management of acute variceal bleeding. WJG. 2014;20(21):6481-94.
6. Ferri PM, Ferreira AR, Fagundes EDT, Liu SM, Roquete MLV, Penna FJ. Portal vein thrombosis in children and adolescents: 20 years experience of a pediatric hepatology. Arq Gastroenterol (Paediatric Gastroenterology). 2012;49(1):69-76.
7. Van Ommen CH, Peters M. Venous thromboembolic disease in childhood. Semin Thromb Hemost. 2003;29(4):391-404.
8. Parasuraman S, Goldhaber SZ. Venous thromboembolism in children. Circulation. 2006;113: e12-e16.
9. Gerotziafas GT. Risk factors for venous thromboembolism in children. Int Angiol. 2004;23(3):195-205.
10. Sheen CL, Lamparelli H, Milne A, Green I, Ramage JK. Clinical features, diagnosis and outcome of acute portal vein thrombosis. QJM. 2000;93(8):531-4.
11. Erkan O, Bozdayi AM, Disibayaz S, Oguz D, Ozcan M, Bahar K, et al. Thrombophilic gene mutations in cirrhotic patients with portal vein thrombosis. Eur J. Gastroenterol Hepatol. 2005;17(3):339-43.
12. Rajekar H, Vasishta RK, Chawla YK, Dhiman RK. Noncirrhotic portal hypertension. J Clin Exp Hepatol. 2011;1(2):94-108.

13. Fisher NC, Wilde JT, Roper J, Elias E. Deficiency of natural anticoagulant proteins C, S and antithrombin in portal vein thrombosis: A secondary phenomenon? Gut. 2000;46(4):534-9.

14. Weingarz L, Schwonberg J, Schindewolf M, Hecking C, Wolf Z, Erbe M, Weber A, Lindhoff-Loff E, Linnemann B. Prevalence of thrombophilia according to age at the first manifestation of venous thromboembolism: Results from the MAISTHRO registry. Br J. Haematol. 2013;163(5):655-65.
DOI: 10.1111/bjh. 12575. Epub 2013 Oct 8.

15. Salmon O, Steinberg DM, Zivelin A, et al. Single and combined prothrombotic factors in patients with idiopathic venous thromboembolism – prevalence and risk assessment. Arteriol Thromb Vasc Biol. 1999;19:511-18.

16. Hwang S, Kim do Y, Kim M, Chon YE, Lee HJ, Park YN, Park JY, Ahn SH, Han KH, Chon CY. Deficiencies in proteins C and S in a patient with idiopathic portal hypertension accompanied by portal vein thrombosis. Korean J Hepatol. 2010; 16(2):176-81.

17. Rodriguez-Leal GA, Moran S, Corona-Cedillo R, Brom-Valladares R. Portal vein thrombosis with protein C-S deficiency in a non-cirrhotic patient. World J Hepatol 2014;6(7):532-7.

18. Qi X, De Stefano V, Wang J, Bai M, Yang Z, Han G, Fan D. Prevalence of inherited antithrombin, protein C, and protein S deficiencies in portal vein system thrombosis and Budd-Chiari syndrome: A systematic review and meta-analysis of observational studies. J Gastroenterol Hepatol. 2013;28(3):432-42.

19. Nowak-Gottl U, Junker R, Kreuz W, von Eckardstein A, Kosch A, Nohe N, Schobess R, Ehrenforth S. (The Childhood Thrombophilia Study Group). Risk of recurrent venous thrombosis in children with combined prothrombotic risk factors. Blood. 2001;97(4):858-62.

20. Turnes J, Garcıa-Pagán JC, Gonzalez M, et al. Portal hypertension-related complications after acute portal vein thrombosis: Impact of early anticoagulation. Clin Gastroenterol Hepatol. 2008;6:1412-7.

21. Chawla Y, Duseja A, Dhiman RK. Review article: The modern management of portal vein thrombosis. Aliment Pharmacol Ther. 2009;30:881-894.

22. Confer BD, Hanouneh I, Gomes M, Chadi Alraies M. Is anticoagulant appropriate for all patients with portal vein thrombosis? CCJM. 2013;80(10):611-613.

28

Epidemiological and Biological Parameters of Monoclonal Plasma Cell Dyscrasias in Thirty One Patients Consulting a Moroccan Pasteur Institute

Ilham Zahir[1*] and Abderahman Bellik[2]

[1]Department of Biology, Faculty of Sciences and Technical, University Sidi Mohamed Ben Abdellah, BP 2202, Road of Immouzer, Fez, Morocco.
[2]Department of Biology, Laboratory of Immunochemistry, Pasteur institute, Casablanca, Morocco.

Authors' contributions

This work was carried out in collaboration between both authors. Author IZ designed the study, collected the data, interpreted results and wrote the first draft of the manuscript. Author AB planned the study, supervised the work and critically revised the manuscript for important intellectual content. Both authors read and approved the final manuscript.

Editor(s):
(1) Ricardo Forastiero, Department of Hematology, Favaloro University, Argentina.
(2) Anamika Dhyani, Laboratory of Biochemistry & Molecular and Cellular Biology Hemocentro-UNICAMP, Brazil.
(3) Dharmesh Chandra Sharma, Incharge Blood Component and Aphaeresis Unit, G. R. Medical College, Gwalior, India.
Reviewers:
(1) Anonymous, Brazil.
(2) Anonymous, Bulgaria.
(3) Anonymous, Nigeria.

ABSTRACT

Aims: To describe epidemiological and biological features of patients with monoclonal plasma cell dyscrasias. The patients were seen at the Moroccan Pasteur Institute in Casablanca during a period of two years and four months.
Place and Duration of Study: Laboratory of immunochemistry, Pasteur institute, Casablanca, Morocco. From April 2006 to July 2006.
Methodology: Thirty one case notes of patients who had a serum or urine monoclonal gamma or beta globulin spike were assessed.
Results: The mean age of the patients was 54.7 ± 10.7 years (range, 26–72 years) and there were more females with a sex ratio 0.82. 66.7% of the patients had a monoclonal gamma globulin peak revealed by electrophoresis. According the results of performed agar gel immuno-electrophoresis,

*Corresponding author: E-mail: ilham_biologie@hotmail.fr

48% of them had monoclonal immunoglobulin G (IgG) antibodies, followed by class IgA with 29% of cases. Moreover, 55% of the patients were Kappa-chain positive, while 45% were Lambda-chain positive. Assessment of prognostic factors of some patients demonstrated an increased erythrocyte serum rate (66.7% of cases), anemia (50% of cases), a raised of calcium serum levels (37.5% of cases) and β2-microglobulin serum levels were higher than 3.5 mg/l (33.3% of cases). In addition, the mean concentration of proteins was 91 g/l (58.6% of cases), low levels of albumin below 36 g/l were observed (63% of cases) and the monoclonal component levels were above 30 g/l (55.6% of cases).

Conclusion: Some of our records were different from those of other series: our patients were younger with a slight predominance of female individuals. Others were consistent mainly with the more frequently observed monoclonal gamma-globulin peak, and also with the assessed levels of IgG, which is known as the most common isotype in plasma cell disorders. On the other hand, a rise of prognostic factors levels was also noted except for C-reactive protein. Nevertheless, our study pointed out that the majority of patients didn't have a rigorous monitoring of their disorders by carrying out hematological and serological examinations.

Keywords: Plasma cell dyscrasias; electrophoresis; immuno-electrophoresis; prognostic factors.

ABBREVIATIONS

PCD: Plasma Cell Dyscrasias, MM: Multiple Myeloma, WM: Waldenström Macroglobulinemia, MGUS: Monoclonal Gammopathy of Undetermined Significance, CLL: Chronic Lymphocytic Leukemia CRP: C-reactive protein, Ig: Immunoglobulin, β2-m: beta-2-microglobulin.

1. INTRODUCTION

Plasma cell dyscrasias (PCDs) are a variety of disorders characterized by monoclonal proliferation and accumulation of lymphoplasmacytic cells in the bone marrow and, sometimes, with a tissue deposition of monoclonal immunoglobulins or their components [1]. These disorders include a wide range of hematological conditions ranging from benign disorders such as monoclonal gammopathy of undetermined significance (MGUS) to malignant pathologies for example, multiple myeloma (MM), smoldering multiple myeloma (SMM), Waldenström macroglobulinemia (WM), amyloid light-chain (AL) amyloidosis, POEMS syndrome, non-Hodgkin lymphoma (NHL) and B-cell chronic lymphocytic leukemia (B-CLL) [1-3].

These diseases may be difficult to diagnose because they affect many tissues and exhibit generally non-specific symptoms [4]. Thus, the bases of the diagnosis are the presence of bone marrow plasmacytosis and the detection of an abnormal monoclonal paraprotein in the serum and/or urine, by means of electrophoresis and immuno-electrophoresis [2]. Since then, the definitive diagnoses of PCDs require a multidisciplinary approach including clinical assessment, radiology and clinical laboratory assays [4]. Furthermore, plasma cell labeling index, karyotypic abnormalities molecular alterations, analysis of beta-2-microglobulin and C-reactive protein levels are laboratory prognostic parameters, related to the intrinsic malignancy of the plasma cells, which indicate the risk of transformation from benign to malignant forms, and, therefore designate the follow-up and treatment of each individual patient [5].

In the current retrospective study, we reviewed the epidemiological and biological features of patients with plasma cell dyscrasias, established during the period between January 2004 and April 2006 in the Moroccan Pasteur Institute (Casablanca).

2. MATERIALS AND METHODS

2.1 Study Location and Patients

This retrospective study was conducted at Pasteur Institute, Casablanca, Morocco, by reviewing case notes of patients consulting immunochemistry laboratory during the period from 1 January 2004 to 30 April 2006.

This laboratory received requests for urine or serum protein electrophoresis and immuno-electrophoresis for various diseases: myeloma, immune deficiencies, hepatic insufficiency, systemic diseases and rheumatology, etc.

One of the first steps in the laboratory evaluation of a patient with a suspected PCD has been electrophoresis of serum or urine. Thus, only patients who had a gamma or beta (rarely alpha 2) monoclonal peak and a monoclonal immunoglobulin demonstrated by urine or serum protein electrophoresis and immuno-electrophoresis, respectively, were retained.

During the period of study, 1758 electrophoreses and 99 immuno-electrophoreses were gathered.

Any double immuno-electrophoresis or non-coupled to electrophoresis was excluded. Thus, our population was limited to 31 patients. Their distribution was done by taking in consideration the age, sex, nature of spike, as well as the type of immunoglobulin heavy and light chains.

Moreover, to detect whether patients had followed-up the evolution of their diseases, some prognostic factors were also evaluated such as erythrocyte sedimentation rate (ESR), C-reactive protein (CRP), serum levels of calcium, $\beta2$-microglobulin ($\beta2$-m), hemoglobin and some other proteins.

It should be noted that bone marrow biopsies were performed in the clinic that sent the patients' sera for testing in the laboratory. We didn't get the results of these analyses.

Statistical analysis was performed by calculation of percentages and arithmetic averages.

3. RESULTS

Our current investigation was a retrospective study that included 31 Moroccan patients having a risk to develop plasma cell dyscrasias consulting Pasteur Institute, Casablanca, between January 2004 and April 2006.

Detailed epidemiological and clinical characteristics of 31 patients are shown in Table 1.

3.1 Epidemiological Data

The mean age was 54.7±10.7 years with extremes ranging from 26 to 72 years. Fifty-five percent of the patients were female and forty-five were male with a sex ratio 0.82.

The two third of our study population were located in the range between 40 and 60 years with equality of reaching for both sexes. However, a female predominance in patients over 60 years was observed. It's noteworthy to mention that the data about the age of one patient had not been found.

3.2 Immunochemical Data

According to the electrophoresis results, 66.7% of patients had a gamma-globulin monoclonal peak, against 33.3% had a monoclonal peak in beta-globulin zone.

The data from immuno-electrophoresis confirmed that the tested population in the current study had a monoclonal band in serum. In fact, we found that immunoglobulin G monoclonal antibody (Ig G) was placed in the forefront. It was observed in 15 patients (48%), Ig A was found in the second place with 9 cases (29%) followed by 4 patients (13%), who had free light-chains and 3 patients (10%) had Ig M, while in none of them Ig D and Ig E were detected (Fig. 1).

Besides that, 17 of the patients (55%) were Kappa-chain positive and 14 (45%) were Lambda-chain positive.

3.3 Biological Data

In some patients, prognostic factors as ESR, CRP, serum levels of calcium, $\beta2$-microglobulin, hemoglobin and other proteins, were also taken in consideration. According the data in Table 2, the majority of patients didn't follow-up the progression of their malignant disorders by biological tests.

Nevertheless, patients requesting for these analyzes demonstrated an elevation of ESR (66.7% of cases), anemia (50% of cases), a raised of serum level of calcium (37.5% of cases) and $\beta2$-microglobulin serum level was greater than 3.5 mg/l (33.3% of cases). Moreover, the mean concentration of proteins was 91 g/l ranged in values varying from 58 to 121 g/l (normal values of serum proteins are between 60 and 80 g/l). It was noted that serum protein electrophoresis had been performed only for 29 patients, while the others had urine electrophoresis. Thus, we found that 58.6% of patients had a hyperproteinemia against 38% having normal levels of serum proteins, whereas 3.4% of cases having a hypoproteinemia, corresponding to a patient with a monoclonal light Lambda chain.

Table 1. Epidemiological and clinical characteristics of 31 patients

P	A	S	Type of protein ep and iep	M. Ig type	Proteins Level (g/l)	Protein fractions levels (g/L): Al	A1	A2	B	G	ESR (mm): FH	SH	CRP (mg/l)	Levels of: Hg (g/dl)	ß2m (mg/l)	Ca (mmol/l)
1	45	M	ser prot	IgM/K	90	33.12	3.96	8.82	29.52	14.58	NP	NP	NP	NP	NP	NP
2	55	M	ser prot	IgG/L	80	40.64	2.65	10.08	11.84	14.88	10	22	<6	14.6	1.56	2.35
3	60	F	ser prot	IgM/K	110	41.25	2.86	8.8	8.47	48.62	NP	NP	NP	NP	1.31	NP
4	46	F	ur prot	LLC	0.4	-	-	-	-	-	NP	NP	NP	NP	NP	NP
5	57	M	ser prot	IgA/K	76	37.012	2.356	7.524	23.408	5.7	NP	NP	NP	NP	NP	NP
6	59	F	ser prot	IgG/K	106	NF	NF	NF	NF	NF	NP	NP	NP	NP	NP	NP
7	50	F	ser prot	IgG/L	84	38,163	2.772	9.072	8.148	25.878	64	105	NP	12.8	1.05	2.24
8	71	M	ser prot	IgG/L	80	23.2	4.16	14.88	3.68	34.08	NP	NP	NP	NP	NP	NP
9	56	F	ser prot	IgG/L	84	39.06	2.856	9.576	8.232	24.276	26	54	NP	11.6	NP	NP
10	61	F	ser prot	IgG/L	120	30.72	2.4	6.96	5.28	74.64	NP	NP	NP	NP	NP	NP
11	NF	M	ser prot	IgG/L	120	34.92	2.88	7.56	6.96	67.68	NP	NP	NP	NP	NP	NP
12	52	M	ur prot	IgG/K	2	-	-	-	-	-	NP	NP	NP	NP	NP	NP
13	56	M	ser prot	IgG/L	80	36.24	3.12	12.88	13.04	14.72	8	18	<6	11.5	1.56	2.3
14	50	F	ser prot	IgA/K	116	29	1.6	5.68	3.9	74	NP	NP	NP	NP	7.76	NP
15	63	F	ser prot	LLC	72	36.43	3.24	12.96	11.304	8.064	NP	NP	<6	12.4	NP	2.54
16	72	F	ur prot	KLC	1.85	-	-	-	-	-	NP	NP	NP	NP	NP	NP
17	49	M	ser prot	KLC	70	35.42	3.08	13.44	9.31	8.75	42	80	<6	NP	14.16	NP
18	67	F	ser prot	IgG/K	94	36.472	3.478	10.81	9.776	33.464	NP	NP	NP	NP	NP	NP
19	71	M	ser prot	IgA/L	120	29.64	3.12	4.44	80.04	2.76	NP	NP	NP	7.9	7.98	NP
20	54	F	ser prot	LLC	58	32.712	3.306	7.424	9.744	4.814	NP	NP	NP	NP	NP	NP
21	45	M	ser prot	IgA/K	110	26.29	2.09	7.04	9.13	65.45	NP	NP	NP	6.4	2.25	NP
22	66	F	ser prot	IgA/L	90	41.58	3.42	10.89	9.45	24.66	NP	NP	NP	NP	NP	NP
23	30	F	ser prot	IgM/K	74	30.118	2.738	7.844	19.092	14.208	NP	NP	NP	10.8	NP	NP
24	58	M	ser prot	IgG/K	102	31.212	2.652	6.834	8.772	52.53	NP	NP	NP	10.8	NP	NP
25	45	F	ser prot	IgG/K	80	31.28	4.08	9.2	8.72	26.72	81	115	NP	9.6	NP	NP
26	51	F	ser prot	IgA/K	72	37.152	2.52	7.92	9	15.408	105	132	NP	12.3	1.05	2.24
27	59	M	ser prot	IgG/L	74	33.152	2.738	9.102	8.51	20.498	64	105	NP	NP	6.77	2.65
28	44	F	ser prot	IgA/K	96	35.424	2.016	6.528	49.344	2.688	NP	NP	NP	NP	NP	2.92
29	57	M	ser prot	IgG/K	106	29.468	3.922	12.508	6.996	53.106	NP	NP	<6	14.2	NP	2.35
30	66	F	ser prot	IgA/K	70	30.87	4.2	12.11	9.94	12.88	10	22	NP	NP	1.56	NP
31	26	M	ser prot	IgA/K	84	33.768	2.268	8.4	31.08	8.484	NP	NP	NP	NP	1.07	NP
				IgA/K	121	NF	NF	NF	NF	NF	NF	NF				

P: patient; A: age; S: sex; Ep: electrophoresis; IEP: immuno- electrophoresis; M: monoclonal; Ig: immunoglobulin; Al: albumin; A1: alpha 1; A2: alpha 2; B: beta; G: gamma; ESR: Erythrocyte sedimentation rate; FH: first hour; SH: second hour; CRP: C-reactive protein; Hg: Hemoglobin; ß2m: ß2-microglobulin; Ca: serum calcium; Ser prot: serum protein; Ur prot: urine protein; M: male; F: female; K: kappa; L: Lambda; LLC: Lambda light chain; KLC: Kappa light chain; NP: not performed; NF: not found

Table 2. Number and percentage of patients requesting for prognostic analyzes

Prognosis factor	Erythrocyte serum rate	CRP	Level of:		
			Calcium	β2-microglobulin	Hemoglobin
Number of patients who requested for each analysis divided by total number of the studied population (%)	9/31 (29%)	5/31 (16.1%)	8/31 (25.8%)	12/31 (38.7%)	12/31 (38.7%)
Number of patients having anomalies in analysis divided by number of patients requesting for prognostic factors (%).	6/9 (66.7%)	0/5 (0%)	3/8 (37.5%)	4/12 (33.3%)	6/12 (50%)

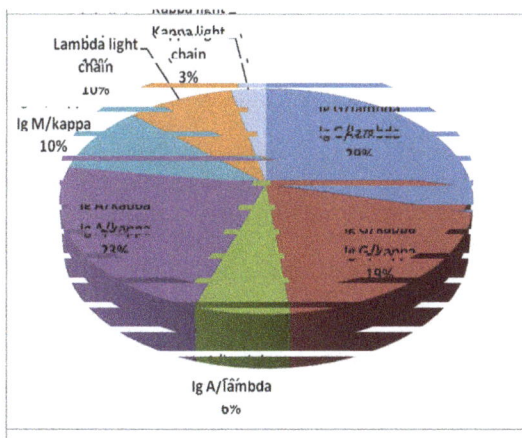

Fig. 1. Percentage of different immunoglobulin subtypes of monoclonal plasmaproliferative disorders (n=31)

With respect to the spike size, 44.4% of the cases were below 30 g/l, and 55.6% above 30 g/l, respectively. The mean concentration of the monoclonal component was 37 g/l.

On the other hand, the average level of albumin was 33.86 g/l with extremes ranging from 23.2 g/l and 41.58 g/l.

In seventeen patients (63%) having low levels of albumin, 15 patients had higher serum monoclonal protein levels. The remaining two patients had normal concentrations of beta- or gamma- globulin fractions, which were probably associated with light chain PCD. However, there was a moderate negative correlation between low levels of albumin and higher serum monoclonal protein concentrations (Pearson's correlation, r = -0.37, n = 17, p=0.12).

4. DISCUSSION

The presented investigation was the first study conducted in 2006 at Pasteur Institute in Casablanca (Morocco) aimed to highlight the epidemiological and biological features of thirty one patients having a risk to develop plasma cell dyscrasias.

Few years later, many studies, performed in Morocco and other countries, were directed to the same target. Some of the results from those investigations were consistent with our data, but others were different. In fact, our patients were younger (54.7 years), in comparison with the data, which were reported by other surveys. Beginning with a Moroccan investigation which had been executed in Mohamed V Military Hospital of Rabat [6], the mean age was 60.21 years. In other countries, the average age was a bit closer to that found by Moroccan institutions. For instance, in India [7], Egypt [1], Tunisia [8] Lebanon [9] and Saudi Arabia [10], it was 56, 58.5, 62.7, 65 and 65.6 years, respectively. However, it was much higher in Western nations especially in Iceland [11], Spain [12] and France [13], with mean ages of 70, 73 and 79 years, respectively. The observed differences in mean ages of patients with PCD between Eastern and Western nations, may be due to the quality of life, health services and medical scientific researches, which are different in the developed and underdeveloped countries.

Besides that, our outcomes had demonstrated that 93.3% of our patients were above 40 years old, but it was important to underline that only two patients were 26 and 30 years. These results were corroborated with the study by Kassem et al. [1], who showed that 96% of patients having PCD were the older age group. This confirmed some literature data [1,4,7,14,15], according which PCDs as MM and MGUS are diseases of older adults.

Similarly the results of other studies showed that the prevalence of PCD increased with the age [1,7,13,15-17]. Nevertheless, the main difference between the cited and our data was that we noted a slight predominance of female individuals with a sex ratio 0.82 and an equality of reaching for both sexes in patients aged between 40 and 60 years, meanwhile, other authors found that men were affected more frequently than women by PCD with different sex ratios 1.08 [11], 1.2 [13,18], 1.24 [9], 1.43 [1,10], 1.71 [8], 1.94 [14] and 2.3 [6], respectively. The established predominance in female individuals can be explained by the eventual influence of geographical distribution of Casablanca population, which was presented by 50.7% of females and 49.3% of males according to 2005 and 2006 statistics performed in Casablanca [19].

On the other hand, the most frequent type of immunoglobulin in the current study was IgG. It was found in 48% of patients, followed by Ig A (29%), monoclonal light chains (13%), and the isotype Ig M (10%) which came in the last place. This distribution coincided with that reported by the clinical oncology department of Cairo University (Egypt) [1], not in point of view the percentage, but the order. In the latter inquiry, 63.6% of the patients were assessed with prevalence of IgG against 17.5% of IgA, while 13.4% had monoclonal light-chains and 5.5% had an Ig M monoclonal band. Nonetheless, our findings were not in concord with those reported by French studies [13]. Effectively, the first investigation was led in internal medicine department of Rennes university hospital [13], which revealed that isotypes repartition was: Ig G (42.8%), Ig M (31.9%), Ig A (8.9%), biclonal gammopathy (9.8%) and monoclonal light chains (6.6%), respectively. Whereas, the second research, conducted in all the department s of General Hospital of Blois [13], showed that this distribution was Ig G (59.7%), Ig M (27.5%), Ig A (11.8%) and monoclonal light chains (2.7%), respectively. In contrast, no monoclonal light chain was detected in an Indian investigation [18], while in Singh et al. survey [7], no IgM type paraprotein was observed.

Moreover, electrophoresis showed a monoclonal peak in gamma globulin fraction in 66.7% of the

patients. Our current findings were in agreement with those previously reported [8,18,20], outlining a monoclonal spike in the gamma zone in 78%, 84.8% and 85.5% of cases, respectively. These observations could be explained by the fact that the gamma fraction contains the largest portion of immunoglobulins. Therefore, PCDs are the most frequently encountered in this portion of the electrophoresis. Additionally, since most IgG monoclonal proteins are cationic, they migrate to the gamma zone of the electrophoretic gel [21]. This statement may justify the predominance of the isotype IgG in all the studies, discussed above.

In addition, the association of IgG with the lambda light chain was established in 29% of cases. In the opposite, the study of Dasse et al. [22] conducted in Abidjan (Ivory Coast), indicated that the association Ig G/kappa was the most found monoclonal form in 60% of cases.

Alternatively, analysis of the association between heavy and light chains revealed that kappa light chain was more linked than was lambda light chain (55% against 45%, respectively). This statement joined the outcomes of many researches [1,7,20,22].

In this series of 31 patients, all the detected heavy chains were associated to light chains (intact immunoglobulin). This result was compatible with the data presented by Dasse et al. [22]. Nevertheless, the presence of immunoglobulin free light chains had been proven in 13% of cases.

With respect to biological tests, the hyperproteinemia touched 58.6% of our patients. A similar result was obtained from the study of Gaougaou et al. [23], in which increased serum protein levels in 63% of the cases with MM have been noticed. It was pointed out that PCDs were not always related with hyperproteinemia. Indeed, cases of PCD, presented in the current investigation, indicated free light chains with normal or low levels (hypoproteinemia) of serum proteins. A similar finding was described in another study [21] reporting that the mean serum total protein concentration was significantly higher in IgG, IgA, and IgM, compared with free light chain PCDs, where this value was within normal limits. This could be explained by the effect of low molecular weight of the light-chain secreted by malignant plasma cells about 22500 Dalton versus 40000 to 70000 Dalton, which shows the variation of molecular weight of the heavy chains. It was important to mention that 17 of 21 patients (80.9%), having total protein level above or equals to 80 g/l, had monoclonal paraprotein concentration above 20 g/l. There was a strong positive relationship between total protein level and monoclonal paraprotein concentration (Pearson's correlation, r = 0.712, n = 21, P<0.001). As was previously reported, in a study, performed by van Hoeven et al. [21], monoclonal proteins often increase serum total protein level. In fact, it was found that paraprotein levels were reflected in significantly increased mean serum total protein in IgG, IgA, and IgM [21].

An increase in β2-micro-globulin levels in 33.3% of cases was as well noted. It has already been reported that this molecule is a small membrane protein, associated with the heavy chains of class I major histocompatibility complex proteins. It's a powerful prognostic factor, correlating with the survival in monoclonal disorders [24]. Indeed, according to the results of Di Giovanni et al. [25], in the group of patients suffering from MM or WM, the mean level of the same protein has been assessed to be significantly higher than in the group with MGUS. Values above 3 mg/L were highly indicative of a neoplastic process. They were observed in all the WM patients and in greater than 90% of myeloma patients. It was noticed, in the current study, that the patients having β2-m concentrations above 5.5 mg/l, had albumin levels below or equals to 35 g/l. This finding is in keeping with a previous investigation [26], demonstrating that serum β2m values had a negative correlation with serum albumin. However, there was a weak negative correlation between albumin and β2-m serum levels (Pearson's correlation, r = -0.34, n = 12, P = 0.309). This, maybe, was due to the small number of patients carrying out the biological test β2-m. Therefore, the current data should be proven by investigating the involvement of both β2-m and albumin serum levels in PCD in a large-scale of Moroccan patients. In this series, patients had as well serum levels of monoclonal protein above 30 g/l except for one patients suffering from kappa light chain PCD. There was a strong positive association between monoclonal component (MC) above 30 g/l and serum β2m levels (Pearson's correlation, r = 0.703, n=5).Our data were in concordance with those recorded by Charafeddine et al. [9], demonstrating that β2-m levels were related to spike size. This correlation could be explained by the fact that β2-m reflects the tumor mass [24], which is detected by hyperproteinemia due to the elevation of serum monoclonal protein in beta- or gamma- globulin zone. In contrary, normal or low (hypoproteinemia) levels of proteins were associated with normal concentrations of beta- or gamma- globulin fractions in patients suffering from light chain PCD, but presenting high levels of β2-m. This result joined that reported by Charafeddine et al. [9], finding that most of the patients, diagnosed with light chain PCD had a spike size below or equals to 20 g/l.

In assessment of serum calcium levels, according to the results of the current study 37.5% of patients had hyper-calcemia, leading to an increased risk of bone lesions and collapse of the vertebral. This was supported by the deduction reached by Pagano et al. [27], who noted that 27% of patients suffering from plasma cell leukemia had an elevation in serum calcium level. Hyper-calcemia is one of the important factors besides renal insufficiency, anemia, and lytic bone lesions (CRAB criteria), that can distinguish between MM and MGUS [1,28,29], since patients with the pre-malignant plasmatic cell disorder are known by absence of hyper-calcemia [20]. However, because MGUS is a condition of the elderly, concomitant diseases can confound the distinction [30]. For instance, hypercalcemia may be caused by hyperparathyroidism that should be considered in the absence of skeletal lesions [30]. It was also made out in the current investigation that the patients with hyper-calcemia had high values of β2-m serum concentrations, albumin levels below or equals to 35 g/l and serum levels of monoclonal protein above 30 g/l, with exception of one patient, suffering from kappa light chain PCD. Statically, there was a moderate negative correlation between albumin levels and calcium concentrations (Pearson's correlation, r = -0.48, n = 8, P = 0.226).

It was also established that the emergence of anemia was more thrust. It was perceived that 50% of patients had a drop in rate of hemoglobin which may reveal the impact of the plasma cell infiltration on the bone marrow production. In other surveys [7,27,18], anemia features were also detected, but only in 48%, 25%, and 7.2% of patients, respectively. It should be noticed that our six patients with anemia might not be affected by solitary plasmacytoma. In fact, the decrease of serum hemoglobin level isn't a criterion for this disease, which is also characterized by a low serum or urinary level of monoclonal immunoglobulin [31]. In contrast, these patients could have MM or WM, for which the anemia is a common complication [4]. In the current study, it was also observed that 4 of 6 patients with anemia had albumin levels below 35 g/l, but had variable levels of serum monoclonal paraprotein (below or above 30 g/l regardless of the immunoglobulin isotype). There was a moderate positive correlation between albumin levels and hemoglobin concentrations (Pearson's correlation, r = 0.606, n = 6). Various studies had demonstrated a positive correlation between hemoglobin and albumin levels in patients with PCD [9,17]. However, according to our investigation, these two factors might not be indicators of the increase of MC levels of non-IgM PCD. In fact, as was previously reported [20,30], anemia may be multi-factorial in the elderly. It could be caused by conditions, different from PCD, such as renal insufficiency, iron deficiency, nutritional imbalance, occult gastrointestinal bleeding, or, less frequently, myelodysplastic syndrome. On the other hand, our observation didn't corroborate with an investigation, performed by Charafeddine et al. [9], carried out in the clinical laboratory of the American University of Beirut Medical Center with 540 patients, in which low serum concentrations of hemoglobin and albumin showed significant correlation with high M spike size above 20 g/l. The difference between the two inquiries resides in the size of the population under study. Thus, our outcome should be confirmed or rejected after study the impact of prognostic factors in a large number of patients.

Furthermore, it was explored that 66.7% of our patients had a higher erythrocyte sedimentation rate (ESR). In others surveys, an elevation of this biological test was observed in all seven reported cases with plasma cell leukemia [32] and in 94.6%, 17.9%, 25.5% of patients with MM [23], MGUS and SMM [33], respectively. In the current investigation, whatever were the ESR levels, MC concentrations were lower than 30 g/L. Probably; there is no clear relationship between ESR levels and the size of MC in patients with PCD as was previously reported [33], suggesting variability in the interaction of individual MCs with red blood cells to create rouleaux formation [33]. Besides that, due to the small number of patients, we can't judge whether or not ERS is a prognostic factor for PCDs.

Unlike the study, performed by Salonen and Nikoskelainen [34], displaying elevated CRP levels in patients with hematological malignancies (around 152 mg/l), all our five patients had a normal CRP, a prognosis index, correlated with survival and activity of proliferative cells [24]. It is also an infection indicator as a cause of death in patients with PCDs [34]. Despite of this positive outcome, the majority of serological and hematological examinations allowing to patients to have a rigorous monitoring of their PCD, had not been carried out by all of them. Additionally, the differential diagnosis between different disorders may not be done. Effectively, findings of Ig M PCD, plasma cell proliferation on bone marrow biopsy and clinical findings consistent with myeloma (CRAB signs) classically distinguished the rare diagnosis of Ig M MM from the more common WM, characterized with a monoclonal Ig M and known by lymphadenopathy, organomegaly, lymphoplasmacytic lymphoma and hyper-viscosity (related to the absolute level and structure of the Ig M pentamer) [28]. Conversely, some patients may not have all of these findings. Both diseases could share clinical and biological manifestations such as hyper-viscosity, which may lead to diagnostic errors [28,35,36]. Recent advances in cytogenetic and immuno-phenotyping of bone marrow plasma cells can help further define the differences between IgM MM and WM [28,37]. Myeloma plasmatic cells lack CD19, CD45, and CD27 expressions and are positive for CD56 (75%), CD117 (30%), and CD20 (30%) according to the report of Rawstrom et al. [38], while in WM, clonal B-cells express CD19, CD20, CD45 [36]. In contrast to WM, MM is characterized by chromosome translocations, which include not only the t(11;14) but also the t(4;14) and t(14;16) located in the genes coding for immunoglobulin heavy chains [37].

Importantly, a definitive diagnostic allows the choice of the adequate treatment for each PCD by taking in consideration age, gender, race and family history.

Our study had several limitations: the laboratory data of the PCD cases were included without their clinical diagnosis (bone marrow biopsy results, radiological studies) and many factors affecting prognosis were not assessed in the univariate and multivariate analyses due to the limited number of patients. Moreover, the current study was Pasteur Institute based and thus cannot be generalized for the entire Moroccan population.

5. CONCLUSION

The purpose of the current study was to evaluate epidemiological and biological characteristics of patients with PCD, detected by the association of electrophoresis and immuno-electrophoresis. Our data were very similar to those reported by others investigations but slightly different in the aspect of mean age and sex ratio. It is also important to mention that biological tests weren't performed by all members of our cohort, probably because of financial constraints, that limit the opportunity for monitoring of their disorders progression and response to the respective treatment.

CONSENT

It is not applicable.

ETHICAL APPROVAL

Ethical committee of Pasteur Institute of Casablanca Morocco approved the study.

COMPETING INTERESTS

Authors have declared that no competing interests exist.

REFERENCES

1. Kassem NM, EL Zawam H, Kassem HA, EL Nahas T, El Husseiny NM, Abd El Azeeim H. A descriptive study of plasma cell dyscrasias in Egyptian population. J Egypt Natl Canc Inst. 2014;26:67–71.
2. Tosi P, Tomassetti S, Merli A, Polli V. Serum free light-chain assay for the detection and monitoring of multiple myeloma and related conditions. Ther Adv Hematol. 2013;4(1):37–41.
3. Kim HS, Kim HS, Shin KS, Song W, Kim HJ, Kim HS, Park MJ. Clinical Comparisons of Two Free Light Chain Assays to Immunofixation electrophoresis for detecting monoclonal gammopathy. BioMed Res Int. 2014;ID647238:1-7.
4. Attaelmannan M, Levinson SS. Understanding and identifying monoclonal gammopathies. Clinical Chemist. 2000;46(8):1230–1238.
5. Boccadoro M, Pileri A. Plasma cell dyscrasias: classification, clinical and laboratory characteristics, and differential diagnosis. Baillieres Clin Haematol. 1995;8(4):705-19.
6. Ouzzif Z, Doghmi K, Bouhsain S, Dami A, El Machtani S, Tellal S, Messaoudi N, Mikdame M, El Maataoui A. Monoclonal gammopathies in a Moroccan military hospital. Rheumatol Int. 2012;32(10):3303-7.
7. Singh K, Singh B, Arora S, Saxena A. Immunological evidence of monoclonal gammopathy in North India: a hospital based study. Pathol Lab Med Int. 2010;2:107–111.
8. Mseddi-Hdiji S, Haddouk S, Ben Ayed M, Tahri N, Elloumi M, Baklouti S, Hachicha J, Krichen MS, Bahloul Z, Masmoudi H. Monoclonal gammapathies in Tunisia: epidemiological, immunochemical and etiological analysis of 288 cases. Pathol Biol. 2005;53(1):19-25.
9. Charafeddine KM, Kaskas HR, Zaatari GS, Mahfouz RA, Hanna TS, Sarieddine DS, Daher RT. Patterns of monoclonal components and their correlation with different analytical parameters. Saudi Med J. 2011;32(3):308-310.
10. Tamimi W, Alaskar A, Alassiri M, Alsaeed W, Alarifi SA, Alenzi FQ, Jawdat D. Monoclonal gammopathy in a tertiary referral hospital. Clin Biochem. 2010;43(9):709-13.
11. Hlif S, Vilhelmìna H, Ísleifur O, Vilmundur G, Helga MO. Monoclonal gammopathy: natural history studied with a retrospective approach. Haematologica. 2007;92:1131-1134.
12. Bergón E, Miravalles E. Retrospective study of monoclonal gammopathies detected in the clinical laboratory of a Spanish healthcare district: 14-year series. Clin Chem Lab Med. 2007;45(2):190-6.
13. Decaux O, Rodon P, Ruelland A, Estepa L, Leblay R, Grosbois B. Epidemiology of monoclonal gammopathy in a general hospital and a university internal medicine department. Rev Med Interne. 2007;28(10):670-6.
14. Ghapanchi J, Rezaee M, Kamali F, Lavaee F, Shakib E. Prevalence of oral and craniofacial manifestations of Hematological Dyscrasias at Shiraz Nemazee Hospital. Middle East J Cancer. 2014;5(3):145-149.
15. Therneau TM, Kyle RA, Melton LJ 3rd, Larson DR, Benson JT, Colby CL, Dispenzieri A, Kumar S, Katzmann JA, Cerhan JR, Rajkumar SV. Incidence of monoclonal gammopathy of undetermined significance and estimation of duration before first clinical recognition. Mayo Clin Proc. 2012;87(11):1071-9.

16. Benson MD. Amyloidosis. Encyclopedia Life Sci; 2001. Nature Publishing Group: 1-8.

17. Cohen HJ, Crawford J, Rao MK, Pieper CF, Currie MS. Racial differences in the prevalence of monoclonal gammopathy in a community-based sample of the elderly. Am J Med. 1998;104(5):439-44.

18. Chopra CG, SM, Gupta, LCP, Mishra LCD. Evaluation of Suspected Monoclonal Gammopathies: Experience in a Tertiary Care Hospital. MJAFI. 2006;62(2):134-137.

19. Benider A, Harif M, Karkouri M, Quessar A, Sahraoui S, Sqalli S, Bendahhou K, Bouchbika Z, Kotbi S, Megrini A, Benchakroun N, Bourezgui H, Haddad H, Eddakaoui H, Machkak S, Ouboutrast A, Bekkali R, Bennani M, Zidouh A, Nejjari C, Chami Y. Cancer registry of greater Casablanca, 2005, 2006, 2007. Association Lalla Salma de lutte contre le Cancer. 2012;1-88.

20. Kyle RA, Therneau TM, Rajkumar SV, Remstein ED, Offord JR, Larson DR, Plevak MF, Melton III LJ. Long-term follow-up of IgM monoclonal gammopathy of undetermined significance. Blood. 2003;102:3759-3764

21. Van Hoeven KH, Joseph RE, Gaughan WJ, McBride L, Bilotti E, McNeill A, Schmidt L, Schillen D, Siegel DS. The Anion Gap and Routine Serum Protein Measurements in monoclonal gammopathies. Clin J Am Soc Nephrol. 2011;6:2814–2821.

22. Dasse SR, Seka SJ, Akre DP, Siransy B, Sombo Mambo F. Study isotype of monoclonal gammopathy in Abidjan. Méd Afr Noire. 2000;47(7):317-318.

23. Gaougaou N, Bahri L, Quessar A, Benchekroun S, El Bakkouri J, Riyad M, Fellah H. Epidemiological, clinical, biological, and prognostic presentation of multiple myeloma in Casablanca (Morocco). J Afr Cancer; 2014. DOI 10.1007/s12558-014-0315-4.

24. Chombart B, Gagneux-Lemoussu L, Eschard JP, Ackah-Miezan S, Novella JL, Brochot P, Pignon B, Etienne JC. Factors useful for predicting survival of myeloma patients in everyday practice. A ten-year study of 148 patients older than 55 years. Rev Rhum. 2005;1299–1305.

25. Di Giovanni S, Valentini G, Ravazzolo E, Carducci P, Giallonardo P, Maschio C. Serum beta 2-microglobulin in patients with monoclonal gammopathies. Int J Biol Markers. 1987;2(3):169-72.

26. Elias J, Dauth J, Senekal JC, Van der Walt P, Joubert HF, Kühn F, Greenacre M. Serum beta-2-microglobulin in the differential diagnosis of monoclonal gammopathies. S Afr Med J. 1991;79(11):650-3.

27. Pagano L, Valentini CG, De Stefano V, Venditti A, Visani G, Petrucci MT, Candoni A, Specchia G, Visco C, Pogliani EM, Ferrara F, Galieni P, Gozzetti A, Fianchi L. De Muro M, Leone G, Musto P, Pulsoni A for GIMEMA-ALWP. Primary plasma cell leukemia: a retrospective multicenter study of 73 patients. Ann Oncol. 2011;22:1628–1635.

28. Schuster SR, Rajkumar SV, Dispenzieri A, Morice W, Aspitia AM, Ansell S, Kyle R, Mikhael J. IgM multiple myeloma: Disease definition, prognosis, and differentiation from Waldenstrom's macroglobulinemia. Am J Hematol. 2010;85:853-855.

29. Merlini G, Seldin DC, Gertz MA. Amyloidosis: Pathogenesis and New Therapeutic Options. J Clin Oncol. 2011;29:1-10.

30. Merlini G, Palladini G. Differential diagnosis of monoclonal gammopathy of undetermined significance. Blood. 2012;595-603.

31. Soutar R, Lucraft H, Jackson G, Reece A, Bird J, Low E, Samson D. Guidelines on the diagnosis and management of solitary plasmacytoma of bone and solitary extramedullary plasmacytoma. Br J Haematol. 2004;124:717–726.

32. Chokshi MH, Baji SN, Gandhi AS. Plasma cell leukemia: A comprehensive analysis of clinical & pathological features of 7 cases. Int J Med Sci Public Health. 2014;1:6-9.

33. Cesana C, Klersy C, Barbarano L, Nosari AM, Crugnola M, Pungolino E, Gargantini L, Granata S, Valentini M, Morra E. Prognostic factors for malignant transformation in monoclonal gammopathy of undetermined significance and smoldering multiple myeloma. J Clin Oncol. 2002;20:1625-1634.

34. Salonen J, Nikoskelainen J. Lethal infections in patients with hematological malignancies. Eur J Haematol. 1993;51(2):102-8.

35. Feyler S, O'Connor SJM, Rawstron AC, et al. IgM myeloma: A rare entity characterized by a CD20-CD56-CD117-

immunophenotype and t(11;14). Br J Haematol. 2007;140:547–551.

36. Cabrera Q, Chantepie S, Salaun V, Levaltier X, Troussard X, Marco M. IgM multiple myeloma: More on a rare and heterogeneous disease. Am J Hematol. 2011;718. DOI: 10.1002/ajh.22067.

37. Owen RG, Feyler S, O'Connor SJM, Bond LR, De Tute RM, Rawstron AC. Defining IgM multiple myeloma. Am J Hematol. 2011;717. DOI: 10.1002/ajh.22061.

38. Rawstrom AC, Orfao A, Beksaec M, et al. Report of the european myeloma network on multiparametric flow cytometry in multiple myeloma and related disorders. Haematologica. 2008;93:431–438.

29

Early Diagnostics of Beta Thalassemia Minor

Archana Singh Sikarwar[1*] and Mohd Farid Bin Dato' Seri Haji Abdul Rahman[2]

[1]*Faculty of Medicine and Health Sciences, Human Biology, International Medical University, Kuala Lumpur, Malaysia.*
[2]*Undergraduate Student, Biomedical Science, International Medical University, Malaysia.*

Authors' contributions

This work was carried out in collaboration between both authors. Author ASS designed the study. Author MFBDSHAR wrote the first draft of the manuscript and managed the literature searches. Both authors read and approved the final manuscript.

Editor(s):
(1) Shinichiro Takahashi, Kitasato University School of Allied Health Sciences, Japan.
Reviewers:
(1) Massimo Berger, Pediatric Onco-Hematology and Stem Cell Transplant Division, Regina Margherita Children Hospital, Italy.
(2) Surajit Debnath, Department of Medical Laboratory Technology, Women's Polytechnic, Hapania, India.
(3) Anonymous, APS University, India.

ABSTRACT

Early diagnosis of disease is highly recommended for the treatment purposes by the clinicians. Thalassemia is a genetic disorder which can be inherited from the parents. Thalassemia is classified into two groups alpha thalassemia and beta thalassemia depending upon the severity of the infants. The methods for early diagnosis of beta Thalassamia which is currently used in some diagnostic labs, for instances, current direct and indirect mutation detection method. Recently, most researchers have been discovered the latest or emerging methods to improve the technology in order to minimize invasive methods that may be used as a routine procedure for the future which is better than current methods, like pre-implantation genetic diagnosis and non-invasive prenatal diagnosis. For current methods, chorionic villi sampling (CVS) and amniocentesis are used whereas blastomere biopsy is used for pre-implantation genetic diagnosis. Hence, non-invasive prenatal diagnosis can be perfomed by using fetal cells which is found in maternal plasma such as trophoblasts, erythrocytes and leucocytes. Emerging methods for early diagnosis of beta thalassaemia minor are much safer than current methods that will minimize the risk and less invasive to the patients.

Keywords: Early diagnosis; thalassemia; chorionic villi sampling; amniocentesis.

*Corresponding author: E-mail: archana_sikarwar@imu.edu.my

1. INTRODUCTION

Thalassemia is a heterogeneous group of genetic disorders of haemoglobin. The causes of thalassemia are due to impaired synthesis of alpha and beta globin chains of haemoglobin. Thalassemia is originated from a Greek word ('thalassa' means sea), which was reported earlier mainly in the Mediterranean population. It was discovered by Thomas Cooley, a paediatrician from Detroit, USA in 1925. Homozygous beta thalassemia or thalassemia major is also known as Cooley anaemia. There are two common types of thalassemia depending upon the lack of synthesis of globin chain such as alpha (α) and beta (β) thalassemia. Alpha thalassemia can be categorized on the basis of clinical severity into 4 types, for example, Hb Bart's Hydrop's fetalis syndrome, HbH disease, thalassemia trait and silent carrier. Beta thalassemia, was further sub classified into B-thalassemia major, B-thalassemia intermediate and B-thalassemia minor [1].

1.1 Pathogenesis of Thalassemia

Thalassemia occurs due to genetic defects caused by decrease or absence of particular globin chain production. There are 4 types of genetic defects that can cause thalassemia, single nucleotide mutation, base substitutions, and large deletion within the alpha globin or beta globin clusters and insertion or deletion mutations within the coding region of the mRNA. The single nucleotide mutation caused by some interferes of messenger RNA (mRNA) production that will decrease the amount of mRNA. Base substitutions can cause changes in the function of promoter, RNA processing or mRNA translation as well as modify a codon into nonsense codon that could lead to premature termination of translation or substitution of an incorrect amino acid. Thus, large deletion with alpha and beta globin clusters by removing one or two gene can cause few changes in regulation of the remaining genes in the clusters. Lastly, the occurrence of insertion or deletion mutation of globin chain may create frame shifts to prevent synthesis of complete normal globin polypeptide. The molecular lesions in thalassemia are complex. The most common cause of beta thalassemia reported by point mutation whereas alpha thalassemia caused by gene deletions [2].

1.2 Diagnosis of Thalassemia

Thalassemia patient can be diagnosed by examining the blood smear and measuring of haemoglobin, haematocrit, red cell count, complete blood count (CBC) and red cell indices [2], followed by using Hb electrophoresis or high performance liquid chromatography for quantifying HBA2 if MCV and MCHC as low [2,3,4]. If HBA2 is more than 3.5%, patient may categorised under beta thalassemia trait, delta beta thalassemia and Hb Lepore trait. If HBA2 is less than 3.5%, it is the alpha thalassemia trait and needs to perform further test for DNA analysis [5]. Other special procedures can be performed by using mass spectrometry. Mass spectrometry can be used to assess the mass of the globin chains by detecting single amino acid substitutions in the globin chain and identify various haemoglobin molecules [6]. Antenatal diagnosis is also used to detect patient's genetic mutation [7].

2. SYNTHESIS OF GLOBIN

Alterations in the sites of erythropoiesis are related to alterations in the type of haemoglobin produced. The synthesis of haemoglobin is maintained by two multigene clusters on chromosome 16 which is encoding of alpha like globin whereas chromosome 11 encodes beta-like globins [8]. The synthesis of globin occurs in three stages, transcription, processing of mRNA and translation as shown in Fig. 1. DNA polymerase enzyme is needed for the synthesis of a single strand of RNA which is originated from DNA template. The base sequence of RNA is complementary to the base sequence of transcription. The promoter will bind to the RNA polymerase for the beginning of translation. RNA molecule assembled when RNA polymerase move along the DNA strand in a 5' to 3' direction. The transcription may proceed through exons and intron. RNA polymerase will be isolated from the DNA strand when comes into contact with chain terminating sequence. RNA strands have been formed known as messenger RNA (mRNA) [8]. This process is followed by the processing of mRNA by addition of a cap structure and poly-A-tail and by the removal of introns. Cap structure is attached at 5' end of mRNA for beginning of translation. Polyadenylation is needed for stability of the transcript and its transport to the cytoplasm. AAUAAA sequence at the 3' end alerts the addition of poly-A tail about 20 bases downstream from the polyadenylation site. The removal of introns and attached together of exons in the mRNA transcript are prerequisite before mRNA is transported from the nucleus to the cytoplasm [8].

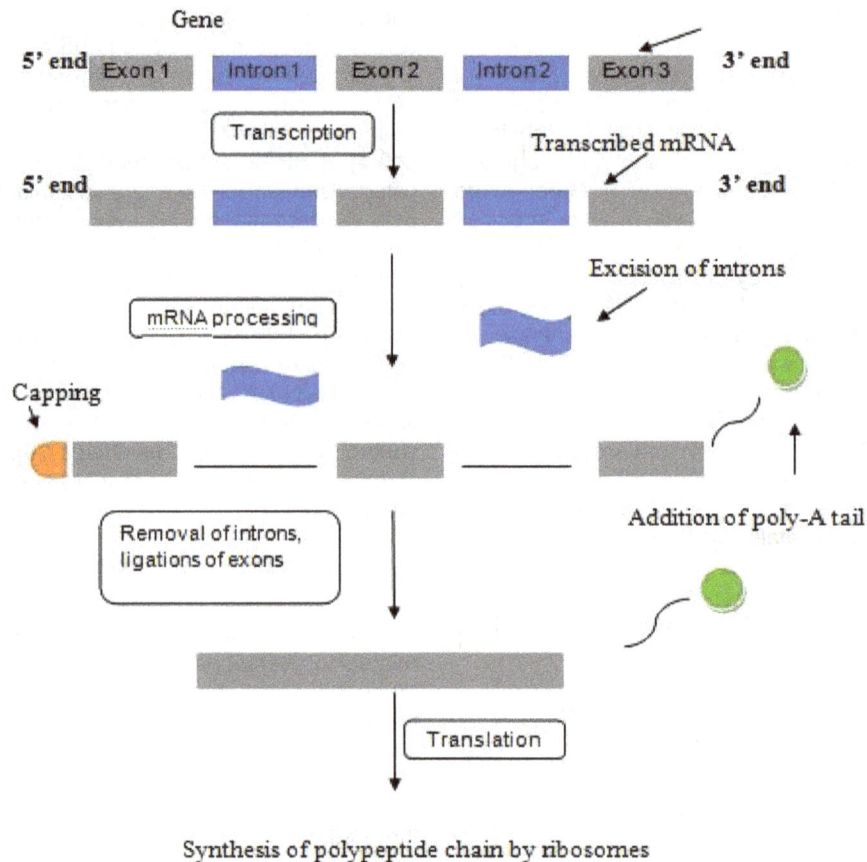

Fig. 1. Globin chain synthesis [9]

Translation takes place in ribosomes to synthesis polypeptide chain according to the directions supplied by mRNA template. Messenger RNA (mRNA), transfer RNA (tRNA) and ribosomal RNA (rRNA) are involved in the synthesis of polypepetides. The DNA template will be transcribed into mRNA where transfer of genetic code occurs from the nucleus to the cytoplasm of erythroblasts to regulate the sequence of amino acids in the formation of polypeptide. Transfer RNA plays an important role where specific amino acids transported from cytoplasm to the specific locations (codons) along with mRNA strand. After translation process and synthesis of polypeptide chain by ribosomes, it transform into globin chain.

Globin gene expression may alter during development to build different haemoglobin tetramers such as embryonic such as Hb Gower I ($\zeta 2\epsilon 2$), Hb Gower 2 ($\alpha 2\epsilon 2$) and Hb Portland ($\zeta 2\gamma 2$), Hb fetal ($\alpha 2\gamma 2$) and adult Hb A ($\alpha 2\beta 2$) and Hb A2 ($\alpha 2\delta 2$). An appearance of clinical manifestation in hemoglobinopathies plays an important role in developmental alteration of globin genes expression. Alpha thalassemia can be identified at birth whereas beta thalassemia can be detected a few months after the birth [8].

3. EPIDEMIOLOGY

Statistical data of the number of patients with alpha and beta thalassemia in seven regions are shown in Fig. 2. Beta thalassemia has the highest number in Asia and South East Asia, reaching 32665 patients and 21693 patients respectively. Beta thalassemia in Eastern Mediterranean has higher number than Pacific region about 9716 patients. Alpha thalassemia is also high in Asia region approximately 17708 patients, followed by Pacific region were 8267 patients. African region has high number of beta thalassemia about 1520 patients, followed by American and Europe region about 534 and 498 patients respectively. Alpha thalassemia has the lowest number in African, with 11 patients and Eastern Mediterranean about 1 patient only [10].

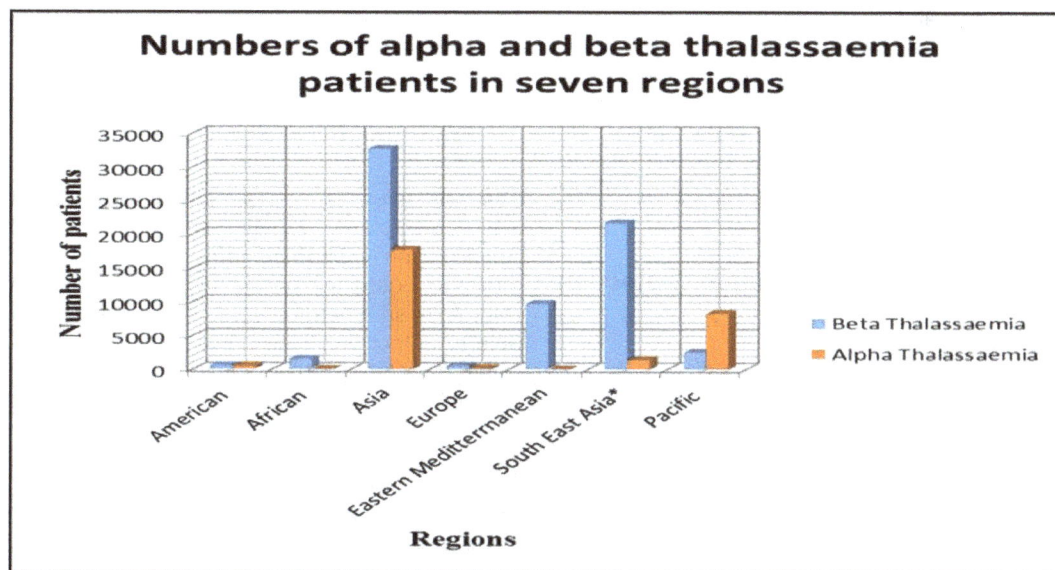

Fig. 2. Number of patients with different types of thalassemia in seven regions [11]

4. DIAGNOSTIC METHODS

Diagnosis of disease is a main challenge for clinicians. It is always recommended that early diagnostics is always better to start treatment and preventive measures for disease.

4.1 Prenatal Diagnosis

Prenatal diagnosis is a method used to monitor human couples and either if these patients have genetic disorder. It also helps them to detect the patient's condition in order to avoid any risk to a child affected with severe haemoglobin disorder. There are four basic parameters of prenatal diagnosis for thalassemia such as timely discovering of couples at risk for an affected pregnancy, the description of their disease causing mutation, acquire the fetal material properly and examine the genotype of the fetal DNA on the basis of parental mutation. Recently, the developments of an early diagnostic are designed and it has been routinely used in many countries. Researchers had discovered the new methods to diagnose and determine the haemoglobin disorder on a prenatal. Moreover, some researchers had discovered the latest version of genetic diagnosis for haemoglobin disorders such as pre-implantation genetic diagnosis and non-invasive prenatal diagnosis which can contribute with some major advantages to the patient with thalassemia disease [12]. For current methods, chorionic villi sampling (CVS) and amniocentesis are routinely

use for the detection of genetic disorder. Chorionic villi sampling can be collected when the patient is 10 to 12 weeks of pregnancy whereas amniocentesis can be collected after 15th weeks of pregnancy [12].

4.2 Current Direct Mutation Detection Methods

There are two types of current methods being used in the research lab such as current direct and indirect mutation detection methods. Current direct mutation detection methods are type of tests used to detect specific known mutation in the population group and mutation detection in carriers of beta thalassemia [13,14], for example, Reverse dot blot and Amplification Refractory mutation system (ARMS) [11]. The researchers have found reverse dot blot targeted only for common mutation of a peculiar ethnic group in Thailand and cause some difficulties to detect less common mutation. Thus, they had created a reverse dot blot strip for the 10 beta-thalassemia mutations, including beta-thalassaemic hemoglobinopathies Hb E and Hb Malay that had been reported about ninety six percent of beta thalassemia in Thailand and other strip for six less common Thai mutations. The second strip avoids requirement of more technically challenging methods. They made multiple copies and identifiable beta globin DNA like two shorter fragments that include all known Thai mutations in order to keep from happening trouble involve with secondary structure of amplified full-length target DNA [9]. Reverse dot-blotting is a rapid method, specific for identification of beta-thalassemia mutations. Amplification refractory mutation system (ARMS) can be used to identify the presence of small deletions of the beta-globin gene and doubt the truth of a very high HbA2 levels if a mutation is not discovered by DGGE analysis [15,16].

4.3 Current Indirect Mutation Detection Methods

Current indirect mutation detection methods are used to examine for the presence of genes regions to identify of sequence variation within each region and specific for unknown mutation after family studies [11,12]. Denaturing Gradient Gel Electrophoresis (DGGE) and denaturing High-Performance Liquid Chromatography (dHPLC). Researchers suggested that DGGE is better than Polymerase chain reaction (PCR) amplified beta globin DNA since they had encountered some problem with Allelic-specific oligonucleotide ASO probes." PCR amplified genomic DNA showed a very diverse spectrum of beta thalassemia in Netherlands with the result about 20% of the beta thalassemia mutation cannot be identified with this problem. DGGE was preferred and they made multiple copies with certain regions of the beta globin gene. On the basis of reported result researchers concluded that several of these mutations to specific regions of the gene rapidly which they were again amplified and sequenced promptly [17]. Denaturing high-performance liquid chromatography (dHPLC) is a method that are applied to identify of known and unknown point mutations which is highly sensitivity and dependable. Coupling heteroduplex and primer extension analysis on the basis of dHPLC is highly specific for beta-thalassemia identification [18,19]. Researchers have developed dHPLC where different compound with diverse in character, identical alleles of human beta globin (HBB) gene mutation and heteroduplex elution profile were detected. Somehow, they also had developed by combining dHPLC and multiplex primer extension analysis for the genotyping of common disease causing mutations in the HBB gene [20]. In Southern Italy, the researchers have done this by using dHPLC where direct sequence analysis was utilized to identify common and rare mutations within beta globin gene. It even identified beta globin gene mutation if standard mutation detection method failed to reveal the result. By this, parental chromatography is dependable because it is

suitable for genetic screening of prenatal and postnatal individual to diagnose beta thalassemia [21].

4.4 Emerging Detection Methods

The examples of emerging detection methods are Multiplex Ligation-dependent Probe Amplification (MLPA) and Real-time PCR. Mutilplex ligation-dependent probe amplification (MLPA) is an emerging detection method that are able to detect duplicate number genomic variant within a targeted region, designated replacement for Southern blot analysis and Fluorescene in situ hybridization (FISH) or second method to gap-PCR in order to examine known and unknown deletions that can cause alpha, beta or delta beta-thalassemia. MLPA is mainly on ligation of multiple probe-pairs combined across a region of interest. The universal-tag PCR primers are used with quantitative PCR to make multiple copies of all ligated probe pairs. It allows fragments analysis of PCR products [22,23]. The usage of PCR primers were carried out with ligated probe pairs in PCR steps which are semi-quantitative and permit to identify deletions or duplications across the locus. The advantages of MLPA is amenable, well regulated and make your own oligonucleotide probe-pairs. The utilization of probe pair with varied lengths, dissimilar tags and fluorescent labels can investigate 50 probe sets across a large region of interest. Other than that, commercial kits are readily available for identifying copy number variations across alpha and beta globin gene clusters, for example: MRC-Holland and Service [XS] available in most diagnostic laboratories but it is not common for prenatal diagnosis. Real-time PCR combine with microvolume rapid-cycle PCR with fluorometry that will enable the real-time fluorescent checking of the amplification reaction for measuring by the quantity of PCR or describing the qualities of PCR products or rapid investigate of genotype, blocking the action of manipulating of any-post–PCR sample. The identifications potential sequences to investigate the genotype applications such as single nucleotide polymorphisms, utilizes the use of two fluorescent probes which combine to near internal sequences within target amplified DNA, regions expected to contain the mutations [24,25].

4.5 Pre-implantation Genetic Diagnosis

Pre-implantation genetic diagnosis is the most common genetic material currently obtained from blastomere biopsy. Oocyte or zygote biopsy can be performed for genetic analysis. The example of pre-implantation genetic diagnosis is Mini sequencing or real-time PCR. This method is capable to discover of the mutation which is rapid and free from error. It is linked to Single Nucleotide polymorphism (SNPs) for the accuracy of the PGD. The amplification of small DNA is more productive with minimum effort than the larger fragment of DNA when beginning from a single cell. Minisequencing is suitable for single cell PCR and combined with microcapillary systems which are used for disease mutation analysis and informative linked SNPs [26]. The methods that are used for genotyping single cells for PGD with rapid and accurate result are Real-time PCR with hybridization probes. It is appropriate for PGD of Beta–thalassaemic hemoglobinopathies because of minute size of the beta gene that allows multiplex genotyping in some cases [27].

4.6 Non–invasive Prenatal Diagnosis

Researchers have reported in their studies that fetal cells such as trophoblasts, erythrocytes and leucocytes can be found in maternal cells [28,29,30]. Beginning from 1960s to 1990s, modus operandi was examined for the separation of fetal nucleated cells from maternal plasma [31,32,33]. The example of non-invasive prenatal diagnosis is Matrix-assisted laser desorption ionization time of flight mass spectrometry (MALDI-TOF MS) related to conventional homogenous Mass EXTEND (hME) assay or a nucleotide specific single allele base extension reaction (SABER) assay, possible for identification of fetal-specific alleles in maternal plasma [15,34,35,36]. This was applied to prevent the occurrence of the fetal inheritance of the four most prevalence Southeast Asian beta-thalassemia mutations in at-risk pregnancies within 7 to 21 gestation. Fetal haplotype analysis was related to single polymorphism joined beta-globin locus, HBB in maternal plasma is capable to exhibit the result which is suitable for couples sharing identical mutations [37]. Mass spectrophotometer is vulnerable to high output automated analysis. The disadvantages of these methods are expertise is needed to handle complication of method and high cost to purchase automated analysis in some diagnostic or research laboratories.

5. CONCLUSION

Thalassemia is a genetic disorder which is inherited from the parents. Thalassemia can be classified into two groups; alpha and beta thalassemia depends on the severity of the infants. Some infants cannot survive if it is severe thalassemia but some infants may survive with asymptomatic (carrier). There are some lab diagnostics that can be detect thalassemia by using different techniques for early diagnosis such as current method which is frequently used in the laboratory nowadays. Some researchers had discovered that the latest or emerging methods to improve the technology in order to minimize invasive methods that may be used as routine procedure for the future which is better than current methods.

CONSENT

It is not applicable.

ETHICAL APPROVAL

It is not applicable.

COMPETING INTERESTS

Authors have declared that no competing interests exist.

REFERENCES

1. Essential of Haematology, published by Jaypee Brothers Medical Publishers (P) Ltd New Delhi in 2006, 1st edition. Authored by Shirish M. Kawthalkar, Chapter 4: Anaemias due to excessive red cell destruction. 140-141.

2. Essential of Haematology, published by Jaypee Brothers Medical Publishers (P) Ltd New Delhi in 2006, 1st edition. Authored by Shirish M. Kawthalkar, Chapter 4: Anaemias due to excessive red cell destruction. 141-147.

3. Essential of Haematology, published by Jaypee Brothers Medical Publishers (P) Ltd New Delhi in 2006, 1st edition. Authored by Shirish M. Kawthalkar, Chapter 4: Anaemias due to excessive red cell destruction. 159-160.

4. Lab Test Online; Thalassemia: Tests; [Serial on the internet]; [Last modified 2013 March 2013, Last reviewed: 2011, May 26];
    Available:http://labtestsonline.org/understanding/conditions/thalassemia/start/2

5. Essential of Haematology, Published by Jaypee Brothers Medical Publishers (P)

Ltd New Delhi in 2006, 1ˢᵗ edition. Authored by Shirish M. Kawthalkar, Chapter 4: Anaemias due to excessive red cell destruction. 3:130-131.

6. Gribbles pathology; Medical Articles; Thalassemia; [Homepage of the internet] [2007 Nov, 1]; Available:http://www.gribbles.com.my/new smaster.cfm?&menuid=24&action=view&r etrieveid=1

7. Peter Kleinert, Marlis Schmid, Karin Zurbriggen, Oliver Speer, Markus Schmugge, Bernd Roschitzki, Silke S. Durka, Urs Leopold, Thomas Kuster, Claus W. Heizmann, Hannes Frischknecht, Heinz Troxler. Mass spectrometry: a tool for enhanced detection of hemoglobin variants. Clinical Chemistry; 2008;54(1): 69-76. Available:http://www.clinchem.org/content/ 54/1/69.long

8. Australian prescriber an independent review, Screening for Thalassemia, D.K. Bowden, Associate Professor, Thalassemia Service, Monash Medical Centre, Melbourne; Testing in Australia: Antenatal Testing. 2001;24:5. Available:http://www.australianprescriber.c om/magazine/24/5/120/3/

9. Cornelis L Harteveld, Marina Kleanthous, Joanne Traeger-Synodinos. Prenatal diagnosis of hemoglobin disorders: Present and future strategies. Clinical Biochemistry. 2009;42(18):1767-1779.

10. Essential of Haematology, published by Jaypee Brothers Medical Publishers (P) Ltd New Delhi in 2006, 1ˢᵗ edition. Authored by Shirish M. Kawthalkar, Section 1- Chapter 1: Overview of physiology of blood. 9-13.

11. Sutcharitchan P, Saiki R, Fucharoen S, Winichagoon P, Erlich H, Embury SH. Reverse dot-blot detection of Thai beta Thalassemia mutations. British Journal of Haematology. 1995;90(4):809-816.

12. Bernadette Modell, Matthew Darlison; Global epidemiology of Haemoglobin disorders, Bulletin of the World Health Organization (WHO). 2008;86(6):480-487. Available:http://www.who.int/bulletin/volum es/86/6/06-036673-table-T2.html

13. Chiu RW, Lau TK, Leung TN, Chow KC, Chui DH, Lo YM. Prenatal exclusion of beta Thalassemia major by examination of maternal plasma. Lancet. 2002;360(9338): 998-1000.

14. Essential of Haematology, published by Jaypee Brothers Medical Publishers (P) Ltd New Delhi in 2006, 1ˢᵗ edition. Authored by Shirish M. Kawthalkar, Chapter 4: Anaemias due to excessive red cell destruction. Prenatal diagnosis. 162-168.

15. Cornelis L. Harteveld, Marina Kleanthous, Joanne Traeger-Synodinos. Prenatal diagnosis of hemoglobin disorders: Present and future strategies. Clinical Biochemistry. 2009;42(18):1768-1769.

16. Antonio Cao, Renzo Galanello, M. Cristina Rosatelli. 8 Prenatal diagnosis and screening of the haemoglobinopathies. Bailliere's Clinical Haematology. 1998; 11(1):215-238.

17. Antonio Cao, Maria Cristina Rosatelli. Screening and prenatal diagnosis of the hemoglobinopathies. Bailliere's Clinical Haematology. 1993;6(1):263-286.

18. Losekoot M, Fodde R, Harteveld CL, van Heeren H, Giordano PC, Bernini LF. Denaturing gradient gel electrophoresis and direct sequencing of PCR amplified genomic DNA: A rapid and reliable diagnostic approach to beta Thalassemia. British Journal of Haematology. 1990; 76(2):269-274.

19. Li Q, Li LY, Huang SW, Li L, Chen XW, Zhou WJ, Xu XM. Rapid genotyping of known mutations and polymorphisms in beta globin gene based on the dHPLC profile patterns of homoduplexes and heteroduplexes. Clinical Biochemistry. 2008;41(9):681-687.

20. O'Donovan MC, Oefner PJ, Roberts SC, Austin J, Hoogendoorn B, Guy C, Speight G, Upadhyaya M, Sommer SS, McGuffin P. Blind analysis of denaturing high-performance liquid chromatography as a tool for mutation detection. Genomics. 1998;15;52(1):44-49.

21. Su YN, Lee CN, Hung CC, Chen CA, Cheng WF, Tsao PN, Yu CL, Hsieh FJ. Rapid detection of beta globin gene (HBB) mutations coupling heteroduplex and primer-extension analysis by DHPLC. Human Mutation. 2003;22(4):326-336.

22. Colosimo A, Guida V, Scolari A, De Luca A, Palka G, Rigoli L, Meo A, Salpietro DC, Dallapiccola B. Validation of dHPLC for molecular diagnosis of beta-Thalassemia in Southern Italy. Genetic Test. 2003;7(3): 269-275.

23. Harteveld CL, Voskamp A, Phylipsen M, Akkermans N, den Dunnen JT, White SJ,

Giordano PC. Nine unknown rearrangements in 16p133 and 11p15.4 causing alpha and beta Thalassemia characterised by high resolution multiplex ligation dependent probe amplification. Journal of Medical Genetics. 2005;42(12): 922-931.

24. Schouten JP, McElgunn CJ, Waaijer R, Zwijnenburg D, Diepvens F, Pals G. Relative quantification of 40 nucleic acid sequences by multiplex ligation dependent probe amplification. Nucleic Acids Research. 2002;30(12):e57.

25. White SJ, Vink GR, Kriek M, Wuyts W, Schouten J, Bakker B, Breuning MH, den Dunnen JT. Two colour multiplex ligation dependent probe amplification: Detecting genomics rearrangements in hereditary multiple exostoses. Human Mutation. 2004;24(1):86-92.

26. Harteveld CL, Kriek M, Bijlsma EK, Erjavec Z, Balak D, Phylipsen M, Voskamp A, Di Capua E, White SJ, Giordano PC. Refinement of the genetic cause of ATR-16, Human Genetics. 2007;122(3-4):283-292.

27. Fiorentino F, Magli MC, Podini D, Ferraretti AP, Nuccitelli A, Vitale N, Baldi M, Gianaroli L. The mini sequencing method an alternative strategy for preimplantation genetic diagnosis of single gene disorders. Molecular Human Reproduction. 2003; 9(7):399-410.

28. Vrettou C, Traeger-Synodinos J, Tzetis M, Palmer G, Sofocleous C, Kanavakis E. Real time PCR for single genotyping in sickle cell and Thalassemia syndromes as a rapid, accurate, reliable and widely applicable protocol for pre-implantation genetic diagnosis. Human Mutations. 2004;23(5):513-521.

29. Schroder J. Transplacental passage of blood cells. Journal of Medical Genetics. 1975;12:230-242.

30. Zipursky A, Hull A, White FD, Israels LG. Foetal erythrocytes in the maternal circulation; Lancet. 1959;1:451-452.

31. Cohen F, Zuelzer WW. The transplacental passage of maternal erythrocytes into the fetus. American Journal of Obstetrics and Gynecology. 1965;93:566-569.

32. Cheung MC, Goldberg JD, Kan YW. Prenatal diagnosis of sickle cell anaemia and Thalassemia by analysis of fetal cells in maternal blood. Nature Genetics. 1996; 14(3):264-268.

33. Kolialexi A, Vrettou C, Traeger-Synodinos J, Burgemeister R, Papantoniou N, Kanavakis E, Antsaklis A, Mavrou A. Non-invasive prenatal diagnosis of beta-Thalassemia using individual fetal erythroblasts isolated from maternal blood after enrichment. Prenatal Diagnosis. 2007;27(13):1228-1232.

34. Lo YM, Corbetta N, Chamberlain PF, Rai V, Sargent IL, Redman CW, et al. Presence of fetal DNA in maternal plasma and serum. Lancet. 1997;350:485–487.

35. Ding C Maldi-TOF mass spectrometry for analyzing cell-free fetal DNA in maternal plasma. Methods Molecular Biology. 2008; 444:253-267.

36. Chunming Ding, Rossa W. K. Chiu, Dennis Lo YM. MS analysis of single-nucleotide differences in circulating nucleic acids: application to non-invasive prenatal diagnosis. Proceedings of the National Academic Sciences USA. 2004;101(29): 10762-10767.

37. Li Y, Di Naro E, Vitucci A, Zimmermann B, Holzgreve W, Hahn S. Detection of paternally inherited fetal point mutations for beta-thalassemia using size-fractionated cell-free DNA in maternal plasma. JAMA. 2005;293(7):843-849.

Prevalence of HIV Infection among Blood Donors at a Tertiary Care Centre in Gwalior, India

Dharmesh Chandra Sharma[1*], Arun Jain[2], Poonam Woike[2], Sunita Rai[2], Lokesh Tripathi[2], Savita Bharat[3] and Rajesh Gaur[2]

[1]*Blood Bank, Component and Aphaeresis Unit, Department of Pathology, G. R. Medical College, Gwalior, India.*
[2]*Department of Pathology, G. R. Medical College, India.*
[3]*Department of Microbiology, G. R. Medical College, Gwalior, India.*

Authors' contributions

This work was carried out in collaboration between all authors. Authors DCS and AJ designed the study, wrote the protocol, and wrote the first draft of the manuscript. Authors PW and SR managed the literature searches, analysis of the study performed and the spectroscopy analysis. Authors LT and SB managed the experimental process. Author RG supervised the research work. All authors read and approved the final manuscript.

Editor(s):
(1) Armel Hervé Nwabo Kamdje, University of Ngaoundere-Cameroon, Ngaoundere, Cameroon.
Reviewers:
(1) Simeon Achunam Nwabueze, Nnamdi Azikiwe University, Nigeria.
(2) Anonymous, Buenos Aires University, Argentina.
(3) Prabhuswami Hiremath, Krishna Institute of Medical Sciences University, India.
(4) Kadima Ntokamunda Justin, University of Rwanda, Rwanda.
(5) Mbirimtengerenji D. Noel, University of Malawi, Malawi.
(6) Anonymous, State Health and Family Welfare Institute, Himachal, India.

ABSTRACT

Background: Transfusion Transmitted Infections (TTIs) threaten safety of the recipients and the community as a whole and are the subject of real concern worldwide. Human immunodeficiency virus (HIV) causes Acquired Immunodeficiency Syndrome (AIDS) which can affect people of any age group. It can be transmitted by sexual intercourse, sharing of needles, transfusion of blood and blood products and vertical transmission from mother to child. There's no complete cure for HIV till date. Incidence among donors reflects the overall disease burden on the society.

*Corresponding author: E-mail: dr_dharmesh_sharma@yahoo.com

Aims and Objectives: The purpose of this study is to estimate the prevalence of HIV infection among the voluntary blood donors at blood bank, J.A hospital, Gwalior Madhya Pradesh, India for a period of eleven years, *i.e.*, from 2004 to 2014.

Materials and Methods: A retrospective study was carried out at Blood Bank J.A Hospital & G.R Medical college Gwalior and seroprevalence of HIV infection among blood donors who donated blood from 2004-2014 at Blood Bank was compiled.

Results: Out of the total 1, 37,767 donors tested for HIV infection, 266 (0.19%) were found to be HIV sero-positive and prevalence difference of HIV positive according to the year 2004 to 2014 were found to be significantly different. (p=0.000002).

Conclusion: The prevalence of HIV was 0.19% among blood donors of Gwalior region and showed decline pattern from 2004 to 2014.

Keywords: Transfusion Transmitted Infections (TTIs); Blood Donor (BD); Human Immunodeficiency Virus (HIV); Acquired Immunodeficiency Syndrome (AIDS).

1. INTRODUCTION

Transfusion of blood and/or its components is a life saving measure but at the same time it has life threatening hazards also and with every unit of blood, there is 1% chance of transfusion-associated problems including transfusion-transmitted diseases [1,2]. Blood transfusion carries the risk of transfusion transmissible infections (TTI), including HIV, Hepatitis B & C, Syphilis and Malaria. Their tests were made mandatory in the year 2001 in India prior to the issue of compatible blood to the patient [3]. Other infections that can be transmitted through blood transfusion are Toxoplasmosis, Brucellosis and some other viral infections like CMV, EBV and Herpes, which are uncommon in India hence, WHO didn't recommend their tests mandatory before transfusion of blood and blood components For Asia Pacific region. Among all infections, HIV and hepatitis are the most dreadful. India has a population of more than 1.2 billion with 5.7 (reduced to 2.5) million Human Immunodeficiency Virus (HIV) positive, 43 million HBV-positive and 15 million HCV-positive people [4]. Human immunodeficiency virus (HIV) was discovered in 1983 by Barre-Sinoussi et al. [5]. HIV is a lentivirus (a subgroup of retrovirus) that causes HIV infection and acquired immunode-ficiency syndrome (AIDS) [6,7]. The full pathogenic potential of human retroviruses was not realized until HIV was established as the cause of AIDS in 1984 [8]. AIDS is a condition in humans in which progressive failure of the immune system allows life-threatening opportunistic infections and cancers to thrive [6,7]. Without treatment, average survival time after infection with HIV is estimated to be 9 to 11 years, depending on the HIV subtype [9]. The disease is transmitted by sexual intercourse, sharing of needles, transfusion of blood and blood products and vertical transmission from mother to child. HIV is present in body fluids in the form of free virus particles and also within infected immune cells. HIV infects vital cells in the human immune system such as helper T cells (specifically CD4+ T cells), macrophages, and dendritic cells [10]. It leads to lowering the level of CD4 + T cells through a number of mechanisms including apoptosis of uninfected bystander cells [11]. The HIV/AIDS epidemic is one of the largest public health crises of the 21st century, which has evolved from a mysterious illness to a global pandemic in less than 20 years. In 2007, a total of 33.2 million people were living with HIV with global prevalence of 2.5 million. In India, the estimated number of HIV-infected people was 2.4 million in 2007. Although globally, as well as in India, the predominant mode of HIV transmission is through heterosexual contact, the risk of contracting HIV infection from transfusion of a unit of infected blood is estimated to be over 95% [12]. In 1992, Government of India demonstrated its commitment to combat the disease with the launch of the first National AIDS Control Programme (NACP-I) as a comprehensive programme for prevention and control of HIV/AIDS in India [13]. Responding to the immense challenge of the HIV/AIDS threat in India, National AIDS Control Organization (NACO) has a response to increase access to services and effectively communicate for behavior change. With continuous efforts, today we stand at the beginning of NACP IV [14]. In 2010, NACO approved the Teach AIDS curriculum for use in India, an innovation which represented the first time that HIV/AIDS education could be provided in a curriculum which did not need to be coupled with sex education [15].

According to HIV sentinel surveillance (HSS) 2012-2013, the overall HIV prevalence among

ANC clinic attendees, considered a proxy for prevalence among the general population, continues to be low at 0.35% in the country, with an overall declining trend at the national level. The highest prevalence was recorded in Nagaland (0.88%), followed by Mizoram (0.68%), Manipur (0.64%), Andhra Pradesh (0.59%) and Karnataka (0.53%). Also, States like Chhattisgarh (0.51%), Gujarat (0.50%), Maharashtra (0.40%), Delhi (0.40%) and Punjab (0.37%) recorded HIV prevalence of more than the national average. Decline in HIV prevalence has been recorded among Female Sex Workers at national level (5.06% in 2007 to 2.67% in 2011), among Men who have Sex with Men (7.41% in 2007 to 4.43% in 2011)and Stable trends have been recorded among Injecting Drug Users at national level (7.23% in 2007 to 7.14% in 2011) [16].

2. MATERIALS AND METHODS

This study was carried out at Blood Bank, Department Of Pathology, Gajra Raja Medical College, Gwalior (Madhya Pradesh), India. Donors were screened by trained personnel after satisfactory completion of the donor's questionnaire, their physical examination and hemoglobin (Hb %) estimation. A total of 1, 37,767 blood units from the selected donors were collected over a period of eleven years (1st January 2004 to 31st December 2014). These donors were Voluntary Donors (VD) and Replacement Donors (RD). Replacement donors were those donors who donated blood for ailing patients and were family members, close relatives and friend's of recipient. The Voluntary donations were obtained from walk in donors and in voluntary blood donation camps organized by different institutions, neighboring colleges, different social and political organizations. Professional and paid donors were carefully eliminated. Written consent from the donor was also taken prior to blood donation. Three ml blood in plain vial and 2 ml blood in EDTA (ethylene diamine tetra acetic acid) vial taken from the satellite bag. All samples were screened for HIV and other Transfusion transmitted diseases. Test for HIV I and II was performed by following commercially available ELISA and card test kits in last 11 years:

1. Rapid card test HIV: an immunochromatography method (J. Mitra & Co. Pvt. Ltd.)
2. Rapid card test HIV: Alere true line, make: Standard Diagnostic

3. Rapid card test HIV: Alere true line, make Standard Diagnostic
4. Microlisa for HIV I & II: Third Generation (J. Mitra & Co. Pvt. Ltd.).
5. Microlisa for HIV I & II: Third generation (SD Bio Standard Diagnostic Pvt LTD.)
6. Elisa HIV I & II: Fourth generation, antibodies & P24 antigen detection (Meril Diagnostic):

Presently, we are doing fourth generation Elisa and card test for detection of HIV.

Confirmation of all the Positive and every 20th Negative test results was done by State Reference Laboratory (SRL), Department of Microbiology, G. R. Medical College, Gwalior and National Reference Laboratory (NRL), National Institute of Immunohaematology (NIIH), K.E.M. Hospital, Parel, Mumbai, India. The blood unit was discarded as per guidelines of NACO, whenever the pilot donor samples were found positive for any TTI. All HIV positive cases were traced and send to Integrated counselling and testing centre (ICTC) Department of Microbiology, G. R. Medical College, Gwalior for confirmation and counselling. From there Patients refer to anti-retroviral therapy (ART) Centre, Out Patient Department (OPD), J. A. Hospital, Gwalior for CD4 count and antiretroviral therapy.

The HIV data of past eleven years was retrieved and results were analyzed in the present study and have been compared statistically by frequency distribution and percentage proportion. Chi square (X2) test was applied to know the significant (*p value*) ratio of difference statistically.

3. RESULTS

Blood from 1, 37, 767 apparently healthy donors aging 18-60 years was collected during the study period. Male to Female donor's ratio in the study was 96.2% (1, 32,470) and 3.8% (5297). Out of 1, 37,767 donors, 94,092 (68.2%) were Voluntary blood donors while 43,564 (31.6%) were relative blood donors (Table No. 1).

Increasing trend in voluntary blood donation was reported from the year 2004 to 2014 (Table No. 1 and Fig. 1).

A total number 1, 37,767 blood donors were tested out of which 266 (0.19%) were positive for HIV infection (Fig. 2). Decreasing Pattern of seropositivity incidence of HIV was reported in the present study from 2004-2014 (Fig. 3 and Table no. 1).

4. DISCUSSION

It is obvious from the result that blood donation in females is markedly less than males in our study because of the fact that a large population of the females in India are usually underweight and anemic according to the donor's selection criteria. And also due to traditional thinking of Indian society. Many studies in Africa reported a male dominance in blood donation programs (71.2% in Burkina Faso) and (90% in Ghana) [17-18]. Our results are in agreement with previous report among blood donors in India which indicated that female gender is less disposed to blood donation [19]. In our study 96.2% donors were males and 3.8% were females. There's a wide range of male: Female voluntary donation ratio geographically. To minimize the gap between the demand and supply of blood/blood components in India (Blood Demand 8.5 million unit/ year requirement and availability is only 4.4 million units/year; Gap 48%) [20], female gender participation in blood donation should be ensured.

One decade ago i.e. in 2004 our voluntary blood donation was only 15.2%. At that time blood was mostly collected from relative donors or/ & from directed donation which increased drastically in 2014 i.e. 90.9%. There's steep rise between the

years 2007-2009 which was 38.5% to 91.3%. Increase in voluntary donors may be attributed to the increasing public awareness and involvement of Government bodies like NACO that actively propagate voluntary blood donation in our country. Since 2009 voluntary blood donation attained a stabilized percentage which is approximately 90% till date. This effort improved the quality of blood component, blood transfusion services and is one of the major factors in controlling and reducing the prevalence of HIV infection in the society. Overall, voluntary versus relative donors are 68.2% and 31.6% respectively. In 2004 voluntary versus replacement donors were 15.2% & 84.8% which reversed in 2009 to 91.3% and 8.7% while national data is still 52% [20]. It has been accepted internationally that prevalence of transfusion- transmitted diseases is much lower in healthy voluntary non-remunerated blood donors [21]. Voluntary unpaid blood donors are the foundation of a safe blood supply because they are usually assumed to be associated with low levels of transfusion-transmitted infection (TTI), including HIV and hepatitis viruses. Voluntary blood donors consider themselves to be healthy, have no infections to their knowledge and come to the blood bank with the intention of helping someone [22]. Voluntary blood donation was not improved after the efforts of WHO in underdeveloped countries like Kenya which reported 64% voluntary and 36% relative blood donors [23].

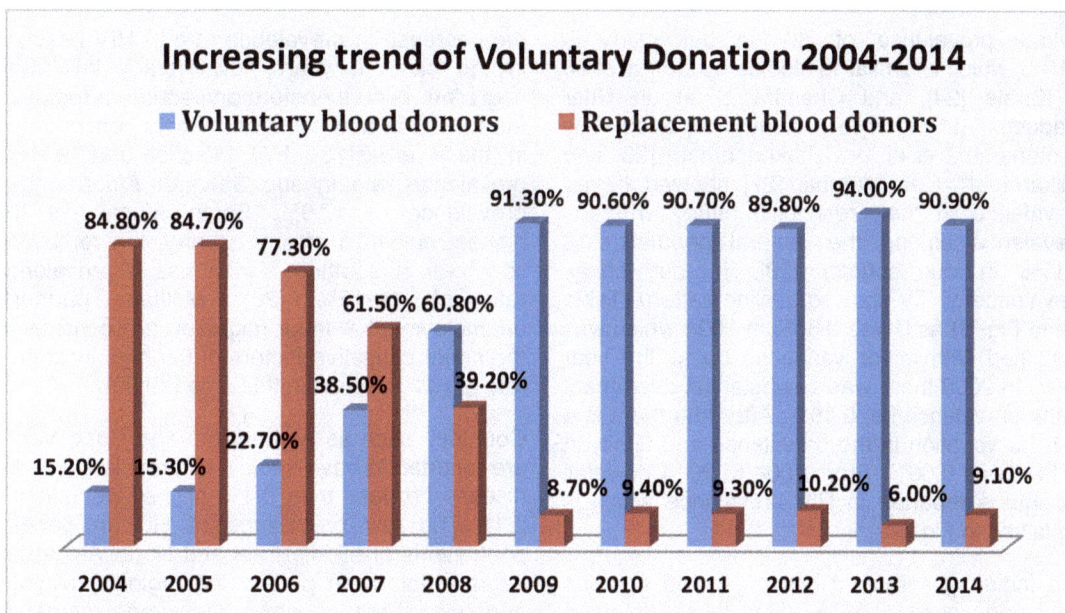

Fig. 1. Trend of voluntary blood donation in past eleven years

Table 1. Blood donations, HIV reactivity and categories of blood donors'

Year	Total blood donations	HIV reactive	Voluntary vs replacement donor	
			Voluntary blood donors	Replacement blood donors
2004	7,900	28(0.35%)	1,201 (15.2%)	6,699 (84.8%)
2005	8,201	30(0.36%)	1,254 (15.3%)	6,947 (84.7%)
2006	11,366	33(0.29%)	2,528 (22.7%)	8,838 (77.3%)
2007	14,461	48(0.33%)	5,580 (38.5%)	8,881 (61.5%)
2008	12,946	25(0.19%)	7,878 (60.8%)	5,068 (39.2%)
2009	12,914	20(0.15%)	11,788 (91.3%)	1,126 (8.7%)
2010	12,638	16(0.12%)	11,449 (90.6%)	1,189 (9.4%)
2011	13,106	17(0.12%)	11,886 (90.7%)	1,220 (9.3%)
2012	14,001	25(0.17%)	12,573 (89.8%)	1,428 (10.2%)
2013	14,473	13(0.09%)	13,613 (94.0%)	860 (6.0%)
2014	15,761	11(0.06%)	14342 (90.9%)	1,308 (9.1%)
Total	137767	266(0.19%)	94,092 (68.2%)	43,564 (31.6%)

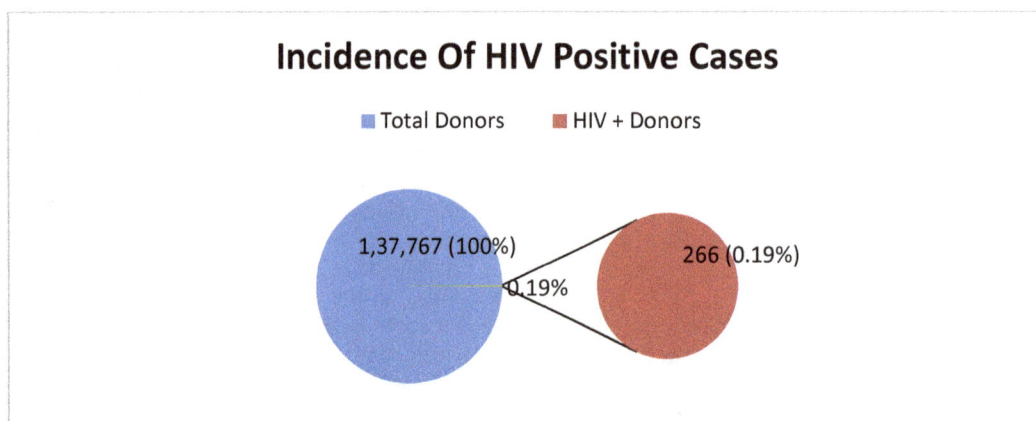

Fig. 2. Prevalence of seropositivity in the study

Overall prevalence of HIV in our study is 0.19%, which is similar to studies by Mathai et al. in Kerala [24], and Chandra et al. in Uttar Pradesh [25] while study reported by Ramanamma et al in Vishakhapatnam [26] and Kulkarni et al. in Mumbai [27] showed higher prevalence in their respective study whereas prevalence among the general population is 0.35% in our country [20]. In our study, prevalence of HIV showed decline pattern (Table 1 and Fig. 3) as it was 0.35% in 2004 which was sustained with minor variations up to the year 2007. In 2008 there was a substantial decrement in the prevalence i.e. 0.19%. After that there is a to & fro variation in the prevalence and finally in 2014 it was 0.06%. From 2004 to 2014 downfall linearity is reported in HIV prevalence which is explained in Fig. 3.

The Indian government has organized rigorous campaigns against AIDS along with numerous awareness and educational programme throughout the country which is responsible for the decrease in prevalence rate of HIV infection in the past 10 years, low literacy level and migration in northeastern and southern region of India HIV is now most commonly concentrated in these areas[13]. HIV infection has a high prevalence rate in sub Saharan Africa with a prevalence of 17.9%. South Africa has the highest epidemic of any country, the remaining countries in southern Africa has a prevalence rate of 10-15% [28]. Multiple partners, unemployment & labor migration are considered the major causative factors of the high incidence rate of HIV infection in this area [29,30].

Countries such as Afghanistan and Cape Verde are reported to have the lowest prevalence of the disease i.e. less than 0.1% of their populations [31]. The low prevalence of HIV in general populations of Middle East and North Africa has been attributed in part to the region's religious and cultural norms, which discourage premarital sex and include the universal practice of male circumcision.

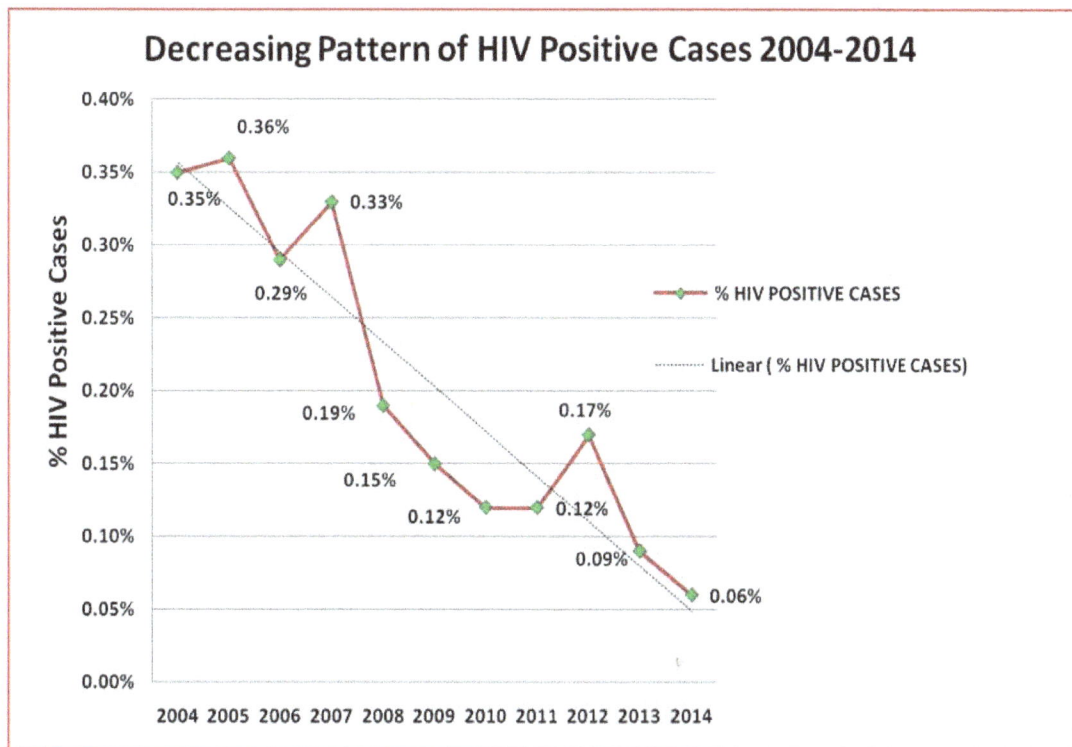

Fig. 3. Decreasing pattern of HIV positive cases from 2004-2014

5. CONCLUSION

From the present study it can be concluded that there is an increasing trend of voluntary donation with a male predominance. It can also be seen from the above data that there's a marked fall in the prevalence of HIV infection in the past decade i.e. from 2004-2014 which could be due to the various awareness, educational programs and campaigns run by The Government of India.

CONSENT

The authors declare that written informed consent was obtained from the patients before being recruited for this research.

ETHICAL APPROVAL

All author(s) hereby declare that all procedure have been examined and approved by the appropriate ethics committee of Gajra Raja Medical College, Gwalior, India and research have therefore been performed in accordance with the ethical standards laid down in the 1964 declaration of Helsinki.

COMPETING INTERESTS

Authors have declared that no competing interests exist.

REFERENCES

1. Fernandes H, D'souza PFm D'souza PM. Prevalence of transfusion transmitted infections in voluntary and replacement donors. Indian Journal of Hematology & Blood Transfusion. 2010;26:89-91.

2. Widmann FK, Technical manual; 9th Edition. American Association of Blood Banks. Aglington USA. 1985;325-44. Available:http://trove.nla.gov.au/version/45297113

3. Dhot PS. Amendments to indian drugs and cosmetics Act and Rules Pertaining to Blood Banks in Armed Forces (MJAFI). 2005;61:264-266. DOI: 10.1016/S0377-1237(05)80170-4

4. Giri PA, Deshpande JD, Phalke DB, Karle LB. Seroprevalence of transfusion transmissible infections among voluntary blood donors at a tertiary care teaching hospital in rural area of India. Journal of

Family Medicine and Primary Care. 2012; 1:48-51.

5. Barre-Sinoussi F, Chermann JC, Rey F, et al. Isolation of a T-lymphocytic retrovirus from a patient at a risk for Acquired Immune Deficiency Syndrome (AIDS). Science. 1983;20(220):4599:868-871.

6. Weiss RA. How does HIV cause AIDS? Science.1993;260 (5112):1273–9. Bibcode:1993Sci...260.1273W. DOI: 10.1126/science.8493571 PMID 8493571

7. Douek DC, Roederer M, Koup RA. Emerging concepts in the immuno-pathogenesis of AIDS. Annu. Rev. Med. 2009;60:471-84.

8. Christopher D, Hillyer Leslie E, Silberstein Paul M, Ness Kenneth C, Anderson John Roback D. Blood banking and transfusion medicine second ed. Churchill Livingstone Elsivier. 600-01.

9. UNAIDS, WHO (December 2007). AIDS Epidemic Update (PDF). 2007;10. (Retrieved 2008-03-12).

10. Kumar Vinay, Abul K. Abbas, Jon C. Aster, editors. Robbins Basic Pathology (9th ed.). Publisher Elsevier. 2012;147.

11. Garg H, Mohl J, Joshi A. HIV-1 induced bystander apoptosis. viruses. 2012;9:4 (11):3020-43. PMC: 3509682. DOI: 10.3390/v4113020 PMID: 23202514

12. Agbovi KK, Kolou M, Fétéké L, Haudrechy D, North ML et al. Knowledge, attitudes and practices about blood donation. A sociological study among the population of Lomé in Togo. Transfus Clin Biol. 2006; 13:260-265.

13. Park JE. Textbook of preventive and social medicine (20th ed.) M/s Banarsidas Bhanot Publishers. 2009;186-302.

14. National AIDS Control Organisation; 1992. Available: www.hivpolicy.org

15. National AIDS Control Organization of India approves Teach AIDS curriculum. Teach AIDS; 2010. (Retrieved 16 December 2010).

16. Annual Report NACO 2014-15. Available:http://naco.gov.in/upload/2015% 20MSLNS/Annual%20report%20 NACO 2014-15.pdf

17. Nébié KY, Olinger CM, Kafando E, Dahourou H, Diallo S, et al. [Lack of knowledge among blood donors in Burkina Faso (West Africa); potential obstacle to transfusion security]. Transfus Clin Biol. 2007;14:446-452.

18. Allain JP, Sarkodie F, Boateng P, Asenso K, Kyeremateng E, et al. A pool of repeat blood donors can be generated with little expense to the blood center in sub-Saharan Africa. Transfusion. 2008;48:735-741.

19. Uma S, Arun R, Arumugam P. The knowledge, attitude and practice towards blood donation among voluntary blood donors in Chennai, India. J Clin Diagn Res. 2013;7(6):1043-1046.

20. Access to Safe blood – NACO National AIDS Control organization. Updated On: 08 Sept, 2015. Available:http://www.naco.gov.in/NACO/N ational_AIDS_Control_Program/Services_f or_Prevention/Access_to_Safe_blood/

21. Asif N, Khokhar N, Ilahi F. Seroprevalence of HBV, HCV and HIV infection among voluntary non remunerated and replacement donors in northern Pakistan. Pak J Med Sci. January-March. 2004; 20(1):24-28.

22. Choudhury LP, Tetali S. Ethical challen-ges in voluntary blood donation in Kerala, India. J Med Ethics. 2007;33(3):140–142. DOI: 10.1136/jme.2005.015644

23. Kimani D, Mwangi J, Mwangi M, Bunnell R, Kellogg TA, Oluoch T, et al. Blood donors in Kenya: A comparison of voluntary and family replacement donors based on a population-based survey. Vox Sanguinis. 2011;100(2):212–218. DOI: 10.1111/j.1423-0410.2010.01376.x (Epub 2010 Aug 25)

24. Mathai PVJ, Sulochana S, Satyabhama PK, Nair R, et al. Profile of transfusion transmissible infections and associated risk factors among blood donors of Kerala. Indian J Pathol Microbiol. 2002;45(3):319-22.

25. Chandra T, Kumar A, Gupta A. Prevalence of transfusion transmitted infections in blood donors: An Indian experience. Trop Doct. 2009;39(3):152-4.

26. Ramanamma MV, Rfamani TV. A preliminary report on the seroprevalence of HIV-2 in Vishakapatnam. Indian J Med Microbiol. 1994;12:212-5.

27. Kulkarni HG, Koppikar GV, Mehta PR, Borges NE. Seroprevalence of HIV-1 infection in Bombay (B321). Abstract Book. 2nd international congress on AIDS in Asia and the pacific; 1992.

28. UNAIDS. Report on the global AIDS epidemic. Technical report, Joint United Nations Programme on HIV/AIDS; 2013. Available:http://www.unaids.org/en/resources/campaigns/globalreport2013

29. Levinsohn JA, McLaren Z, Shisana O, Zuma K. HIV status and labor market participation in South Africa. NBER Working Paper, No. 16901;2011.

30. Hanson BW. Refocusing and prioritizing HIV programmes in conflict and post-conflict settings: Funding recommendations'. AIDS. 22 (Supplement 2). 2008; I:S95-103.
DOI: 10.1097/01.aids.0000327441.66656.da
PMCID: PMC2853944

31. Central Intelligence Agency (CIA). CIA World Factbook - HIV/AIDS adult prevalence rate; 2011. Available:https://www.cia.gov/library/publications/the-world.../2155rank.html

A Case Report of Pregnant Woman with Aplastic Anemia: Diagnosis and Management through Subsequent Pregnancy

Harshini Vana[1*], J. B. Vidyashree[1], Mangala Gowri[1] and Renuka Ramaiah[1]

[1]*Department of Obstetrics and Gynecology, RGUHS, ESICMCPGIMSR, Bangalore, India.*

Authors' contributions

The work had been carried out in collaboration between all authors. Authors HV and JBV have designed the article, managed literature searches and managed the patient. Authors RR and MG had taken responsibility of managing the patient, planning and discussing treatment with multidisciplinary approach also edited this article. All authors read and approved the final manuscript.

Editor(s):
(1) Johnson M. Liu, Steven and Alexandra Cohen Children's Medical Center of New York, Division of Pediatric Hematology/ Oncology & Stem Cell Transplantation, USA And Hofstra University School of Medicine in Partnership with North Shore-LIJ Health System, USA.
(2) Tadeusz Robak, Medical University of Lodz, Copernicus Memorial Hospital, Poland.
(3) Dharmesh Chandra Sharma, Incharge Blood Component and Aphaeresis Unit, G. R. Medical College, Gwalior, India.
Reviewers:
(1) Anonymous, USA.
(2) Golam Hafiz, Pediatric Hematology and Oncology, Bangabandhu Sheikh Mujib Medical University, Dhaka, Bangladesh.
(3) Anonymous, Czech Republic.

ABSTRACT

Introduction: Aplastic anemia is characterized by decreased bone marrow function with inadequate production of erythrocytes, granulocytes, and platelets. Marrow failure may be caused by absence of or defects in hematopoietic stem cells, abnormalities of the bone marrow microenvironment, or immune disorders. There are no clear guidelines for the management of aplastic anemia during pregnancy.
We report a case of pregnant woman in whom anemia was evaluated and diagnosed as Aplastic anemia, managed through the pregnancy and followed her up until subsequent pregnancy with good outcome.
Case: A 19 year teenage girl, primigravida at 36 weeks of gestation presented to our hospital complaining with generalized weakness since 1 month during her antenatal check up. She was

Corresponding author: E-mail: vharshini84@gmail.com

evaluated wherein Hb-5.8g/dL, platelet count 11,000, peripheral smear – Megalocytic Anemia with Leucopenia and Thrombocytopenia and no other abnormal cells, was managed conservatively. She had underwent Vaccum assisted vaginal delivery and was third stage of labor was uneventful without any post partum hemorrhage or other bleeding manifestations. During post-partum period, she developed severe anemia and thrombocytopenia with HB-5g/dL, platetlet count of 21,000 and so bone marrow aspiration was done, found to have hypocellular marrow with atypical lymphoid cells, bone marrow biopsy showed hypocellular marrow with decrease in all 3 hematopoietic cell lines, few lymphoid cells with hyper chromatic nucleus and scant eosinophilic cytoplasm, few megakaryocytes. CMV IgM, IgG were found to be positive, ANC was 150 cells /ml and the diagnosis of severe aplastic anemia was confirmed. As her sister was HLA identical sibling, donor stem cell transplantation was performed. She conceived spontaneously, in this subsequent pregnancy had uneventful antenatal, intrapartum and post partum period, delivered live term baby. **Conclusion:** Women with severe anemia and thrombocytopenia are to be thoroughly evaluated so as to make timely diagnosis of the disease.

Keywords: Pregnancy; anemia; aplastic anemia; bone marrow transplant; gvhd prophylaxis; mycophenolate moefetil.

ABBREVIATIONS

AA – Aplastic Anemia ;CY- Cyclophosphamide; IST- Immunosuppressive Treatment or Therapy; CsA - Cyclosporin A; ATG- Anti-thymocyte Globuline; ECG – Electrocardiography; ECHO- Echocardiography; SGOT- Serum Glutamic Oxaloacetic Transaminase; SGPT - Serum Glutamic Pyruvic Transaminase; HBsAg - Hepatic B Surface Antigen; SDP- Single Donor Platelet obtained by apheresis; ANC - Absolute Neutrophil Count.

1. INTRODUCTION

Aplastic anemia [AA], is characterized by decreased bone marrow function with inadequate production of erythrocytes, granulocytes, and platelets. Marrow failure may be caused by absence of or defects in hematopoietic stem cells, abnormalities of the bone marrow microenvironment, ineffective cell-to-cell interactions, or immune disorders. Although most patients with aplastic anemia have normal immunity, some have abnormalities of T- and B-lymphocytes. Rare patients have an immune cause of marrow failure [1]. Our understanding of the molecular basis for these disorders has progressed in recent years and the genetic defects have been mapped to DNA damage repair mechanisms (Fanconi Anemia) [2], telomerase dysfunction (Dyskeratosis Congenita) and ribosomal function (Schwachman–Diamond syndrome) [3]. Acquired AA is usually the result of an autoimmune attack that appears to be directed at hematopoietic stem/progenitor cells [4]. Depending on affected cell lines, AA is associated with fatigue, bleeding due to thrombocytopenia and recurrent infections due to neutropenia [2]. The diagnosis of 'Aplastic Anemia' is confirmed by hypocellularity of the bone marrow. The remaining cells are morphologically unaffected without malignant infiltration. Potential triggers for the onset of AA include T-cell mediated auto-immune disease, iatrogenic agents, viral infection and pregnancy [3]. There is, however, no causal relation between pregnancy and the onset of AA [5]. This notion is supported by the similar incidence of AA in men and women. A complete blood count, leukocyte differential, reticulocyte count and a bone marrow aspirate and biopsy can establish the diagnosis. Peripheral blood flow cytometry to detect cells missing Glycosyl Phosphatidyl Inositol anchored proteins (GPI-AP) [4], bone marrow karyotyping and FISH to help exclude hypoplastic Myelodysplastic syndromes (hMDS) should be performed on all patients. GPI-AP deficiency is a hallmark of Paroxysmal Nocturnal Hemoglobinuria (PNH); however, small-to-moderate populations of GPI-AP deficient cells (usually 0.1-15%) can be found in most of the patients with acquired AA at diagnosis [6]. Finding PNH excludes congenital form of the disease.

Distinguishing between AA and hMDS is often challenging, the percentage of CD34$^+$ cells in the bone marrow is often helpful [7]. The percentage of CD34$^+$ cells is usually <0.3% in AA, whereas the CD34$^+$ percentage is either normal (0.5-1.0%) or elevated in hMDS.

Pregnancy associated AA is a rare association. Patients with established AA should avoid pregnancy [8]. During pregnancy bone marrow transplantation is contraindicated because of potential embryo toxicity [9]. There are no clear guidelines for the management of AA during pregnancy.

We report a case of pregnant woman in whom anemia was evaluated and diagnosed as AA managed through the pregnancy and followed her up until subsequent pregnancy with good outcome.

2. CASE

A 19 year teenage primigravida at 36 weeks of gestation presented to our hospital with complaints of generalized weakness since 1 month during her antenatal check-up. She was evaluated, wherein Hb- 5.8%, platelet count 11,000, peripheral smear - megalocytic anemia with leucopenia and thrombocytopenia and no other abnormal cells, serum vitamin B12-242 pg/ml, serum folate level -8ng/ml, Dengue IgM & IgG were negative. As she had spontaneous rupture of membranes, we had conservatively transfused packed cells and platelets. She had underwent Vaccum assisted vaginal delivery and third stage of labor was uneventful without any post-partum hemorrhage or other bleeding manifestations. During post-partum period, as she had again developed severe anemia and thrombocytopenia with Hb-5g/dL, platetlet count of 21,000 bone marrow aspiration was done, found to have hypocellular marrow with atypical lymphoid cells, bone marrow biopsy showed hypocellular marrow with decrease in all 3 hematopoietic cell lines, few lymphoid cells with hyperchromatic nucleus and scant eosinophilic cytoplasm, few megakaryocytes. So she was further evaluated. On further investigating, she had normal coagulation profile, liver and renal function tests, chest X ray, ECG, ECHO, abdominal ultrasound. No growth on blood, urine and vaginal swab culture was found, serology was negative for Malaria, Dengue, HIV, HBsAg, Antiplatelet antibody titer. CD55, CD59 and HAM test were advised. HAM test is performed to diagnose Paroxysmal Nocturnal Hemoglobinuria. CMV IgM, IgG were found to be positive, ANC was 150 cells/ml and the diagnosis of Severe Aplastic Anemia was confirmed. As her sister was HLA identical sibling, donor stem cell transplantation was performed after 17 days of diagnosis of AA. Conditioning was done with Fludarabine 30 mg/m 2/day [270 mg] and

cyclophosphamide 120 mg/kg/day [6240mg], transplantation cell dose – 5.7*108 nvbc cells / kg. As engraftment 1 pint of packed cells, 10 pint platelet, 1/2 SDP were given, ANC >500 on day 14, platelet >20000 on day 17 was present. As GVHD prophylaxis Methotrexate 5 mg/m2 on day1 with Folinic acid rescue was administered. She had grade 1 mucositis and acute GVHD diagnosed by raised SGOT, SGPT. It was managed with corticosteroids and Mycophenolate moefetil. She had no signs of hemorrhagic cystitis, pneumonitis, nor chronic GVHD. She was followed up for 18 months every 3 months for history of infections or abnormal bleeding, physical examination and complete blood count. She conceived spontaneously, in this subsequent pregnancy had uneventful antenatal, intrapartum and post partum period, delivered live term baby.

3. DISCUSSION

Aplastic Anemia is classified as non-severe (NSAA), severe (SAA) and very severe based on the degree of the peripheral blood cytopenias (Table 1) [10]. The 2-year mortality rate with supportive care alone for patients with SAA or very severe AA approaches 80% Patients with severe cytopenia require urgent support with blood products. Blood products should be irradiated to prevent transfusion associated GVHD [11], and filtered to reduce the incidence of viral infections and prevent alloimmunization. Transfusions from family members should be avoided to decrease sensitization to potential bone marrow donors. The initial goal of transfusion therapy for anemia should be to correct or avoid cardiopulmonary complications. Platelet transfusions are indicated when platelet levels are below 10,000/ul or if the patient is experiencing bleeding. Granulocyte transfusions remain controversial in AA and should be used judiciously. There may be a limited role for Granulocyte colony stimulating factor (G-CSF) administration in an attempt to stimulate a neutrophil response in the presence of severe infection.10In young non-pregnant patients first choice therapy for AA is allogenic stem cell transplantation with a five-year survival of 70 to 80%.A recent report from the EBMT of over 1500 patients confirmed that predictors of survival following BMT included matched sibling donor, age of less than 16 years, early transplant (time from diagnosis to transplant of less than 83 days) and a non-radiation conditioning regimen [11]. Most patients achieve full donor chimerism after BMT. However, Stem Cell transplantation is not feasible during pregnancy because of the teratogenic effects of the immunotherapy and radiotherapy for the unborn child [12]. Pregnancy termination to start bone marrow transplantation was not recommended because of the relatively good prognosis for both mother and child. During pregnancy supportive therapy with erythrocyte and platelet transfusions is a widely used, reasonable alternative.

Table 1. Aplastic anemia: Definitions and diagnosis [10]

Severe AA
- Any two of three required for diagnosis
- – Absolute neutrophil count <500/mm^3
- – Platelets <20,000/mm^3
- – Reticulocyte count <1.0% corrected or <60,000/mm^3

Very severe AA
- Meets criteria for severe disease and absolute neutrophil count <200/mm^3

Non-severe AA
- Does not meet criteria for severe AA

Transplant of hematopoietic stem cells obtained from alternative sources, such as fetal liver cells or stem cells from long-term, in-vitro cultures, also may be useful [1]. Graft rejection is a greater obstacle for unrelated transplants. Over recent years GVHD prophylaxis with various drugs are being proposed. The combination of Methotrexate (MTX) and Cyclosporin A (CsA), as well as the combination of MMF and CsA have been successfully used for GVHD prophylaxis. [10] Interest has recently turned towards high-dose CY as GVHD prophylaxis. Another highly effective therapy for SAA is ATG and CsA IST and is generally first-line therapy for SAA patients who lack matched sibling donors or are not good candidates for BMT. The hematopoietic response rate after ATG/CsA is 60-70% and the probability of survival at 5 years ranges from 60 to 85%13. However, up to 40% of patients eventually relapse [11]. There are currently no standard criteria to deem IST a treatment failure. Many institutions use 4 months of IST without response to deem that treatment was ineffective before moving to a secondary treatment. Prognostication for response to IST is an ongoing area of research. The determination of telomere length is useful for the characterization of many bone marrow failure disorders, including SAA, by the quantitative (q) PCR method [13]. With modern therapies, the 5-year survival rate for SAA exceeds 85%. BMT offers the best

chance for cure, but its use is restricted by the relatively high morbidity and mortality, especially in older patients and those who lack an HLA-matched sibling donor. IST remains the standard of care and leads to meaningful remissions in up to 75% of patients, but the high rate of relapse and secondary clonal diseases makes this therapy less attractive, especially for young patients with SAA [10].

4. CONCLUSION

Women with severe anemia and thrombocytopenia are to be thoroughly evaluated so as to make timely diagnosis of the disease. The accurate management of the patient can improve prognosis and also helps in early recovery. Pre pregnancy counseling and regular follow up of these women play pivotal role in the maternal and fetal outcome.

CONSENT

All authors have obtained written consent from the patient for publication of this case report.

ETHICAL APPROVAL

It is not applicable.

ACKNOWLEDGEMENTS

We thank our patient, hospital and hospital staff for all their cooperation. We also appreciate the support we had received from various departments without which we could not have been able to manage the case to the best of our efficiency.

COMPETING INTERESTS

Authors have declared that no competing interests exist.

REFERENCES

1. Gale RP, Champlin RE, Feig SA, Fitchen JH. Aplastic anemia: Biology and treatment. Annals of Internal Medicine. 1981;95(4):477-494.
2. Nakanishi K, Taniguchi T, Ranganathan V, et al. Interaction of FANCD2 and NBS1 in the DNA damage response. Nat. Cell Biol. 2002;4(12):913-920. [PubMed]
3. Uechi T, Nakajima Y, Chakraborty A, Torihara H, Higa S, Kenmochi N.

Deficiency of ribosomal protein S19 during early embryogenesis leads to reduction of erythrocytes in a *Zebrafish* model of diamond–blackfananemia. Hum. Mol. Genet. 2008;17(20):3204-3211. [PubMed]

4.   Brodsky RA, Mukhina GL, Li S, et al. Improved detection and characterization of paroxysmal nocturnal hemoglobinuria using fluorescent aerolysin. Am. J. Clin. Pathol. 2000;114(3):459-466. [PMC free article] [PubMed]

5.   Young NS, Calado RT, Scheinberg P. Current concepts in the pathophysiology and treatment of aplastic anemia. Blood. 2006;108(8):2509-2519. [PMC free article] [PubMed]

6.   Mukhina GL, Buckley JT, Barber JP, Jones RJ, Brodsky RA. Multilineage glycosylphosphatidylinositol anchor deficient hematopoiesis in untreated aplastic anemia. Br. J. Haematol. 2001;115:476-482. [PubMed]

7.   Matsui WH, Brodsky RA, Smith BD, Borowitz MJ, Jones RJ. Quantitative analysis of bone marrow CD34 cells in aplastic anemia and hypoplastic myelodysplastic syndromes. Leukemia. 2006;20(3):458-462. [PubMed]

8.   Aitchison RG, Marsh JC, Hows JM, Russell NH, Gordon-Smith EC. Pregnancy associated aplastic anaemia: a report of five cases and review of current management. BrJ Haematol. 1989;73:541-45. PubMed Abstract. Publisher Full Text.

9.   Young NS. Acquired aplastic anemia. Ann Intern Med. 2002;136:534-546.

10.   Amy E DeZern[1], Robert A Brodsky[2]. Clinical management of aplastic anemia. Expert Rev Hematol. 2011;4(2):221-230.

11.   Locasciulli A, Oneto R, Bacigalupo A, et al. Outcome of patients with acquired aplastic anemia given first line bone marrow transplantation or immunosuppressive treatment in the last decade: A report from the European Group for Blood and Marrow Transplantation (EBMT) Haematologica. 2007;92(1):11-18. [PubMed] ••Guidance for immunosuppressive therapy or bone marrow transplantation as first-line therapy.

12.   Young NS, Calado RT, Scheinberg P. Current concepts in the pathophysiology and treatment of aplastic anemia. Blood. 2006;108(8):2509-2519. [PMC free article] [PubMed]

13.   Pavesi E, Avondo F, Aspesi A, et al. Analysis of telomeres in peripheral blood cells from patients with bone marrow failure. Pediatr. Blood Cancer. 2009;53(3): 411-416. [PubMed]

Permissions

List of Contributors

Nahla Ahmad Bahgat Abdulateef
Laboratory and Blood Bank Department, King Abdullah Medical City, Makkah, Kingdom of Saudi Arabia

Nahla Ahmad Bahgat Abdulateef, Manar Mohammad Ismail and Essam Hamed Abdou
Clinical Pathology Department, National Cancer Institute, Cairo University, Cairo, Egypt

Manar Mohammad Ismail
Laboratory Medicine Department, Faculty of Applied Medical Science, Um Al-Qura University, Makkah, Kingdom of Saudi Arabia

Soha Aly Elmorsy
Pharmacology Department, Faculty of Medicine Cairo University, Egypt Research Center, KAMC, Makkah, Kingdom of Saudi Arabia

Aziza F. ALswayyed
Laboratory and Blood Bank , KFMC, Riyadh, Kingdom of Saudi Arabia,

Omima Elemam
Oncology Center, KAMC, Makkah, Kingdom of Saudi Arabia Medical Oncology, Oncology Center, Mansoura University, Mansoura, Egypt

Essam Hamed Abdou
Clinical pathology Consultant, SGH, KSA, Jeddah, Kingdom of Saudi Arabia

Feryal Karaca
Department of Radiation Oncology, Van Regional Training and Research Hospital, Van, Turkey

Cigdem Usul Afsar
Department of Medical Oncology, Tekirdag Corlu State Hospital, Tekirdag, Turkey

Fatma Sert
Department of Radiation Oncology, Faculty of Medical, Ege University, Izmir, Turkey

SebnemIzmir Guner
Department of Hematology, Bahcelievler Medical Park Hospital, Istanbul, Turkey

Vehbi Ercolak
Department of Medical Oncology, Faculty of Medical, Harran University, Sanlıurfa, Turkey

Erkut Erkurt and Candas Tunali
Department of Radiation Oncology, Faculty of Medicine, Cukurova University, Adana, Turkey

Basma Doro
Department of Microbiology and Immunology, Faculty of Pharmacy, University of Tripoli, Tripoli, Libya

Wajdi M. Zawia, Nagi Meftah Gerbil Abdalla, Adam M. Rifai, Fatma J. Amar and Abdulwahab N. Aboughress
Central Blood Bank, Tripoli, Libya

Walid M. Ramadan Husien
Department of Microbiology and Immunology, Medical Faculty, University of Tripoli, Central Blood Bank, Tripoli, Libya

Enase Dourou
Department of Community Medicine, Medical Faculty, University of Tripoli, Libya

Ademola S. Adewoyin
Department of Haematology and Blood Transfusion, University of Benin Teaching Hospital, P.M.B.1111, Benin City, Edo State, Nigeria

Olayinka A. Oyewale
Department of Anaesthesiology, University of Benin Teaching Hospital, P.M.B.1111, Benin City, Edo State, Nigeria

Daisy Ilagan-Tagarda
Department of Medicine, Fellow in Training, University of Santo Tomas Hospital, Section of Infectious Diseases, Philippines

Flordeluna Zapata-Mesina
Department of Medicine, Fellow in Training, University of Santo Tomas Hospital, Section of Adult Clinical Hematology, Philippines

John S. Delgado
Department of Medicine, University of Santo Tomas Hospital, Section of Infectious Diseases, Philippines

Jomell C. Julian
Department of Medicine, University of Santo Tomas Hospital, Section of Adult Clinical Hematology, Philippines

Ngwu Amauche Martina and Obi Godwin Okorie
Department of Hematology and Immunology, Enugu State University of Science and Technology, Enugu, Enugu State, Nigeria

Anigolu Miriam Obiageli
Department of Chemical Pathology, Enugu State University of Science and Technology, Enugu, Enugu State, Nigeria

Eluke Blessing Chekwube
Department of Medical Laboratory Science, University of Nigeria, Enugu Campus, Enugu State, Nigeria

K. A. Fasakin, C. T. Omisakin and A. J. Esan
Department of Haematology, Federal Teaching Hospital, Ido Ekiti, Nigeria

O. D. Ajayi
Department of Pharmacology and Therapeutics, College of Medicine and Health Sciences, University of Afe Babalola, Ado Ekiti, Nigeria

Otu E. Etta and Emma Etuknwa
Department of Anaesthesia, University of Uyo Teaching Hospital, Uyo, Akwa Ibom State, Nigeria

Laurence Adlai B. Morillo, Flordeluna Zapata-Mesina and Ma Rosario Irene D. Castillo
Section of Hematology, University of Santo Tomas Hospital, Manila, Philippines

Mestewat Debasu
Department of Biochemistry, St. Paul's Hospital Millennium Medical College, P.O.Box 1271, Addis Ababa, Ethiopia

M. K. C. Menon, Yididya Belayneh and Daniel Seifu
Department of Medical Biochemistry, School of Medicine, Faculty of Health Sciences, Addis Ababa University, P.O.Box 9086, Addis Ababa, Ethiopia

Workeabeba Abebe
Department of Pediatrics and Child Health, School of Medicine, Faculty of Health Sciences, Addis Ababa University, P.O.Box 1176, Addis Ababa, Ethiopia

Degu Jerene
Department of Preventive Medicine, School of Medicine, Faculty of Health Sciences, Addis Ababa University, P.O.Box 1176, Addis Ababa, Ethiopia

Sunitha Dontha, Hemalatha Kamurthy and Nandakishora Chary Madipoju
Department of Pharmaceutical Chemistry, Malla Reddy College of Pharmacy, Maisammaguda, Secunderabad-14, Telangana, India

Mohamed Kaled A. Shambesh
Department of Community Medicine, Medical Faculty, University of Tripoli, Libya

Ezzadin Areaf Franka
Department of Community Medicine, Faculty of Medicine, University of Tripoli, Libya

Faisal Fathalla Ismail
Department of Medical Science, Faculty of Medical Technology, Omar Al Mukhtar University, Tobruk, Libya

Nagi Meftah Gebril, Kamel Ahmed Azabi and Fatma Amar
Department of Community Medicine, University of Tripoli, Central Blood Bank, Tripoli, Libya

J. B. Borges, T. Sakurada Jr, S. Lautenschlaugher and A. R. T. Pupulin
Department of Basic Health Sciences, State University of Maringa, Maringá, P.R. Brazil

N. C. S. Santana and N. A. Lima
Post Graduate Program in Pharmaceutical Sciences, State University of Maringa, Maringá, P.R. Brazil

Susana Perez, Irma Bragós, Mariana Raviola, Arianna Pratti, Germán Detarsio, Maria Eda Voss, Irma Acosta and Mara Ojeda
Departamento de Bioquímica Clínica, Cátedra de Hematología, Facultad de Ciencias Bioquímicas y Farmacéuticas, Universidad Nacional de Rosario. Suipacha 531. Rosario. Santa Fe, Argentina

Sandra Zirone and Luciano Verón
Departamento de Hematología, Instituto Davoli. Laprida 1061. Rosario. Santa Fe, Argentina

Hazizi Abu Saad, Aina Mardiah Basri and Zahratul Nur Kalmi
Department of Nutrition and Dietetics, Faculty of Medicine and Health Sciences, Universiti Putra Malaysia, 43400 UPM Serdang, Selangor, Malaysia

S. Adewoyin Ademola
Department of Haematology and Blood Transfusion, University of Benin Teaching Hospital, PMB 1111, Benin City, Edo State, Nigeria

Jerold C. Alcantara and Ann P. Opiña
Saint Louis University, School of Natural Sciences, Baguio City, Philippines

Rhashani Arjay M. Alcantara
Lorma Medical Center, Clinical Laboratory Department, San Fernando City, Philippines

Azita Chegini
Blood Transfusion Research Center, High Institute for Research and Education in Transfusion Medicine, Tehran, Iran

Alireza Ebrahimi
Department of Hematology, Faculty of Medical Sciences, Tarbiat Modares University, Tehran, Iran

Amirhossein Maghari
Department of Biostatistics, New Hearing Technologies Research Center, Baqiyatallah University of Medical Science, Tehran, Iran

I. O. George and P. N. Tabansi
Department of Paediatrics, University of Port Harcourt Teaching Hospital, Nigeria

C. N. Onyearugha
Department of Paediatrics, Abia State University Teaching Hospital, Nigeria

Orkuma Joseph Aondowase and Onoja Anthony Michael
Department of Hematology, College of Health Sciences, Benue State University, Makurdi Benue State, Nigeria

Gomerep Simji Samuel
Department of Internal Medicine, Faculty of Medical Sciences, University of Jos, Plateau State, Nigeria

Egesie Julie Ochaka
Department of Hematology and Blood Transfusion, Faculty of Medical Sciences, University of Jos, Plateau State, Nigeria

Orkuma Jenifer Hembadoon
Department of Laboratory, College Clinic, Federal School of Forestry, Jos-Plateau state, Nigeria

Mbaave Tsavyange Peter
Department of Internal Medicine, College of Health Sciences, Benue State University, Makurdi Benue State, Nigeria

Haile Nega Mulata, Natesan Gnanasekaran, Umeta Melaku and Seifu Daniel
Department of Medical Biochemistry, School of Medicine, College of Health Sciences, Addis Ababa University, Ethiopia

Ashraf Elghandour, Hashem Naenaa, Mohamed Eldefrawy and Hadeer Mohammed
Internal Medicine, Alexandria University, Egypt

Magdy Elbordeny
Clinical Pathology, Alexandria University, Egypt

O. E. Iheanacho
Department of Haematology and Blood Transfusion, University of Benin Teaching Hospital, Benin City, Nigeria

I. O. George and A. I. Frank-Briggs
Department of Paediatrics, University of Port Harcourt Teaching Hospital, Nigeria

Ijioma Solomon Nnah
Department of Veterinary Physiology, Pharmacology, Biochemistry and Animal Health, College of Veterinary Medicine, Michael Okpara University of Agriculture, Umudike, Nigeria

Imoru Momodu
Department of Haematology, Aminu Kano Teaching Hospital/Bayero University, P.M.B. 3452, Kano, Kano State, Nigeria

Olutayo Ifedayo Ajayi
Department of Physiology, School of Basic Medical Sciences, University of Benin, P.M.B. 1154, Benin-City, Nigeria

F. A. Fasola and F. O. Fowodu
Department of Haematology, University College Hospital, Ibadan, Nigeria

A. Akere
Department of Medicine, University College Hospital, Ibadan, Nigeria

Ilham Zahir
Department of Biology, Faculty of Sciences and Technical, University Sidi Mohamed Ben Abdellah, BP 2202, Road of Immouzer, Fez, Morocco

Abderahman Bellik
Department of Biology, Laboratory of Immunochemistry, Pasteur institute, Casablanca, Morocco

Archana Singh Sikarwar
Faculty of Medicine and Health Sciences, Human Biology, International Medical University, Kuala Lumpur, Malaysia

Mohd Farid Bin Dato' Seri Haji Abdul Rahman
Undergraduate Student, Biomedical Science, International Medical University, Malaysia

Dharmesh Chandra Sharma
Blood Bank, Component and Aphaeresis Unit, Department of Pathology, G. R. Medical College, Gwalior, India

Arun Jain, Poonam Woike, Sunita Rai, Lokesh Tripathi and Rajesh Gaur
Department of Pathology, G. R. Medical College, India

Savita Bharat
Department of Microbiology, G. R. Medical College, Gwalior, India

Harshini Vana, J. B. Vidyashree, Mangala Gowri and Renuka Ramaiah
Department of Obstetrics and Gynecology, RGUHS, ESICMCPGIMSR, Bangalore, India

www.ingramcontent.com/pod-product-compliance
Lightning Source LLC
Chambersburg PA
CBHW080246230326

41458CB00097B/3997